## *Advance Praise for*
## MY GLUTEN-FREE FAMILY KITCHEN

"Packed with such love and deliciousness, Vanessa Weisbrod has created another gluten-free winner, and a must for every family's kitchen!"

—MARILYN GELLER, CEO, Celiac Disease Foundation

"Anyone who knows Vanessa also knows that she does this out of love for her community and also with the deep understanding of what it takes to be gluten-free. This book will inspire all family members to participate and enjoy the process of helping loved ones stay safe and gluten-free."

—DR. EDWIN LIU, Director of the Celiac Disease Center at Children's Hospital Colorado

"Vanessa's recipes get kids and families into the kitchen together, while encouraging sharing with gluten-free and non-gluten-free friends and family. This book makes it easy to invite your friends and family (gluten-free or not) over for an undeniably delicious gluten-free meal. These recipes are kid AND whole-family friendly (trust me, I've tried a bunch) and help educate even the youngest children about their important dietary needs. Your kids will come away from using this book as strong self-advocates and inspired little chefs."

—JULIE LEPORE, Publisher, *Macaroni Kids*

"For years and years we gluten sufferers were stuck labeling foods as PGFGF or 'pretty good for gluten-free.' Our specialty foods were fine but they were seldom GOOD. Everything I've tried in *My Gluten-Free Family Kitchen* is just plain great, no qualifier needed. Whether it's Peach Blueberry Yogurt Muffins or Chai Spiced Chocolate Chip Apple Bread for the newsroom, or the Creamy Cilantro Lime Dressing or Thai Pumpkin & Apple Soup I made at home, my glutinous colleagues in the newsroom nor three kids at home never had a clue they were eating gluten-free. Fooling the people you love has never been so fun, or delicious."

—DAVE BRIGGS, Co-host of CNN's *Early Start*

"Make room on your shelf for this recipe collection that sets a new standard for gluten-free cooking. Curated with love and attention to detail, these recipes taste even better than they look and will please the pickiest gluten-eaters and gluten-avoiders in your family."

—DR. JOCELYN SILVESTER, MD, PhD, FRCPC, Director of Research for the Celiac Disease Program at Boston Children's Hospital

# MY GLUTEN-FREE
*Family Kitchen*

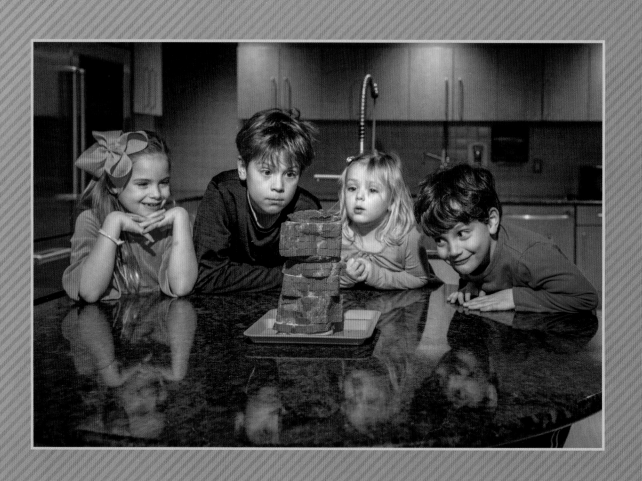

# MY GLUTEN-FREE
## Family Kitchen

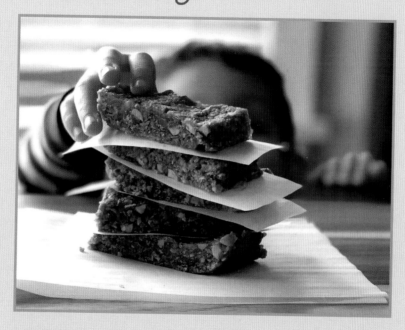

*151 Fast, Fun, and Flavorful Recipes*

# Vanessa Weisbrod

**Celiac Disease Program at Children's National Medical Center**

Post Hill
PRESS

A POST HILL PRESS BOOK

*My Gluten-Free Family Kitchen:*
*151 Fast, Fun, and Flavorful Recipes*
© 2019 by Vanessa Weisbrod, Celiac Disease Program at Children's National Medical Center
All Rights Reserved

ISBN: 978-1-64293-294-2

Cover design by Cody Corcoran
Photography by Vanessa Weisbrod
Photography by Kenson Noel: pages iv, 8, 9, 10, 16, 18, 21
Content organization, interior design, and composition by Greg Johnson, Textbook Perfect

**Post Hill Press**
New York • Nashville
posthillpress.com

Published in the United States of America
Printed in China

*In loving memory of Dr. John Snyder.*
*We will forever miss his smile and*
*hugs but will always remember his*
*passion and dedication to his patients*
*and their families.*

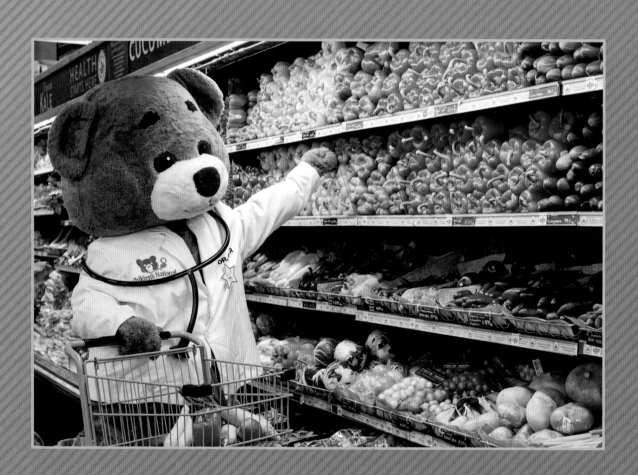

# CONTENTS

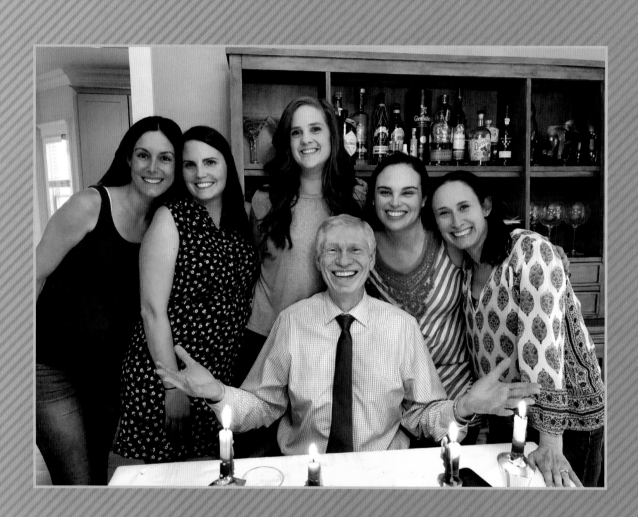

# INTRODUCTION

# It Takes a Village...

My mommy friends have decided that I'm not allowed to sign up for one more committee. At our regular Mom's Night Out last week, Jackie, Julie, and Heather threatened not to refill my glass of Wente Morning Fog Chardonnay if I signed up to fill the room parent slot for our kids' class. I reluctantly agreed and chugged my glass of wine, only to go home and immediately commit to be the *chair of the entire parents' committee.* Darn! My mom tribe is not going to be happy.

"The rabbi is coming!" I screamed into the phone, letting my husband know that our spiritual leader is coming to Shabbat dinner at our house. It's my own Mrs. Maisel moment. As a proud culinary school graduate, it's game time. The brisket must be perfect.

How did I get roped into this you ask? As the chair of our parents' committee, I was tasked with building community. My kids go to a Jewish preschool, so my brilliant idea was to have small groups of families host Shabbat dinners in their homes so the families can get to know one another better. The first one will be at

my house and Rabbi Stu will come to show his support for the initiative.

I'm beyond excited. I immediately order a new apron and placemats. I'll make my famous cider-braised brisket, roasted eggplant and spinach salad, charred Brussels sprouts with green apples, mashed sweet potatoes with a crispy oatmeal topping, key lime parfaits and chocolate chip cookies for desserts and, of course, challah. Then I remember that my house is entirely gluten-free.

I was diagnosed with celiac disease fifteen years ago, and my oldest son, Brandon, was diagnosed in 2016 when he was three years old. My mom also has celiac disease. Don't feel bad for us. We're doing great. We're all extremely active, healthy, and proud of our commitment to a gluten-free lifestyle.

But oh my…what am I going to do about the challah? Will the rabbi eat it gluten-free? Gluten-free challah is not soft and fluffy like the challah they give out on Fridays at Temple. Gluten-free challah is most often crumbly and only good if served right out of the oven or sufficiently warmed. Even my recipe (which I adore), is best served fresh and warm.

For a hot second, I panicked about challah. But thankfully, my husband calmed me down and lovingly said, "Vanessa…the challah is the first thing people will eat. Five seconds later, they'll eat the brisket and forget that challah was ever on the table."

"Fine," I said and went back to the kitchen. I'm not going to lie, I was anxious for days leading up to this dinner, mostly because I couldn't stop thinking about what the rabbi would think of the gluten-free challah.

I invited four families to join us for dinner and asked everyone to bring an appetizer or beverage. The big night was here! As my friends and their kids began to arrive, festive platters started covering the counter. Even though everyone knows that Brandon and I are gluten-free, I still did my normal dance of making little food ID tags to identify food that contains gluten. I do this mostly for Brandon so he will easily know what he can and cannot eat.

Jackie walked in with her son, husband, a bowl of sweet potato hummus with sliced veggies, and her famous cheese platter that comes with our favorite, Drunken Goat Cheese. Heather arrived with her two girls, husband, and a bag full of gluten-free crackers to go with the cheese platter. She picked the herb and seed crackers that we can't stop talking about. Amy and her husband walked in with their son (sans newborn twin girls) accompanied by a basket full of gluten-free cookies. And, of course, Julie came in loaded with her two vivacious boys and a case of Justin Vineyards Cabernet Sauvignon.

I looked at the table and started laughing with tears in my eyes. I didn't need those labels—all of my friends showed up with gluten-free food. Julie looked at my tears and blurted out, "What the heck is wrong with you?" I didn't say anything in response. I just gave her a hug and bustled back to the kitchen to finish dinner.

Ding Dong. The rabbi is here! I quickly pull the challah out of the oven and cover it with a beautiful napkin my mom gave me as a hand-me-down from my grandma, Lela Mae. She was an incredible cook. I'll never forget seeing her buzz around the kitchen, pulling pies and snickerdoodles out of the oven like she was a magical fairy baker. In the language of my kids, she is the star of Nick Jr.'s hit show, Butterbean's Café. I know my Mamaw would be proud.

Back to Butterbean for a second. Butterbean's Café is an animated series designed for young children. The fairy (Butterbean) opens a magical neighborhood bakery and café with her sister and fairy friends. They have magical whisks, kind spirits, healthy treats, and a slew

of animal friends. They cook together, help their neighbors, overcome kitchen disasters, and always end the episodes with lots of high fives and hugs. You can judge me for allowing my kids screen time, but I wholeheartedly believe that letting my kids watch television shows about food and friends eating together has helped them broaden their horizons, try new things, and get excited about helping me in the kitchen. (No, they didn't pay me to say that!) My kids watch an episode and then bounce around my kitchen dancing and singing the theme song.

We sit down to dinner in our dining room with Rabbi Stu at the head of the table, light the candles, and say the blessings over the wine. The kids start singing the Hamotzi prayer in unison: "...we give thanks to God for bread, our voices join in song together as our joyful prayer is said." Here it comes…. Rabbi Stu takes the cover off of the challah, pulls off a piece, and puts it into his mouth. I watch him chew as though it's happening in slow motion. Please don't crumble! I silently beg the challah.

"Fresh out of the oven! Vanessa, this is—" But before he can finish his sentence, Rocco, Julie's boisterous and delightfully starving little one, grabs the challah and shoves a giant piece into his mouth.

"Beee-NESSA," Rocco says to me adoringly, "it's deeeelicious!"

Anxiety gone. Sweaty palms gone. Pure joy from the mouth of a two-year-old who has somehow managed to lose his pants before dinner even started. And Rocco had no idea the challah was gluten-free.

I sit down in my chair and look around the table as my family, friends, and Rabbi Stu pass around the platters of my home-cooked food and load up their plates. Bite after bite, yum after yum. Everyone is eating the food and loving it. I look at their smiling faces and squeeze my husband's hand under the table. These aren't just our friends. They are our friends who feel like family.

— · —

I don't sign up for these committees because I like seeing my name on every email or because I have a crazy need to be in charge. I sign up so I have a role in building a community that is thoughtful, kind, and inclusive for kids and families, regardless of how they need to eat. By showing people that gluten-free food can be beautiful, creative, and absolutely delicious, it helps bring them into my gluten-free circle and, in turn, become a source of support for my son, me, and others like us.

In our Multidisciplinary Celiac Disease Program Clinic at Children's National Medical Center in Washington, D.C., we see families every single day who are struggling with the gluten-free diet, most often because of the cost of products or lack of support from family and friends. Recent data show that children and adolescents with celiac disease often report problems with stigma, social activities, and social relationships, particularly while attending school activities, parties, sporting events, or visiting other people's homes. More than one-third of our patients report anxiety and anger surrounding their need to be on a gluten-free diet, and more than a quarter report depression. Limitations on the food children eat can affect normal social and emotional development and can lead to their withdrawal from very normal life activities involving food.

The community we've built around us helps Brandon and me stay strong on the gluten-free diet. We never spend a moment feeling excluded from social, school, or basic life activities. That's not to say that our lives are completely rosy. In fact, just a few weeks ago we had some families over for a playdate. One mom walked in handing me a basket of muffins. She smiled and said, "I made you muffins, but they are not gluten-free. Sorry."

Ummmm, OK, I thought to myself. She brought non-gluten-free muffins to a playdate hosted by a mom and child who she knew couldn't eat them. That was thoughtful….

I could have said something not so flattering, but instead I just smiled, took the muffins and thanked her for bringing me something to feed my non-celiac husband for breakfast the next morning. Look at the bright side—more gluten-free pancakes for Brandon and me!

You will encounter experiences like this. There will be times that someone in your family or a close friend forgets to have a gluten-free option. There will be times you're at a wedding, baby shower, or pre-school fundraiser and are starving. Don't be naive about it. It will happen. Expect it. Plan for it by always having an extra snack in your bag and then when it happens, brush it off. Dwelling on it only makes things even worse.

Helping our patients and families achieve normalcy in their gluten-free lives has always been my goal. I've found that normalcy most often comes from learning to own their gluten-free diet and building a supportive community around them. Sometimes our patients find such support in our peer mentorship and support group activities or through meeting friends at our annual Gluten-Free Education Day and Expo. But most often, support and normalcy happen through educating their family and friends about how the gluten-free diet is helping them to grow up stronger.

This is the fourth cookbook I've written, and I have to say that it is, by far, my favorite. It's the first one that I really wrote for my family and me. I've made every recipe in this book for my kids Brandon (five) and Leo (two and a half), and they've eaten and liked each one! Some of the recipes are ones that I've made for decades. Others came from Mom's Nights Out when we've brainstormed how to recreate restaurant dishes (particularly brussels sprouts), and still others are favorites shared by friends. You'll hear more about them later.

The tips and tricks are all things I've done with my own kids to get them to eat new foods, especially the suggestions on Plating with Purpose. The hands you see in recipe photos throughout the book are my kids and their best buds who came over after school to help with photo shoots. They genuinely dug their hands and hearts into the food I was photographing. Some of the placemats you'll see throughout the book is artwork done by my kids and their classmates at the Temple Sinai Early Childhood Education Program. I'm inspired every day by the creativity that comes from these kids, and I hope you'll be inspired, too, as you cook your way through this book.

I am beyond blessed to have the love and support of the most amazing people. Family, DC/Children's National friends, UCLA friends, high school/college friends, mommy friends, Temple Sinai friends… The list is long. You know who you are. In case I haven't said it enough, thank you. Your kindness, generosity, and support for gluten-free eating is more than I ever could have asked for.

All I've ever wanted in my life and in my kid's lives is a village that welcomes us with open arms, joins us at the gluten-free table, and once in a while, brings over a gluten-free bagel. And I think I've got it. I hope you find this in your life too.

P.S. Rabbi Stu loved the challah.

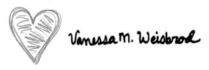 Vanessa M. Weisbrod

# About the Celiac Disease Program at Children's National Medical Center

The Multidisciplinary Celiac Disease Clinic at Children's National Medical Center allows children diagnosed with celiac disease and their families the opportunity to schedule one integrative multidisciplinary appointment. Our approach is to care for not only the gastrointestinal symptoms and concerns associated with celiac disease but to also look into the neurological and psychological problems that may arise as a result of gluten intolerance.

All patients have:

- The benefit of a care coordinator dedicated to ensure an optimum experience in the clinic and attention to execution of needed investigations, receipt of results, and ongoing instruction.

- Care in accordance with "best practice guidelines" recently published by John Snyder, MD, and leading experts in the field to include gastroenterology, neurology, and neuropsychology consultations.

- The opportunity to consult with a nutritionist specialized in ensuring a well-balanced, gluten-free diet.

- A psychologist available to teach patients skills such as coping, adjustment, and adherence to the gluten-free lifestyle and resolve tensions related to having a chronic condition.

- Extensive educational resources including nutrition education classes, a bi-weekly podcast, web-based cooking videos, peer mentor activities for varying age groups and parents, and several other recurring activities to help patients live a happy and healthy gluten-free lifestyle.

- In partnership with the Global Autoimmune Institute, patients and their families have the opportunity to participate in clinical research projects including:

  > Better understanding the connection between celiac disease and neurological symptoms.

  > Establishing prevalence rates of psychological health issues in children with celiac disease.

  > Evaluating new devices to measure levels of gluten in urine and stool.

  > Developing tools to measure knowledge and risk of gluten exposure.

  > Testing common school supplies to determine the likelihood of gluten transfer to a child with celiac disease.

Go to **www.childrensnational.org/celiac** to learn more.

*Part 1*

# Eating Gluten-Free

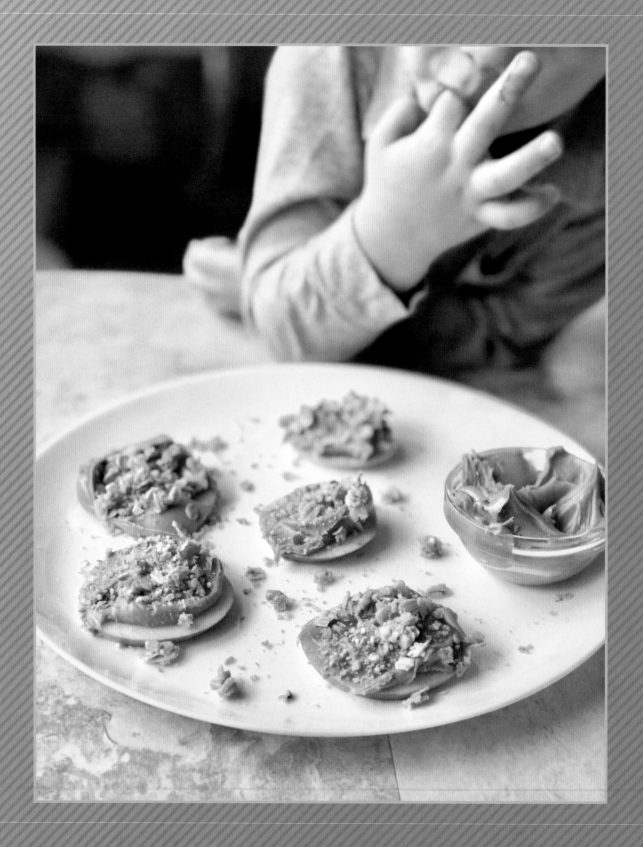

# 1

# The Gluten-Free Diet Guide

## Why Eat Gluten-Free?

There are a number of reasons to start a gluten-free diet. For the patients and families we see at Children's National Medical Center in Washington, D.C., it's most frequently because they have a genetic autoimmune disease called **celiac disease**. When these patients eat **gluten (a protein found in wheat, rye, and barley)**, antibodies form, and a reaction occurs that causes inflammation and damage to the nutrient-absorbing villi in the small intestine. In turn, this damage to the gut prevents absorption of nutrients from food and can lead to severe complications.

Celiac disease was first thought to exist in young patients, ages six to eighteen months, who showed signs of malnutrition, bloating, abdominal pain, and diarrhea. Until recently, this "classic" presentation was the only one described in medical textbooks. However, recent research has uncovered a much more extensive list of subtle signs and symptoms of celiac disease in both pediatric and adult populations. Today, there are hundreds of recognized symptoms of this autoimmune disease that can affect any system of the body. I could go on and on about this, but you're probably not reading this cookbook to learn about the systems of the body, so if you're interested in more information about the symptoms and testing for celiac disease, please visit the Children's National website at www.childrensnational.org/celiac.

About one in one hundred people in the United States has celiac disease, which translates to about three million individuals. However, there are about eighteen million people in America who are living a gluten-free lifestyle for reasons other than celiac disease. Some of them have a true **allergy to wheat**. If they are exposed to wheat, they may require treatment with antihistamines or an EpiPen. Others are diagnosed with **non-celiac gluten sensitivity (NCGS)**, which means they may feel considerable discomfort when they eat gluten. However, patients with NCGS do not have a defined immune reaction to eating gluten and have no damage to the small intestine.

Finally, there are some individuals who choose to eat gluten-free because they believe it is a **healthier lifestyle**. There are mixed opinions on whether or not this is true. I believe that if you choose to eat gluten-free in a natural way, it is an excellent and nutrient-filled diet. I'm talking about filling your diet with naturally gluten-free foods like fresh fruits and vegetables, lean proteins (chicken, beef, fish, shellfish, etc.), dairy, and whole grains like quinoa, brown rice, and sorghum. It's when you add the processed and packaged gluten-free foods that the diet becomes significantly less wholesome. But more about that later.

# Ten Tips for Managing a Gluten-Free Diet

## 1. Understand the Definition of Gluten

It's really important to understand what gluten is. You'd be surprised how many families come to our clinic and can't answer that question. So, to make sure we're all on the same page, gluten is the protein found in wheat, rye, and barley. It's most often found in food, but also in some medications, vitamins, makeup, and school supplies like Playdoh and paper maché.

**Common Ingredients that Contain Gluten**

| Barley | Barley Extract | Barley Grass | Barley Malt | Barley Pearls |
|---|---|---|---|---|
| Bran | Bleached Flour | Bulgur | Bulgur Wheat | Couscous |
| Durum | Einkorn | Emmer | Farina | Fu |
| Graham | Hordeum Vulgare | Hydrolyzed Wheat Protein | Kamut | Macha |
| Malt | Malt Flavoring | Malt Syrup | Malt Vinegar | Matzo |
| Mir | Rye | Seitan | Spelt | Semolina |
| Sprouted Wheat | Tabbouleh | Triticale | Wheat | Wheat Starch |

If you're on a gluten-free diet, you must avoid all forms of wheat, rye, and barley, including any derivatives of these grains. (See the chart opposite, page 4).

## 2. Know Safe Gluten-Free Ingredients

Having a deep understanding of safe ingredients will help you breeze through the grocery store and quickly identify foods that are suitable for the gluten-free diet. A brief list is shown in the chart below, but please refer to the **Gluten-Free Ingredient Glossary** on page 335 for a full description of each ingredient.

## 3. Prevent Cross-Contact

One of the most common questions I'm asked in our Multidisciplinary Celiac Disease Clinic is "does my entire house need to be gluten-free?"

My answer? A strict gluten-free diet means avoiding any chance of cross-contact with gluten-containing products, but you do not need a sterile, 100 percent gluten-free home to be safe. Some families keep their homes entirely gluten-free to make things a little easier, but by no means is this a requirement. By taking a few precautions, it's very possible to have both gluten-free and gluten-containing foods in the same household. Let me explain:

**If you can prevent bacteria from contaminating your kitchen, you can also prevent gluten cross-contact.** If you prepare gluten-containing foods, just make sure to clean with the same rigor that you would if you had just prepared raw chicken in the same space. For example, wash pots, pans, utensils, and countertops with hot soapy water before bringing out gluten-free foods.

### Gluten-Free Foods

| | | | | |
|---|---|---|---|---|
| Acorn Flour | Almond Flour | Amaranth | Arborio Rice | Arrowroot |
| Basmati Rice | Bean Flours | Brown Rice Flour | Buckwheat | Calrose Rice |
| Canola | Cassava | Channa | Chickpea Flour | Coconut Flour |
| Corn Flour | Corn Meal | Cornstarch | Cottonseed | Dal |
| Dasheen Flour | Enriched Rice | Fava Bean Flour | Flax | Flax Seed |
| Flaxseed Meal | Garbanzo | Glutinous Rice | Guar Gum | Hominy |
| Kasha | Lentils | Millet | Peanut Flour | Potato Flour |
| Potato Starch | Quinoa | Red Rice | Rice Bran | Rice Flour |
| Risotto | Sesame | Sorghum | Soy | Soybeans |
| Sunflower Seeds | Sweet Rice Flour | Tapioca | Tapioca Flour | Taro Flour |
| Teff | White Rice Flour | Xanthan Gum | Yeast | Yuca |

If you're making **pasta**, cook the gluten-free first. Remove it from the water and strain, then transfer it to a bowl. Now, cook and strain your gluten-containing pasta. Or, use two separate pots and strainers for each type of pasta.

For **frying**, always think: "fresh oil." Do not fry gluten-free foods in the same oil used to fry gluten-containing foods. Even if the oil looks clear, there may be gluten that could stick to your gluten-free foods. Either fry your gluten-free foods first or use separate oil.

When it comes to **food storage**, I always recommend designating an area of your kitchen to keep all of your gluten-free products. But this isn't always feasible, so if you can't have a separate section, then always store gluten-free foods above gluten-containing foods just in case any flour or food particles fall from an open package. While we hope that there is never falling food of any sort in your pantry or cabinets, if it does happen, you'll be able to rest assured that no gluten will contaminate your gluten-free products.

Any **condiment** that requires you to dip should not be used for both gluten-free and gluten-containing ingredients. My best advice is to always buy condiments in squeeze bottles. The good news is that most condiments like mayonnaise, mustard, ketchup, relish, honey, and maple syrup are easily found in squeeze bottles. For condiments like butter, cream cheese, peanut butter, and Nutella that typically come in tubs, consider having separate containers and label one set as gluten-free. If buying double isn't an option for your family, make sure that everyone in the household uses

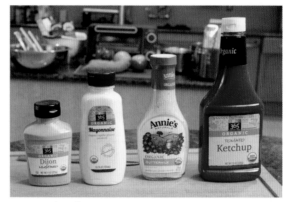

*Squeeze bottles prevent contamination.*

these items in a way that is safe for someone with celiac disease to eat.

**Here's an example to avoid cross-contact:** Using a clean knife or spoon, scoop a portion of peanut butter or Nutella onto your plate and return the knife or spoon to the jar (without touching the gluten-containing food). Using a different knife, spread the condiment onto your gluten-containing toast. This way there is no chance of the crumbs from the toast getting back into the full container.

Until recently, it was thought that a pop-up toaster was a major source of cross-contact as they are almost impossible to clean. A recent study by our Celiac Disease Program found that pop-up toasters may not be the major source of cross-contamination they were thought to be. Best to err on the side of caution, so if you love your pop-up toaster, I recommend having two toasters and dedicating one as the gluten-free toaster. However, if you have a toaster oven, it's easier to share. Simply line the rack with foil when toasting gluten-free foods and remember to frequently clean out the crumb tray.

**Serving utensils** cannot be used for gluten-free and gluten-containing foods at the same time. If you're serving both types of food, use separate serving utensils for each dish. For example, it's Thanksgiving dinner and you have two dishes of stuffing. One is made from gluten-containing bread, and the other is made from gluten-free bread. If you dip a serving spoon into the gluten-containing stuffing, you can no longer use it to serve the gluten-free stuffing without causing cross-contamination. Studies show that even a small amount (⅛ teaspoon) can cause a reaction for a person with celiac disease.

## 4. Understand Food Labeling Laws

There are no federal laws requiring that a product be labeled as gluten-free. However, in 2013, the U.S. Food and Drug Administration (FDA) announced the Gluten-Free Labeling Rule. According to the rule, when a manufacturer chooses to label a product as gluten-free, it must contain less than 20 parts per million (ppm) gluten. It's very important to note that this rule is voluntary, so a manufacturer does not have to label a product as gluten-free, even if it is.

So, how do you use this information? Let's take a look…

First of all, don't get confused by differing gluten-free labels and certification marks. There is no nationally-accepted certification for gluten-free. There are lots of third-party companies that charge manufacturers fees to test their products, and if they are deemed satisfactory, the manufacturer is able to use the certifier's chosen gluten-free symbol. Or, a manufacturer can do their own in-house gluten testing or send their products to an independent lab for testing. Assuming the product tests below the 20ppm threshold, the manufacturer can choose to use any form of the words "gluten-free" on their product if it meets their brand standard. Here are some of the most commonly seen gluten-free symbols:

**The Take-Home Message:** If you see the words "gluten-free" on a food package, it must meet the FDA rule.

Another point of confusion is when you see products like sparkling water or apples that have a gluten-free sticker on them. Use common sense and good judgement when it comes to tactics like this. Many companies use the "gluten-free" label as a marketing strategy, but all water and all apples in their natural form are gluten-free. Don't get roped into buying a more expensive product just because it says "gluten-free" on the label.

During our clinic education sessions, one of the most common questions we receive is, "Why are you telling me to stay on a strict gluten-free diet, but the FDA says that I can eat 20ppm?"

The bottom line is that 20ppm is a very, very tiny amount. Take a look at this photo of my hand holding approximately one million granules of sugar. That tiny little pile on the end of my palm is twenty pieces of brown sugar. The big glob is 999,980 pieces of sugar. So think about this proportion as your 20ppm.

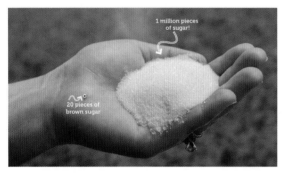

But where did the 20ppm threshold come from? The FDA relied on celiac disease experts from around the world to arrive at this threshold. It's a combination of the sensitivity of the tests to measure gluten in food and data from evidence-based research from clinical trials and analytical studies.

**Tests to Measure Gluten:** The most accurate tests reliably measure gluten in food at the 20ppm level. Tests that claim to measure lower levels have a very high margin of error.

**Evidence-Based Research:** Leading researchers at the Center for Celiac Research conducted trials that found that the majority of people with celiac disease can tolerate up to ten milligrams (mg) of gluten per day with no reaction, meaning they did not develop antibodies or have damage to the gut. So, what does this mean in parts per million and everyday life?

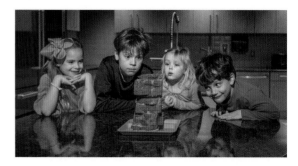

In order to reach the ten milligrams of gluten threshold, you would need to eat approximately eighteen slices of gluten-free bread, with each slice containing 20ppm gluten. That's an awful lot of gluten-free bread!

Conversely, let's say you want to cheat and have a bite of food that you know contains gluten. To reach the 10mg level, you would only need to eat about ⅛ of a teaspoon of that food. It's a tiny amount, right? Ingesting such a small amount of gluten can set off a cascade of unpleasant symptoms, so just stick to gluten-free. I guarantee you will never feel satisfaction from ⅛ teaspoon of pizza.

**Reading Food Labels:** It's very important that you're able to read food labels properly, especially if a product does not clearly show a gluten-free stamp. If you are left to sort through the ingredients list you're going to be looking for the words wheat, rye, and barley (plus all of their derivatives). Make sure to refer to that list of unsafe and safe ingredients.

**The Good News:** The Food Allergen Labeling and Consumer Protection Act (FALCPA) went into effect in January 2006 and requires consumer-friendly labeling on packages of the eight most common food allergen items: wheat, milk, soy, eggs, peanuts, tree nuts, fish, and shellfish. You'll most often see these ingredients show up in an "Allergen Statement" that appears right below the ingredients list.

**The Not-So-Good News:** FALCPA makes it easy for people with celiac disease to identify wheat in a product, but unfortunately, barley and rye are not included in the act's rules, so you'll have to read ingredient labels anyway.

Let's take a look at some labels below with our "Gluten-Free Detectives" and discuss the best way to read them.

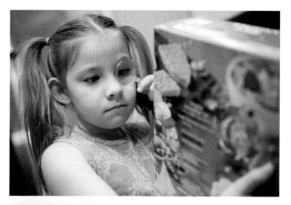

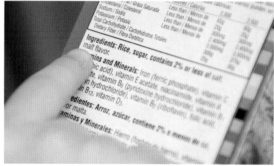

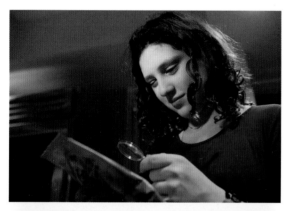

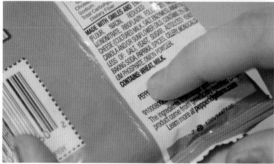

The package of Goldfish above clearly labels the product as containing wheat. This is an easy one. It is **not safe** for a gluten-free diet.

The box above of Rice Krispies is very confusing. It does not say gluten-free, and it also does not say wheat, rye, or barley on the label. The only key word is "**malt flavor**," which is made from barley. This product is unsafe for a gluten-free diet, but the label doesn't make it very clear. That's why it's really important to know the list of unsafe foods.

**Tricky situations.** Sometimes the legal departments at food manufacturers go a little overboard to protect the company and put too many allergen statements on a product. Here's how to navigate these label situations.

**For Products "Made on the Same Equipment as Wheat":** If the product also has a gluten-free label on it, you know the product meets the 20ppm standard regardless of the equipment on which it was manufactured. If the product does not have a gluten-free stamp on it, I recommend checking the company's website. If you don't find a satisfactory answer, call the customer service line or send them an email to find out how the product was made and precautions taken to prevent cross-contamination.

need to dig further before deciding whether or not to eat these nuts.

**For Products "Made in the Same Facility as Wheat:"** If the product also has a gluten-free label on it, you know it meets the FDA standard regardless of the facility in which it was manufactured. If the product does not have a gluten-free stamp on it, I recommend checking the company's website. If you don't find a satisfactory answer, call the customer service line or send them an email to find out how the product was made and precautions taken to prevent cross-contamination.

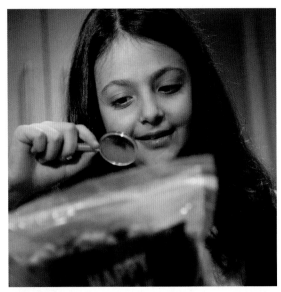

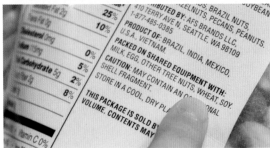

These mixed nuts contain this label but make no mention of their gluten-free status. Our "Gluten-Free Detective" will definitely

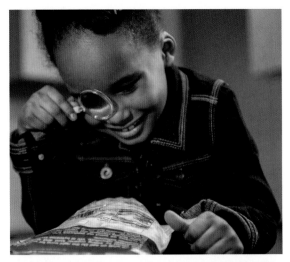

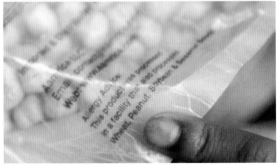

Take a look at that package of crispy garbanzo beans. They are made in the same facility as wheat and several other allergens. Our "Gluten-Free Detective" will need to put her investigation skills to work before deciding whether or not to eat these beans.

**For Products Labeled "May Contain Wheat:"** In the world of food labeling, this statement bothers me the most. How does a manufacturer not know if the product actually contains something? For products with these statements, call the manufacturer's customer service line or email to find out what this actually means before eating the item. Specifically, ask how the product was made and what precautions were taken to prevent cross-contamination.

**To summarize, it's ALWAYS a good idea to check food labels.** If there is a gluten-free label, the product must meet the FDA standard. If there's any question, contact the manufacturer to get more information. When in doubt, go without.

## 5. Keep Your Diet Whole and Clean

The easiest way to manage a safe gluten-free diet is to eat naturally gluten-free foods and forget about eating the processed "junk." Fresh fruits and vegetables, proteins, milk, yogurt, eggs, and whole grains like quinoa, brown rice, and sorghum are all gluten-free in their natural form. If you stick to foods like these, you'll save yourself lots of time reading labels and stressing out about a product's safety.

## 6. Dine Safely in Restaurants

Eating outside of the home, particularly in a restaurant can be one of the most stressful and anxiety-provoking activities for a family with celiac disease. While some families make the choice to limit dining out, I hope I can convince you that going out to eat is a critically important part of social life and that by planning ahead you can still enjoy it.

- **Gluten-Free Menus in Restaurants.** There are no regulations for gluten-free menus. A gluten-free menu in a restaurant simply signifies that the restaurant has food options that they deem to be safe.

- **You Choose the Restaurant.** Be the planner. I know it doesn't come naturally to everyone, but start being the one in your crew who speaks up first and suggests the restaurant. This way you can pick a spot that you know is safe for you or your child.

- **Call Ahead.** When you don't get to pick the restaurant, call ahead and ask the manager or chef about safe gluten-free options. It can be overwhelming to ask a lot of questions when you're sitting at the table in a busy restaurant, so call ahead to ask the questions. This lets you get answers you need in a more relaxed environment, and it gives the restaurant a heads-up that you're coming.

- **Review the Menu at Home First.** I always look over the menu for a new restaurant before I actually go. I want to have an idea of the dishes I like that may need modifications. Doing background research helps the ordering process go faster. Also, I always have a back-up plan if my first choice isn't available gluten-free.

- **Be Prepared to Educate.** When you arrive at the restaurant, don't assume everyone knows what gluten-free means. If your server seems uneasy, it's OK to give them a little back-ground like, "I have celiac disease, and I get really sick when I eat gluten. Can you please make sure that the chef is very careful that my food doesn't touch any gluten?"

- **Apps for Restaurants.** There are lots of companies and apps that offer gluten-free restaurant cards in many different languages. I recommend downloading some of these cards to take to restaurants, particularly those where English is not the first language.

- **Ask for the Chef.** It always helps to speak to the person making your meal, so whenever possible try to speak personally to the chef. I like the chef to remember my son's face and mine while he's making our meal.

- **Don't Be Shy.** Ask as many questions as you need to feel safe.

- **Say Thank You!** While this might seem silly, I always remind families to say "thank you" when they have a great gluten-free meal. These simple words make restaurants feel good about making accommodations and encourages them to continue doing.

**When Something Goes Wrong.** Let's all agree—we don't live in a bubble and mistakes happen. I've been gluten-free for sixteen years, and I know it's a risk to dine out, but I love it! I love experiencing new foods with friends and family and socializing outside of my home is very important to me. So…I keep doing it, understanding that, at some point, my luck will run out, and I will get sick.

I have been badly glutened five times—all in restaurants. In these situations, I waited a day until my symptoms subsided and then I called to discuss the situation. Two restaurants were incredibly apologetic and even offered to provide us with a complimentary meal to prove that they knew how to cook gluten-free. The other three times? They denied the possibility of gluten contamination and told me it must have happened somewhere else.

In your gluten-free journey, you'll see both of these extremes. The important lesson is that when a mistake happens, use your manners and your patience to educate the restaurant so that, hopefully, it won't happen again. Or, if the restaurant isn't cooperative, don't go back.

## 7. Integrating Oats into Your Diet

Oats are naturally gluten-free; however, they are typically grown in fields adjacent to other grain crops including wheat, rye, and barley. This makes for lots of cross contact when oats are grown, harvested, transported, and pro-cessed. But don't worry, there are safe oats for a gluten-free diet. To find them, always look for a gluten-free label on any oat product you purchase. This is very important to confirm that the oats were tested to below the 20ppm threshold set by the FDA.

There are lots of theories floating around about gluten-free oats. At the Celiac Disease Program at Children's National Medical Center, our stance on oats is this: when you are first diagnosed with celiac disease, refrain from eating oats until you feel considerably better and your antibody levels have stabilized. Then, introduce one certified gluten-free oat product into your diet. If you still feel great, go right ahead and continue enjoying gluten-free oats and products made with them. Oats are an excellent source of fiber, iron, and protein, and they make a great addition to cookies, banana bread, granola, and smoothies.

However, if you're one of those individuals who feels sick after eating oats, even if they are gluten-free, it's time to talk to your gastroenterologist or dietitian. Many people with celiac disease also react to oats, even if they are gluten-free. The protein in oats is structured similarly to gluten and, in turn, some people react badly to all forms of oats. There is no reliable test to measure an intolerance to oats, so you'll likely be advised to remove oats from your diet until you feel healthy again and then try a different gluten-free oat product. If you feel bad again with the different product, you're likely intolerant to oats.

## 8. Cheating Is a Bad Idea

It's really tempting to cheat. I'm not going to lie to you. There are times when I've wished I could take a huge bite of a pastry. Don't do it. Just think about those days before you or your child was diagnosed with celiac disease. Today you're healthy and on the path to leading a very normal life. For the momentary satisfaction of biting into a chocolate eclair, you may spend days in the bathroom with diarrhea or a week with a miserable migraine. It's not worth it. And, remember that regular exposure to gluten can lead to lots of long-term health consequences, so don't allow yourself or your child to sometimes cheat.

## 9. Going to School

Particularly for younger children, it's important to have a plan for a safe and inclusive school year. Section 504(a) of the Rehabilitation Act of 1973 prohibits discrimination in all institutions receiving federal financial assistance, including public schools, on the basis of disability, including certain diseases. The law requires that public schools remove barriers to learning, which include accommodating a child's gluten-free diet.

A 504 Plan is the federally-recognized method of detailing all accommodations that need to be made by the school system to assure a child with a disability receives an appropriate education. The plan is developed after diagnosis through meetings between the parents and school officials and is renewed annually to allow for changes and transitions.

The plan stays with a child throughout their entire time in a school district, making transitions to different grade levels easier, and can follow the child if he or she moves to another school within the district.

Our Celiac Disease Program regularly offers trainings for schools and families around the country. If you're interested in learning more, please contact our Celiac Disease Program at celiac@childrensnational.org.

## 10. Don't Believe Everything on the Internet

The internet is flooded with information about living a gluten-free lifestyle. Some of it is excellent, and some of it is bogus. There are a lot of wonderful online forums for patients and families to connect with one another, particularly on Facebook. I always recommend joining these groups, but I make the recommendation with a word of caution. Do not take medical advice from anyone besides your doctor. Oftentimes, well-meaning individuals try to provide commentary on living with a chronic disease that isn't always acceptable or even correct. One comment in an online group can go viral very quickly and lead to lots of misinformation.

For example, in 2018 there was a lot of buzz that vaccines may contain gluten. This rumor flew around the internet so much that researchers at the Columbia University Celiac Disease Center did a study of 1,500 people and found that about 25 percent of people with celiac disease and 40 percent of people with a gluten sensitivity did not believe that vaccines were safe for individuals on a gluten-free diet. Additionally, about 30 percent of these individuals reported forgoing important vaccinations like the flu vaccine.

We've all seen news stories about how deadly the flu can be. Because of rumors online, a large percentage of people living a gluten-free lifestyle could have put themselves at risk for getting a bad case of the flu.

So how do you filter information? Most of the time these online groups are filled with wonderful people who are supporting one another through their gluten-free diets. But when you see information that doesn't seem quite right, check with your doctor or dietitian and get the right answer. Then, share the correct information in the online group to help continue spreading accurate knowledge to the celiac disease community.

— • —

*The gluten-free diet is a journey.* The change doesn't happen overnight. It's a lifetime of learning, exploring, and adapting. I promise, you'll find a rhythm and some incredible gluten-free food along the way.

# 2

# Cooking & Eating with Kids

If you want your kids to learn to eat good food, you have to serve it to them. Forget about store-bought chicken nuggets, boxed mac and cheese, frozen pizza, or bagel bites. *And*, forget about a "Kid's Meal" at restaurants because it reinforces the idea that kids can't eat the same food as grownups.

## Twelve Tips for Success with Little Hands in the Big Kitchen

### 1. Don't Give the Option for "Kid Food." Instead, Plate with Purpose

I advocate for a "Kid's Portion"—serve your kids the same food you eat for dinner with a few modifications. Here's some examples:

- **Better Butter Noodles with Chicken and Zucchini:** I'm not going to lie. My kids are obsessed with butter noodles. To make their butter noodle dinners more nutrient dense, I start by using a quinoa or red lentil-based pasta. You can buy these pastas in pretty (and natural) colors (red, green, and yellow), which they love, and I love that they are packed with protein, fiber, and iron. I make a full box for dinner, toss it with coconut-based butter for the kids, and serve it with rotisserie chicken and roasted zucchini on the side. When I plate these three items for my kids, I put each food group in separate spots on their plates and they devour it! The assembly looks a little different for my husband and me. I heat olive oil and minced garlic in a pan and toss in the rotisserie chicken, roasted zucchini, and cooked pasta, along with a handful of Parmesan cheese. Yum! There's *no* chance my kids would eat this all tossed together, but separate they're A-OK!

- **Brisket Burrito Bowls:** My two boys are obsessed with brisket. If you ask them at breakfast what they would like for dinner that night, they'll probably say brisket and strawberries. However, if I try to serve them **Slow Cooker Brisket Burrito Bowls with Jalapeño Lime Slaw** on page 168, they make faces and (not so politely) decline. But, if I plate the elements separately (brisket, steamed rice, crumbled cheese, and shredded carrots from the slaw), they gobble it up.

## 2. Get the Right Tools and Safety Equipment

- **Kid's Knives:** Search Amazon for kid's knives, and you'll find a variety of kid-safe options that will let them feel big and important while keeping their tiny fingers safe. These knives come in every color imaginable and a set can be purchased for under $10.
- **The Right Grater:** Bigger kids can easily and safely use a box grater, but younger children may not understand keeping their fingers back and end up with a sliced hand. For

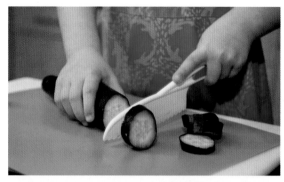

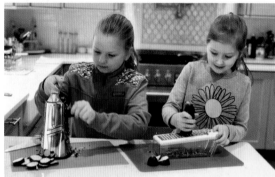

*Kid-friendly knives and graters.*

younger kids, use a grater that lays flat. This will help protect their precious fingers.

- **Long Oven Mitts:** These are key. My five-year-old has started sitting in front of the oven waiting for the timer to go off and begs me to pull the pans of cookies out of the oven. If you're going to let your little one take on this task, be sure to have extra-long oven mitts that go most of the way up their arms to prevent burning. Even with these, stay very close and be perched to assist.
- **Stools for Reaching the Counter:** Investing in a good stool for your kids is critical. Don't just buy one online. Take the time to go to a store like Target or Bed Bath and Beyond,

and let your kids practice standing on them before purchasing. Make sure they are comfortable on the stool so they aren't feeling uneasy while cooking. In some cases, a stool might not be the right option. Despite having three types of stools in our house for my older son to use, my younger son refuses to use anything besides a dining room chair. He likes having the high back to hold on to.

- **Locks on Oven/Stove:** If your kids are toddlers like mine, having safety locks on the oven and stove is crucial. Some oven/stove sets come with them built-in, but if yours doesn't, just Google "stove knob covers." For less than $20, you're ensuring your kids don't turn on the stove and accidentally start a fire or seriously burn themselves.

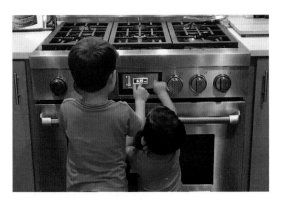

- **Colorful Whisks, Spoons, and Tongs:** Kids love all things colorful, so splurging on some kitchen tools designed for kids is a great way for them to take ownership of their participation in the kitchen. For $22, I purchased a set of silicone cooking utensils and spatulas that came with a rainbow-colored whisk. My kids are obsessed with the tools, and every time

we finish using them, they carefully put them away in their "secret kitchen tool box," so I can't use them if they aren't with me.

### 3. Pick Jobs that Kids Can Do Safely and Successfully

The last thing you want is for your kids to get injured or frustrated while helping you cook. Before starting a cooking project, read the recipe carefully and figure out which steps are safest for your kids. Some ideas include:

- Stirring
- Pouring
- Sifting
- Whisking
- Cracking eggs
- Measuring
- Gather ingredients
- Decorating
- Pushing buttons on equipment

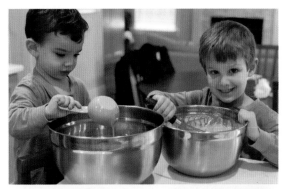

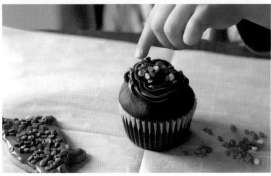

### 4. Sneak Veggies In…

Throughout this book, you'll see lots of places where it seems crazy to toss in a handful of grated zucchini (like in the hamburger recipe on page 223), but guess what? My kids (and all of their friends at our BBQ) ate the burgers and didn't complain, so I consider this a "mom win!" I'm not saying it's easy to get kids to eat veggies. With some kids, it's a nightmare, so I try to sneak them in when possible.

### 5. Story Time in the Cookbook Aisle of a Bookstore or Library

I love reading cookbooks. You probably guessed that since I'm writing one. But I absolutely love reading stories about how others became inspired to cook and looking at their beautiful photos. To me, this suggestion is a double win—I get to sit with my kids and look at cookbooks, and they get to choose what we make for dinner. I love to watch them flip through the pages and get inspired by the photos they come across. Their excitement shows me how important food styling is for kids.

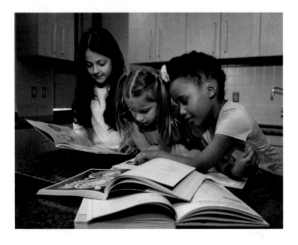

### 6. Don't Be Afraid of the Mess

I'm entirely guilty of only posting adorable photos of my kids cooking on social media. But someday, I promise I'm going to post photos of what the kitchen really looks like after our cooking experience. Being covered in flour and having chunks of dough stuck to my cabinets used to stress me out a lot. But as I cook more with my kids, I remind myself that I'm trading a temporary mess for their long-term love of good-for-you food. I also try different ways to control the mess, such as placing a sheet or tarp under my kids while they cook. This makes the mess much easier to contain and clean up later. If you don't have a sheet or tarp, just tape some parchment paper on the floor beneath them. Always have dish towels or paper towels nearby for accidental spills. And if a spill occurs, I beg you to not get mad. Instead, stop and look at your child's face. The look on a kid's face when they've just made a kitchen mistake is priceless. Follow up with a good giggle and continue on.

### 7. Take Your Kids Grocery Shopping

Until recently, I considered grocery shopping to be my time. I loved taking my time, roaming the aisles and brainstorming my meals for the week. I loved meandering through the produce section savoring the abundance, colors, and textures. Essentially, grocery shopping was an activity I cherished as something to do alone.

Once I had Brandon, I was convinced my "grocery store bliss" days were over. I was convinced it was going to be difficult to share my outings. As we all know, taking little kids

# Substitutions for Dairy Allergies

Kids and grownups with celiac disease sometimes have multiple sensitivities to foods, most often a coexisting dairy allergy. To make this book as accessible as possible for everyone living a gluten-free lifestyle, please find my list of favorite substitutions when using recipes that include dairy.

When my youngest son was diagnosed with a severe dairy allergy, I was devastated. Now I had to figure out how to cook both gluten- and dairy-free. The good news is that I've found incredible substitutions, most notably coconut products, that make most recipes taste just as good, if not better, than their dairy-containing counterparts.

**Milk Replacement Options:** Coconut milk, soy milk, almond milk, rice milk, oat milk, or hemp milk.

*Vanessa's Pick:* There are many brands of coconut milk and each brand has multiple options including sweetened, unsweetened, and flavored. After trying out many types of coconut milk, my favorite for cooking with is the SO Delicious Original Coconut Milk. It has wonderful richness that makes all recipes taste great.

**Butter/Margarine Replacements:** Coconut oil, olive oil, canola oil, or vegetable oil.

*Vanessa's Pick:* Smart Balance Original Dairy-Free Butter with Omega-3 is the only dairy-free butter that my dairy-eating son and husband will eat and not taste the difference. I buy it at Costco and always have it in the house. I bake with it, spread it on gluten-free toast, and use it in sautés and risottos. You'll never know the difference. I also always keep organic coconut spread and organic coconut oil on hand. I actually prefer baking with these because of the wonderful coconut flavor.

**Yogurt/Sour Cream Replacement:** Coconut yogurt, plant-based yogurts, puréed silken tofu, applesauce, soy yogurt, or almond yogurt.

*Vanessa's Pick:* While writing this cookbook, I tested out dozens of dairy-free yogurts in recipes and my absolute favorite was one called Lavva Yogurt. It's made from a blend of coconut cream, plantains and pili nuts. The yogurt had an incredible texture—very similar to traditional yogurt—and reacted well when baked, keeping the foods soft and moist. I also regularly use SO Delicious Plain Coconut Milk Yogurt Alternative.

**Cheese Replacements:** Coconut cheese, soy cheese, rice cheese, or almond cheese. (Note of Caution: Always double-check these labels for casein. Many cheeses are lactose-free but still contain casein, the protein found in milk.)

*Vanessa's Pick:* Call me crazed for coconuts, but once again, our household favorite is the coconut-based cheese shreds. The coconut cheese from SO Delicious is made from coconut milk and coconut cream mixed with navy bean flour and it really does melt well in quesadillas.

shopping can be very stressful. Often, they run off, grab things, and beg to open items before you pay for them. But I encourage all of us to take a deep breath and engage them in the grocery store. Let them walk through the produce section and pick fruits and vegetables that excite them. Take them to talk to the butcher about the kinds of meats that they want to eat. You never know…letting your child pick their own shrimp just may be enough to get them to try seafood.

Now, after a few years of fun (and frustration) shopping with my boys, I experience joy when I see them excited as they take in all the foods of the world. Worth it!

## 8. Plant a Garden and Watch Food Grow

Planting herbs and vegetables has become a highlight of our year. As spring approaches, we visit our local farm and pick out the items we will grow for the summer. Typically, we choose tomatoes, cucumbers, lettuce, sugar snap peas,

zucchini, and a ton of herbs. After each day at camp, the kids rush to the backyard to water the plants and inspect for changes in growth or color. When picking day comes, they are over the moon with their growing accomplishments.

## 9. From the Orchard to Their Mouths

Get a membership to a local orchard and actually go! This provides excitement for about half of the year and allows your kids to see how lots of different fruits and veggies grow. Letting them pick their food right off the vine is exciting! Here's a general outline of when different crops are available in my area of the East Coast, but check your local orchards to see their specific availability:

- Strawberries: Mid-to-late May through June
- Sugar snap peas: Mid-to-late June
- Blueberries: Late June through early August
- Cherries: Late June
- Red raspberries: Mid-August until first frost

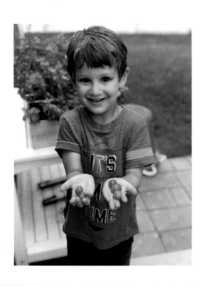
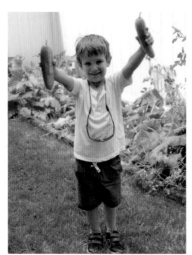
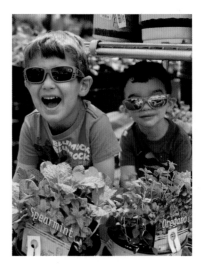

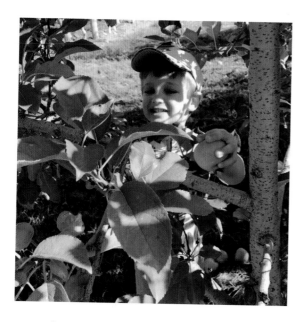

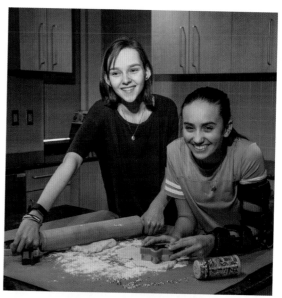

- Apples: September through mid-October
- Pumpkins: Late September through October

## 10. Make Food Artistic

Food is art. Inspire your kids to "play" with their food by having them plate it creatively.

- **Cookie Cutters for Everything:** Cookie cutters should not be reserved just for cookies. Try using fun shapes for waffles, pancakes, eggs, and even scones. You never know…the shape of a food may persuade your child to try it out.

- **Artsy Veggie Platter:** My sister-in-law is the queen of the Thanksgiving Turkey Veggie Platter, and the kids get such a kick out of seeing all of these colorful veggies make up the body of the turkey. This is just one example, but if you check out Pinterest, you'll find lots of great instructions for building beautiful veggie artwork.

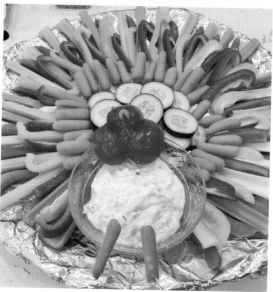

- **Dinner Party Masterpieces:** We get together often with lots of families in our town, and it's always nice for the parents to have some time to chat while the kids are otherwise entertained. One fun trick I've found is setting up appetizers for the kids on a card

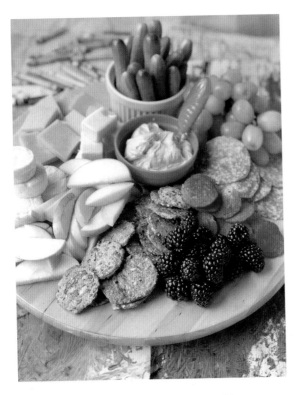

table that's covered with a disposable paper tablecloth. Set up a bunch of crayons and washable markers, and let the kids color on the tablecloth while they snack. At the end of the evening use the tablecloth as the backdrop for a photoshoot.

## 11. Try New Things

Many times, it takes kids lots and lots of tries tasting a new food before they actually love it. So, as parents, we've got to constantly encourage them to try new things. At the risk of being judged, I'm going to share the best mom hack I've come up with: taking my kids to an **all-you-can-eat restaurant where kids eat free.** Now, please don't think I'm promoting wasting food, because that's not the case at all! I'm simply suggesting going to a restaurant where your child can pick small amounts of a variety of foods, and you won't feel frustrated if your kids don't eat everything on their plate.

The first time my husband and I did this was at a sushi restaurant called Sushi Palace. It's $22.95 for adults and kids four and under eat free with a paying adult. Eric and I ordered our usual sushi favorites and, for the kids, we ordered edamame, white rice, grilled chicken, mango avocado rolls, cucumber rolls, and tamago egg rolls. They devoured these kid-friendly foods, and we were shocked when they wanted to taste our food: salmon sushi, seaweed salad, and mushroom soup. Now we go to this restaurant weekly as a family for sushi and love every moment of watching our kids chow down on a sushi platter! (P.S. We always bring our own gluten-free soy sauce).

## 12. Showcase Success

Share a bazillion pictures online, and let your kids be proud of what they created and/or ate. Let them take their creations to school, family gatherings, playdates, wherever…just let them revel in their creativity. It will encourage them to continue engaging with food. After all, isn't this what Instagram is for? **#cookingwithkids**

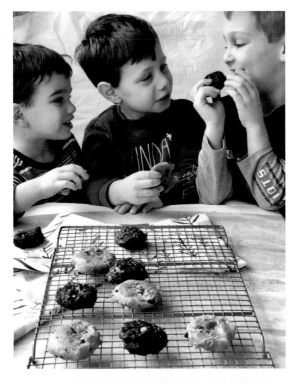

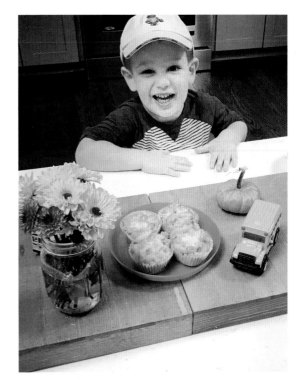

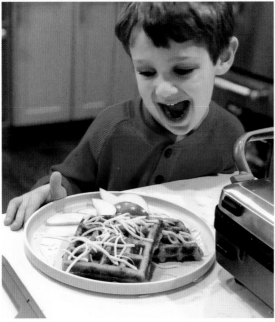

As you look over the recipes in this book, you'll notice that I've included two features that will keep your kids involved in the process.

- **Color-coded text** for kid-friendly recipe participation. Look for method instructions coded in orange that engage kids in food preparation.

- **Dr. Bear Fun Facts!** Dr. Bear is the face of Children's National Health System and will appear throughout the cookbook offering tips for every recipe. Whether it's a dairy- or egg-free substitution or a fun fact about gluten-free whole grains, Dr. Bear will stick with readers throughout most of the recipes.

# 3

# Meal Planning: One Prep, Many Meals

I was never good at meal planning until I had kids. Now that I have two little munchkins bouncing around, I find it harder and harder to plan dinner on a whim. So now, every Saturday, I plan my weekly menu, shop, and prep some items to make those busy week-days a little easier.

***Recipe bases are lifesavers!*** Recipe bases are sauces, vegetable purées, compound butters, or any foundational ingredients that can be used in different recipes. Just make a big batch of them at the beginning of the week. The same base can transform everything from plain risotto to cheese enchiladas into a magical and easily prepared meal.

Some of my favorite bases and how I use them follow. These are easy combinations of dishes that taste so good you'll be getting compliments for days. Once you recognize how much time bases save, experiment with different ingredients to make your own. In the meantime, enjoy these!

# Butternut Squash & Caramelized Onion Mash

Perhaps my favorite creation for a recipe base is the Butternut Squash and Caramelized Onion Mash on page 226. This started out as a spread that my friend Jackie made at a dinner party. She spread the mashed squash onto a sliced baguette and topped it with a spoonful of ricotta cheese. The flavors in the mash were so intensely delightful that I had to come home and immediately figure out how to make it myself. It's simply roasted butternut squash that's mashed together with sweet yellow onions that are caramelized with maple syrup and apple cider vinegar. The first time I prepared the mash, I ate it alone out of a bowl with a spoon…it's that good. I immediately started thinking about all of the ways I could use this purée in many other recipes. The recipe plans below are easy to make, and taste so, so good.

**Day 1: Butternut Squash & Caramelized Onion Mash** (page 226). Serve the mash as a side dish topped with crumbled goat cheese. The mash pairs well with roasted chicken, steaks, and salmon.

**Day 2: Rotisserie Chicken & Butternut Squash Enchiladas** (page 160). Spread the purée on the bottom of corn tortillas. Top with shredded chicken and cheese and roll them up. Pour enchilada sauce over the top and some extra shredded cheese and you've got a sensational supper ready to go.

**Day 3: Butternut Squash & Caramelized Onion Risotto** (page 147). Risotto is one of my favorite meals, rich and delicious. I always have Arborio rice, onions, garlic, and chicken stock on hand, so with the addition of a cup of this mash, I've got a bright-flavored dish that takes little prep time, but tastes like I cooked all day.

**Day 4: Grilled Cheese with Butternut Squash & Gruyère** (page 177). OK, I'll admit—this was a total on-a-whim creation fueled by a starving moment. I had Gruyère cheese in the fridge and some of this butternut squash mash, so I tossed them together on some gluten-free bread and sizzled it in a pan. My oh my, was this a delight!

**Day 5: Baked Squash Macaroni & Cheese Cups** (page 189). What I love about this mash is that it pairs well with so many different flavors. Even after five days of using the same mash, you still feel like you're getting a totally different set of ingredients each time you eat it.

**Weekend Brunch: Roasted Butternut Squash & Goat Cheese Quiche** (page 70). This is probably my favorite recipe in the book. This recipe came to be because I had exactly one cup left of the mash and didn't want to waste it. We had a group of friends coming over for Sunday brunch, so I decided to use it, and oh boy, was that a good decision. I made it the night before and used a gluten-free, puff pastry crust. All I had to do in the morning was put it in the oven. Serve this quiche paired with the **Tossed Arugula Salad with Sweet Lemon Vinaigrette** (page 125). It's literally the easiest combination of dishes.

# Delightfully Dairy-Free Caramel Sauce

I created this recipe (page 258) when my younger son was diagnosed with a dairy allergy, and I found myself no longer able to use store-bought caramel sauce. I had used a date purée as a sweetener in the past, so I decided to try to thin it out and see what happened. The incredible result was a blend of dates, hot water, vanilla extract, and coconut oil.

Blair Raber, the founder of our Celiac Disease Program, was at my house when I struck gold. "It's so good, I just keep taking a spoonful every time I walk past the kitchen!" she said. I totally agreed, so as I was working on recipes for this book, I started using this sauce as a base for lots of others. Add an egg, peanut butter, gluten-free oats, coconut, and gluten-free all-purpose flour and you've got yourself **Peanut Butter Coconut Breakfast Cookies** (page 73). Or, purée this base with an avocado, banana, peanut butter, and cocoa powder, and you've got chocolate pudding found in the recipe for **Cookies & Cream Chocolate Pudding Cups** (page 303). The options are endless, but the base stays the same. Make a batch of this sauce, and keep it in the fridge. You'll use it more than you ever imagined.

## Dressings, Butters & Sauces

Throughout the book you'll see lots of recipes in which I use sauces over and over again. That's why I decided to create an entire section that has all of the sauces, dressings, and compound butters in one place. I love to make lots of these when I have a free day and then freeze them, so when I need something quick, I can pull one out of the freezer to use in recipes. Use them as marinades for meats, dressings on salads, or for a boost of flavor to steamed veggies.

# Rotisserie Chicken

There is no easier meal option than the grab-and-go rotisserie chicken. Not only is it healthy and tasty, it is one of the most versatile products in the grocery store. For years, I've relied heavily on the Costco rotisserie chicken. I buy one and immediately shred it off the bones so I have it ready to go for the week. While I was working on the recipes for this cookbook, I decided to keep track of every rotisserie chicken I bought to see exactly how much chicken could be pulled off the bones. I was shocked. Each of the four Costco chickens yielded ten cups of shredded chicken! My recipes use between two and four cups, so with just one chicken, I can easily make meals for several nights of the week.

In the Family Suppers section of the book, you'll find my tasty recipes using rotisserie chicken including:

- **Basic Roasted Chicken**, page 152.
- **Mexican Pizza with Rotisserie Chicken & Pineapple Avocado Salsa**, page 155.
- **Thai Chili Chicken Pizzas with Rotisserie Chicken & Tangy Cucumber Slaw**, page 156.
- **Lettuce Wraps with Rotisserie Chicken, Creamy Slaw, & Sriracha Mayo**, page 159.
- **Rotisserie Chicken & Butternut Squash Enchiladas**, page 160.
- **Ginger Soy Fried Rice with Rotisserie Chicken & Sugar Snap Peas**, page 163.
- **Citrus and Cilantro Pulled Chicken with Rice & Beans**, page 164.

But before we get to cooking, let's go over a few suggestions for making sure the rotisserie chicken purchased at a grocery store is really gluten-free.

## Safety Tips for Choosing a Rotisserie Chicken

Unfortunately, not all rotisserie chickens are gluten-free. Some stores use spice blends and marinades that include gluten-containing ingredients, so it's important always to check the labels before making a purchase.

Here are some tips to select a safe chicken:

- **Stick to the classic rotisserie chicken that is seasoned with just salt and pepper.** Some flavored varieties (like the Cajun or Teriyaki ones) use spice mixes that contain gluten.
- **Safe Cooking Practices.** Check with a manager in the meat or deli department to make sure the chicken is not prepared in a shared space where cross-contact might occur *or* that the store takes precautions to prevent contamination from gluten.
- **Check to make sure the chicken was not prepared with flour.** Some store brands prepare their chickens with a dusting of flour to make a crispier finished product. These chickens are not safe for a gluten-free diet.

**Make Your Own!** While the store-bought chicken is a quick and easy option, it's also really simple to roast your own chicken at home. Follow my recipe on page 152 for basic roasted and shredded chicken, and in just a short time you'll have freshly roasted chicken.

# 4

# For Better or Worse: Gluten-Free Flours & Mixes

People with celiac disease spend a lot of time discussing why gluten is bad but don't often consider the benefits gluten brings to baked goods. Humor me for a moment, and let's consider why gluten is good.

Gluten is a protein that provides structure, texture, viscosity and thickening properties to food, particularly baked goods. Just think about pizza dough. We've all been to a pizzeria where the chef is tossing dough up in the air to stretch it out to the perfect diameter for the pizza pan. The element of the dough that allows this stretchiness is the gluten in the wheat flour.

Although gluten is found in wheat, rye, and barley, for the purposes of this section, I'm talking about baking with wheat flour. Few recipes use rye or barley flour, so I'm focusing on the issues with replacing wheat flour.

Unfortunately, there is no one-to-one replacement for the structural or nutritional properties that you'll find in gluten-containing wheat flour. So, when home cooks, chefs, or food manufacturers attempt to replace wheat-based flour in recipes, they use a combination of gluten-free ingredients to replicate these important properties. These blends are typically made using combinations of ingredients such as brown rice, sorghum, almond, coconut, buckwheat, and tapioca flours, as well as starches like potato and cornstarch. You'll also need a binder—either xanthan or guar gum.

It's important to understand that not all gluten-free flours are created equal. They each have very different weights, rising abilities, and binding properties. Some are super starchy (brown and white rice flours, cornstarch, potato starch, and tapioca flour). Some are loaded with fiber and protein (millet, teff, sorghum, chickpea, quinoa, and amaranth flours). And some are very low in carbohydrates (almond, soy, and coconut flours).

The nutritional profiles of these gluten-free ingredients look quite different than the nutritional profile of wheat flour. In some cases, the gluten-free ingredients are void of important nutrients like protein and fiber, and in other examples, they are much higher in carbohydrates. On the flip side, some of them are actually significantly better in nutrition than wheat flour. Some are loaded with protein and fiber and are very low in carbohydrates.

Let's take a deeper look. The chart below, shows a listing of fiber, protein, carbohydrates, and fat for the most common gluten-free substitute ingredients with a comparison to whole wheat flour.

The bottom line is that reading the food label goes beyond looking for gluten-containing or gluten-free ingredients. You've got to look at what's actually in the gluten-free products you're purchasing so you can make an informed decision about the quality of your food. If your diet is filled with gluten-free products made from just white rice flour and tapioca flour (which many are), you're risking low nutritional

| Ingredient | Fiber (per ¼ cup) | Protein (per ¼ cup) | Carbohydrates (per ¼ cup) | Fat (per ¼ cup) |
|---|---|---|---|---|
| Almond Flour | 3g | 4g | 6g | 12g |
| Coconut Flour | 11g | 5g | 8g | 3g |
| Brown Rice Flour | 2g | 3g | 31g | 1g |
| White Rice Flour | 1g | 2g | 32g | 0.5g |
| Teff Flour | 5g | 5g | 29g | 1.5g |
| Millet Flour | 4g | 3g | 22g | 1g |
| Sorghum Flour | 3g | 4g | 25g | 1g |
| Tapioca Flour | 0g | 0g | 26g | 0g |
| Soy Flour | 3g | 10g | 8g | 6g |
| Cornstarch | 0g | 0g | 7g | 1g |
| Potato Starch | 0g | 0g | 10g | 0.5g |
| Quinoa Flour | 2g | 4g | 18g | 1.5g |
| Buckwheat Flour | 4g | 4g | 21g | 1g |
| Whole Wheat Flour | 5g | 6g | 27g | 0.5g |

*Nutritional values from Bob's Red Mill Product Packages (www.bobsredmill.com)*

intake, which can lead to health complications and deficiencies.

My advice? Look for gluten-free flour blends that are made from a combination of these flours, especially the ones that are packed with protein and fiber, and are lower on the carbohydrate scale. They give you loads of energy and help keep you full longer.

## Gluten-Free Flours in This Book

Before I had kids I regularly made my own gluten-free all-purpose flour. I made huge batches at a time and stored it in the freezer. I'm sharing my favorite all-purpose flour blend with you.

It's a combination of sweet white sorghum flour, coconut flour, tapioca flour, and xanthan gum. Each ingredient has a purpose for being in the blend. The sorghum flour is packed with protein, iron and fiber. The coconut flour has a slight sweetness which allows you to reduce the amount of sugar in the overall recipe. It's also loaded with fiber and protein and low in carbohydrates. The tapioca flour has little nutritional value, but it gives baked goods an amazing thin and sturdy crust, so I put some in.

But let's get back to reality. Even though it only takes a few minutes to make this flour blend, I rarely go through the trouble to make it myself unless I've thought ahead to buy all of the ingredients. There are dozens of wonderful gluten-free, all-purpose flour mixes in grocery stores and, most often, it's cheaper to buy one of them than the individual ingredients to make my own.

So, how do you pick one?

### Vanessa's Favorite Homemade Gluten-Free Flour Blend

**YIELD: 7 CUPS**
Prep Time: 5 minutes
Total Time: 5 minutes

3 cups sweet white sorghum flour
3 cups tapioca flour
1 cup coconut flour
3 teaspoons xanthan gum

**1.** In a large mixing bowl, whisk all of the ingredients together.

**2.** Store in an airtight container for up to one month, and use as a one-to-one replacement in baking recipes.

# Ready-Made, Gluten-Free All-Purpose Flours

Over the last fifteen years, I've tested nearly every gluten-free, all-purpose flour for sale and each is totally different. As a rainy-day activity, I've picked out four different flours and had my kids make the same recipe of chocolate chip cookies using each of the varieties. You wouldn't believe how different they looked. Some cookies were flat and crispy, some were fluffy and cakey, and others barely stayed together when they were picked up.

To qualify for shelf space in my pantry, a gluten-free flour blend must have a balanced variety of ingredients, including a high starch flour, a high protein flour, and either xanthan or guar gum. If the flour mix does not include xanthan or guar gum, you will have to buy it separately and add it in, so I find no reason to purchase an all-purpose flour that doesn't come with a gum included.

Why xanthan or guar gum? Both xanthan and guar gum provide the "doughy" factor in gluten-free baked goods. A gum mimics the missing gluten in gluten-free flours and helps make the dough elastic. You can use xanthan or guar gums interchangeably in recipes.

I won't spend time telling you about the gluten-free flour blends that I don't like, but I will mention those that I love and regularly keep in my pantry. I've tested all of the recipes in this book using at least three of these blends to make sure the recipes come out the same with different flours. They are listed below with the ingredients they contain as of the publishing date of this book. If you use a different gluten-free, all-purpose flour, don't be alarmed if your recipe doesn't look exactly like the photo. It's likely because the flour blend has very different properties. The good news is that it will likely taste just the same!

- **King Arthur Gluten-Free Measure for Measure Flour:** Whole Grain Brown Rice Flour, Whole Grain Sorghum Flour, Tapioca Starch, Potato Starch, Cellulose, Xanthan Gum, vitamin and mineral blend—calcium carbonate, niacinamide (vitamin $B_3$), reduced iron, thiamin hydrochloride (vitamin $B_1$), riboflavin (vitamin $B_2$).

- **Pamela's Products All-Purpose Gluten-Free Flour:** Brown Rice Flour, Tapioca Starch, White Rice Flour, Potato Starch, Sorghum Flour, Arrowroot Starch, Guar Gum, Sweet Rice Flour, Rice Bran.

- **Bob's Red Mill Gluten-Free 1-to-1 Baking Flour:** Sweet Rice Flour, Whole Grain Brown Rice Flour, Potato Starch, Whole Grain Sorghum Flour, Tapioca Flour, Xanthan Gum.

- **Blends by Orly Gluten-Free Pastry Flour (Manhattan Blend):** Brown Rice Flour, Whole Grain Sorghum Flour, Millet Flour, Long Grain Rice Flour, Potato Starch, Tapioca Starch, Xanthan Gum.

# Decision: Store Bought or Homemade?

I used to make everything from scratch. I like having control over the quality of ingredients and nutritional value of the food I make. But, these days, I just can't always find the time to make everything myself. Don't get me wrong, I do cook a lot, but there are some foods that are just considerably more convenient to buy than to make. So, I've made some concessions.

## Puff Pastry

I made gluten-free puff pastry one time. What a pain! I went for years without using puff pastry because I couldn't bring myself to go through the trouble. I got annoyed anytime I saw a recipe in a magazine that called for one package of puff pastry. Thankfully there are now two manufacturers making gluten-free puff pastry, and it has really changed my life for the better. I now make quiches, tarts, and turnovers galore.

*Vanessa's Picks: Schär Puff Pastry Dough or GeeFree Gluten-Free Puff Pastry*

## Hamburger Buns, Baguettes, Croissant Rolls, and Brioche Rolls

I'm not a huge fan of the commercially-available buns and rolls sold in big grocery stores, but I do love those made by local gluten-free bakeries. I encourage you to Google "gluten-free bakery (your city name)," and go taste lots of different options. Many bakeries ship nationwide, so look online for reviews as well and trying some out. I now stock up on these items and keep them in my freezer for Sunday brunches and BBQs. Sometimes I even take my own bun to restaurants and order just the burger and toppings with no bun and then add my own at the table.

*Vanessa's Picks: Rise Bakery (Washington, DC), Modern Bread and Bagel (NYC), Gluten-Free Gloriously Bakery (Stirling, NJ), Mariposa Baking (San Francisco, CA), Sweet Love Pastry (Hollywood, FL)*

## Pasta, Ravioli, Gnocchi

Someday I'll venture into making my own pasta. But, with the abundance of gluten-free pasta options on the market, for now I'll continue saving time by using store-bought pasta. The vast majority of gluten-free pastas are made with rice flours because rice mimics gluten very well in pasta form. But there are also a lot of pastas made from blends of grains (corn, quinoa, amaranth, buckwheat), beans, and lentils. These pastas are packed with important nutrients, taste great, and some come in pretty (and natural) colors. You'll also find all of the popular pasta shapes in gluten-free varieties including: spaghetti, linguine, penne, lasagna, elbows, rotini, angel hair, fettuccine, shells (large and small), fusilli, manicotti, ziti, farfalle, egg noodles, casarecce, capellini, wheels, ravioli, bucatini, and gnocchi.

*Vanessa's Picks: Jovial (farfalle bow ties and manicotti), Garofalo (casarecce), Ancient Harvest (garden pagodas), Tolerant (red lentil penne), and Tinkyada (large shells).*

## Pizza Dough

Making your own pizza dough is really fun. My kids get a kick out of watching the dough double in size while it rises. But, they also get cranky because they have to wait so long to eat the pizza.

Although it sounds amazing to always make your own pizza dough, in truth, it's just not practical or necessary. There are fantastic pre-made mixes and frozen gluten-free crusts on the market that taste great and are ready to go at a moment's notice.

### Pre-Made Gluten-Free Pizza Doughs

These gluten-free pizza doughs come as a dough ball in a freezer-friendly package. They just needs to be thawed and opened, and they're ready to roll! I always have a package of this dough in my freezer and use it for everything from traditional pizza to calzones, garlic twists, cinnamon rolls, and monkey bread.

*Vanessa's Picks: Wholly Wholesome Gluten-Free Pizza Dough or Gillian's Foods Pizza Dough*

### Gluten-Free Pizza Dough Mixes

If you're looking to still have a dough-making experience without having to worry about collecting all the ingredients, these mixes are the answer! Minimal ingredients are needed and most mixes even come with an included yeast packet. All that's needed is water and an egg.

*Vanessa's Picks: Pamela's Products Pizza Crust Mix or Bob's Red Mill Pizza Crust Mix*

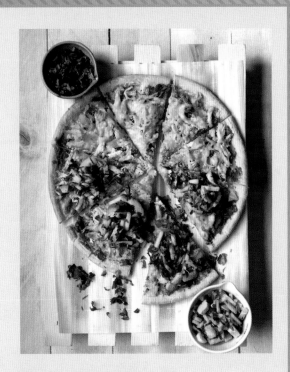

### Ready-Made Gluten-Free Pizza Crusts

By far the easiest version! Just open the package, put on your favorite toppings, and pop it in the oven. There are lots of different varieties to choose from. Some mimic a traditional pizza crust. Others are very cheesy, and some are made using cauliflower as the base. Try out a few and then stock up on your favorite crust just in case you get a pizza craving!

*Vanessa's Picks: Against the Grain Gourmet Gluten-Free Crust (cheesy), Udi's Gluten-Free Crust (traditional thin crust), Schär Gluten-Free Crusts (traditional thick crust), and Caulipower Gluten-Free Crust (cauliflower-based).*

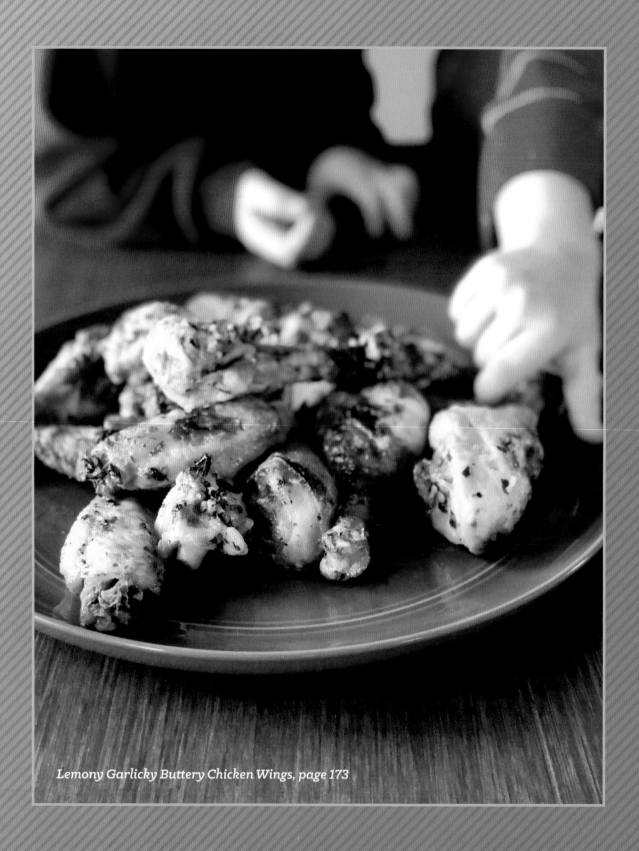

Lemony Garlicky Buttery Chicken Wings, page 173

*Part 2*

# Gluten-Free Recipes

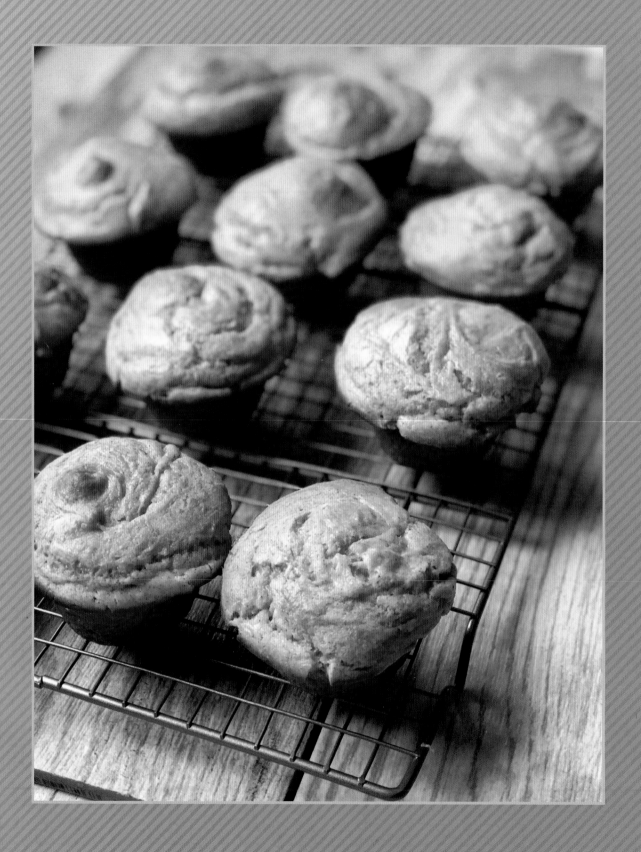

# 5

# Nourishing Breads
# & Breakfasts

Kid-friendly participation steps are printed in **ORANGE**

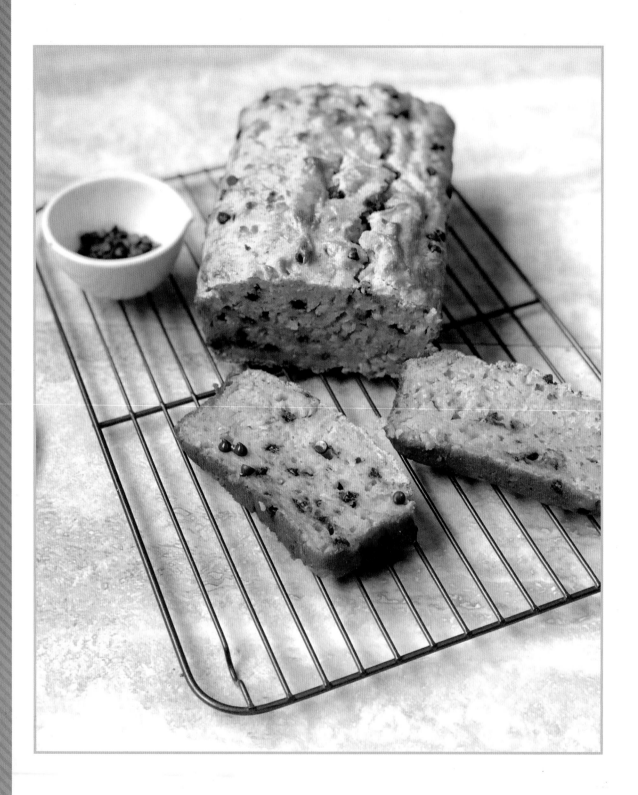

# Chai Spiced Chocolate Chip Apple Bread

*This bread is beyond good. It's one of those recipes where I make it for a playdate, and every mom asks me for the recipe and immediately goes home to make it. If you or your child has a dairy allergy, simply substitute a dairy-free, coconut-based yogurt for the Greek yogurt. You'll never know the difference.*

**YIELD: 1 LOAF (12 SERVINGS)**
Prep Time: 15 minutes
Total Time: 75 minutes

---

2 cups gluten-free all-purpose flour

1 teaspoon ground cinnamon

1 teaspoon ground ginger

½ teaspoon ground allspice

1 teaspoon baking powder

½ teaspoon salt

1 cup sugar

¾ cup coconut oil

½ cup plain Greek yogurt

2 eggs

1 teaspoon vanilla extract

2 apples, core removed and shredded finely

½ cup mini chocolate chips

**1.** Preheat oven to 350°F. Grease an 8x4-inch loaf pan with nonstick cooking spray and set aside.

**2.** In a mixing bowl, whisk together the gluten-free all-purpose flour, cinnamon, ginger, allspice, baking powder, and salt. Set aside.

**3.** In the bowl of a stand mixer, using the paddle attachment, beat together the sugar, coconut oil, Greek yogurt, eggs, and vanilla extract. Mix until smooth.

**4.** Slowly add the dry ingredients into the wet ingredients, mixing well after each addition.

**5.** Gently fold in the shredded apples and mini chocolate chips to the mixture.

**6.** Pour the batter into the prepared loaf pan and bake for 55 to 60 minutes until a toothpick inserted into the center of the loaf comes out clean. Cool before serving.

 **Dr. Bear Fun Fact!** Chai tea is called "masala chai" in India. "Chai" is the Hindi word for "tea," and "masala" means a mix of spices. Chai spices usually include cinnamon, ginger, cloves, and cardamom, but is easily adaptable to mix in other spices.

*Nutritional data reflects one serving, based on a 12-serving yield.*

**PER SERVING** Calories: 336; Total Fat: 17.2g; Saturated Fat: 13.1g; Cholesterol: 29.9mg; Sodium: 160.1mg; Total Carbohydrates: 42.3g; Dietary Fiber: 1.8g; Sugars: 24.3g; Protein: 3.6g

# Zucchini Banana Bread

*My husband's biggest complaint about gluten-free baked goods is that they are dry and crumbly. Over the fourteen years we've been together, I've worked very hard to develop a banana bread recipe that he loves as much as I do. Adding zucchini was the magic touch. It's loaded with water and really helps keep the bread moist.*

**YIELD: 1 LOAF (12 SERVINGS)**
Prep Time: 15 minutes
Total Time: 90 minutes

---

2 cups gluten-free all-purpose flour

1 cup gluten-free quick cook oats

2 teaspoons baking powder

1 teaspoon ground cinnamon

1 teaspoon salt

1 cup lightly packed brown sugar

¾ cup vegetable or coconut oil

1 teaspoon vanilla extract

3 eggs

3 large, ripe bananas, peeled and mashed

½ cup coconut milk

1 cup shredded zucchini, ends removed

1. Preheat oven to 350°F. Spray an 8-by-4-inch loaf pan with nonstick cooking spray and set aside.

2. In a mixing bowl, whisk together the gluten-free all-purpose flour, gluten-free oats, baking powder, cinnamon, and salt. Set aside.

3. In the bowl of a stand mixer, using the paddle attachment, beat together the brown sugar, oil, vanilla extract, and eggs. Mix until well combined.

4. Add in the bananas and coconut milk and mix until well combined.

5. Slowly add the dry ingredients into the wet ingredients, mixing well after each addition.

6. Gently fold in the shredded zucchini.

7. Pour the batter into the prepared loaf pan and bake for 70 to 75 minutes until a toothpick inserted into the center of the loaf comes out mostly clean. Because of the moisture in the zucchini and bananas, you will likely not get a perfectly clean toothpick. Cool before slicing.

 **Dr. Bear Fun Fact!** Zucchini are in the same family as pumpkins!

*Nutritional data reflects one serving, based on a 12-serving yield.*

**PER SERVING** Calories: 340.5; Total Fat: 15.9g; Saturated Fat: 2.9g; Cholesterol: 41mg; Sodium: 299.7mg; Total Carbohydrates: 47.2g; Dietary Fiber: 2.4g; Sugars: 22.6g; Protein: 3.8g

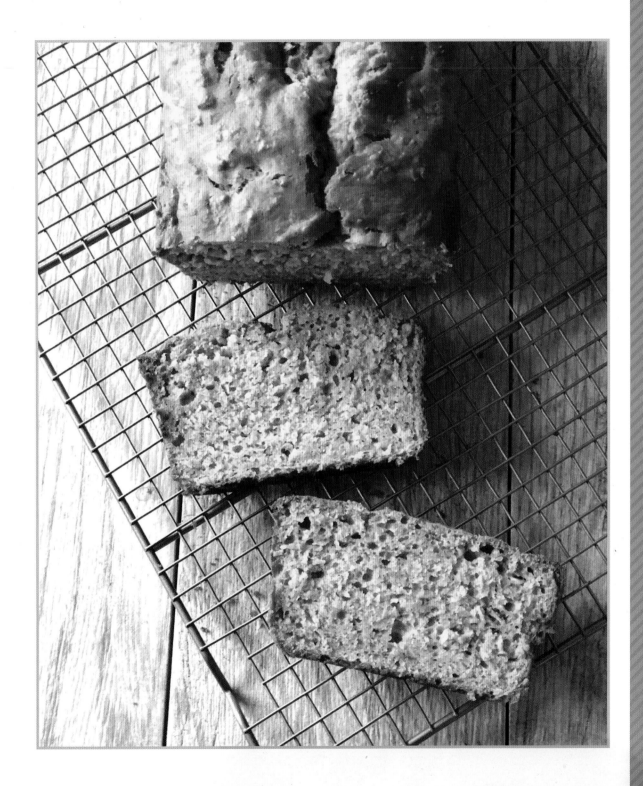

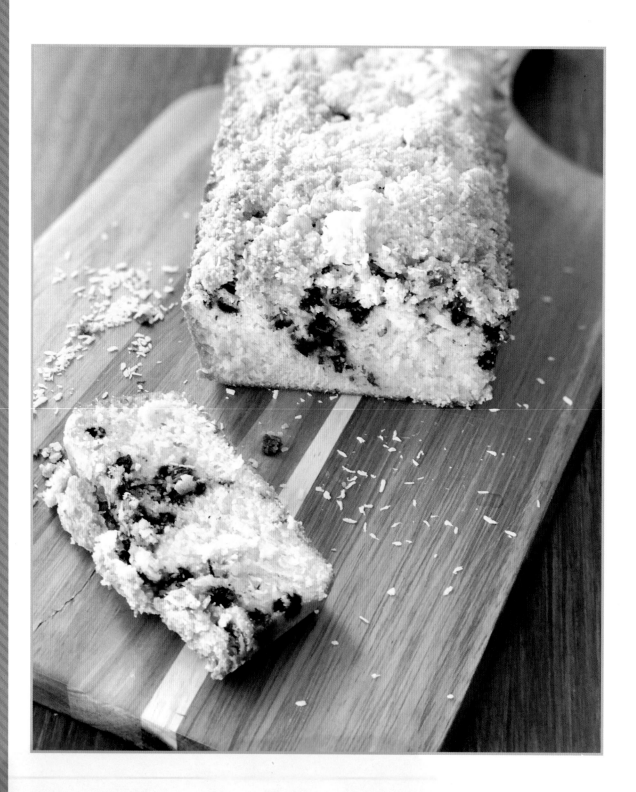

# Lemon Blueberry Coconut Crumble Loaf

*This recipe started out being made with butter, but when I went to test out the dairy substitutes to write this headnote, I decided I liked the bread better with coconut milk and coconut oil! So, if you don't have coconut milk or oil on hand, and you don't need a dairy-free option, feel free to use whole milk and butter to make this delicious loaf.*

**YIELD: 1 LOAF (12 SERVINGS)**
Prep Time: 15 minutes
Total Time: 55 minutes

———————

### For the Batter
2 cups gluten-free all-purpose flour
2 teaspoons baking powder
1 teaspoon salt
1 cup sugar
½ cup coconut oil, melted
2 eggs
⅓ cup coconut milk
¼ cup lemon juice
Zest of 1 lemon
1 cup frozen blueberries

### For the Coconut Crumb Topping
¼ cup sugar
2 tablespoons cornstarch
2 tablespoons very cold coconut butter, cut into small pieces
Zest of 1 lemon
½ cup coconut flakes

1. Preheat oven to 350°F. Spray an 8-by-4-inch loaf pan lightly with nonstick spray and set aside.

2. In a mixing bowl, whisk together the gluten-free all-purpose flour, baking powder, and salt. Set aside.

3. In the bowl of a stand mixer, using the paddle attachment, beat together the sugar, coconut oil, eggs, coconut milk, lemon juice, and lemon zest. Beat until light and smooth.

4. Slowly add the dry ingredients into the wet ingredients, making sure to mix well after each addition. Fold in the blueberries. Set aside.

5. To make the crumb topping, mix together sugar, cornstarch, coconut butter, lemon zest, and coconut flakes in a small bowl until small pea-sized crumbles form.

6. Pour the batter evenly into the prepared loaf pan.

7. Sprinkle the crumb topping evenly across the top.

8. Bake for 50 to 55 minutes until a toothpick inserted into the center of the loaf comes out clean.

 **Dr. Bear Fun Fact!** Coconut is one of the most versatile foods on earth! You can make milk, oil, butter, flakes, water, and flour from the inside, and the husk can be used for inedible things like rope, brushes, nets, mattresses, and floor mats.

*Nutritional data reflects one serving, based on a 12-serving yield.*
**PER SERVING** Calories: 301.3; Total Fat: 14g; Saturated Fat: 11.2g; Cholesterol: 27.4mg; Sodium: 290.9mg; Total Carbohydrates: 42.4g; Dietary Fiber: 2.1g; Sugars: 23.1g; Protein: 2.4g

# Blueberry Peach Yogurt Muffins

*These muffins are super moist thanks to the buttermilk and Greek yogurt. At the time I was writing this cookbook, blueberries and peaches were in season, but you can really make them with any fruits you have in your refrigerator.*

**YIELD: 12 MUFFINS**
Prep Time: 15 minutes
Total Time: 50 minutes

---

2 cups gluten-free all-purpose flour
1 cup gluten-free quick cook oats
2 teaspoons baking powder
½ teaspoon salt
¾ cup sugar
3 eggs
½ cup coconut oil, melted
¾ cup buttermilk
¾ cup plain Greek yogurt
2 teaspoons vanilla extract
¾ cup chopped peaches
¾ cup fresh blueberries, rinsed and patted dry

1. Preheat oven to 350°F. Spray a 12-cup muffin pan with nonstick spray and set aside.

2. In a mixing bowl, whisk together gluten-free all-purpose flour, gluten-free oats, baking powder, and salt. Set aside.

3. In the bowl of a stand mixer, using the paddle attachment, beat together the sugar, eggs, and coconut oil until well combined. Add in the buttermilk, Greek yogurt, and vanilla extract, and mix until well combined.

4. Slowly add the dry ingredients into the wet ingredients, mixing well after each addition.

5. Gently fold in the chopped peaches and blueberries.

6. Pour heaping portions of the batter into the prepared muffin pan.

7. Bake for 30 to 35 minutes until a toothpick inserted into the center of the muffins comes out clean. Cool before serving.

 **Dr. Bear Fun Fact!** Blueberries and peaches pack a nutritious punch in this recipe! Both are high in fiber and great antioxidants.

*Nutritional data reflects one muffin, based on a 12-muffin yield.*
**PER SERVING** Calories: 277.1; Total Fat: 11.8g; Saturated Fat: 8.5g; Cholesterol: 43.9mg; Sodium: 217.6mg; Total Carbohydrates: 37.2g; Dietary Fiber: 1.7g; Sugars: 16g; Protein: 5.4g

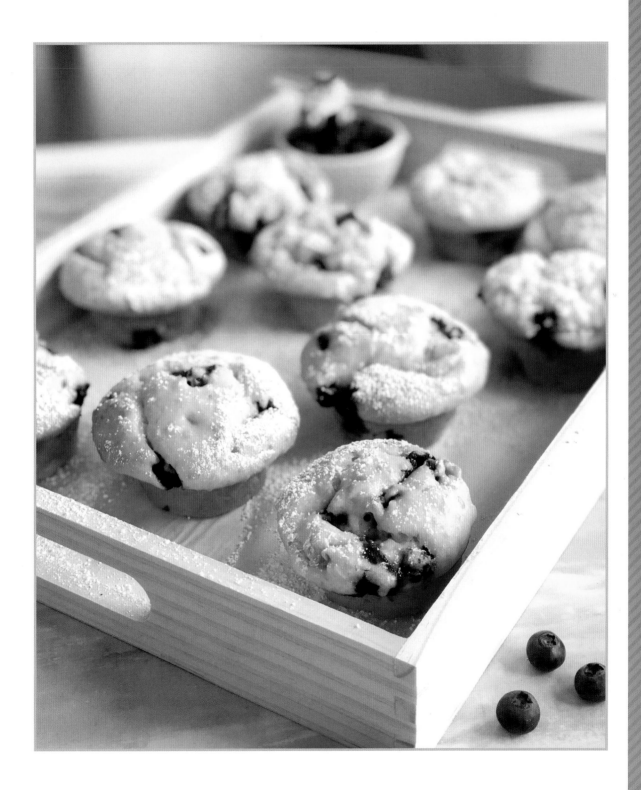

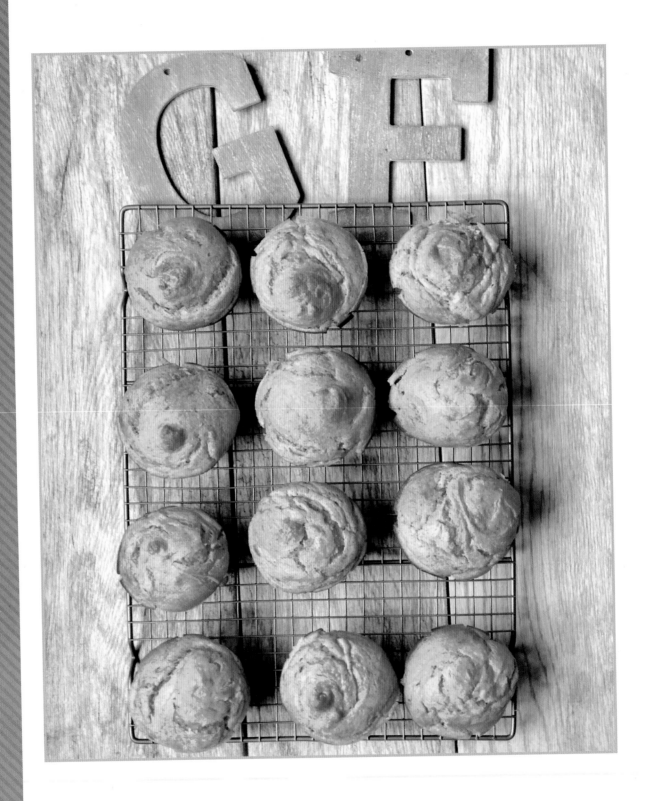

# Pumpkin Goat Cheese Swirl Muffins

*These muffins are packed with warm, fall flavors with a touch of tart from the goat cheese. If you prefer a more mellow muffin, replace the goat cheese with cream cheese.*

**YIELD: 12 MUFFINS**
Prep Time: 15 minutes
Total Time: 50 minutes

---

**For the Filling**
1 cup (8 ounces) goat cheese, softened
1 egg
¼ cup sugar
½ teaspoon ground cinnamon
1 teaspoon vanilla extract

**For the Muffin Batter**
1½ cups gluten-free all-purpose flour
2½ teaspoons baking powder
1 teaspoon pumpkin pie spice
½ teaspoon nutmeg
½ teaspoon salt
1 cup sugar
2 eggs
1 cup pumpkin purée
⅓ cup coconut oil, melted
¼ cup maple syrup
1 teaspoon vanilla extract

*Nutritional data reflects one muffin, based on a 12-muffin yield.*

**PER SERVING** Calories: 264.4; Total Fat: 10g; Saturated Fat: 7g; Cholesterol: 46mg; Sodium: 270mg; Total Carbohydrates: 40g; Dietary Fiber: 1g; Sugars: 26g; Protein: 5g

**1.** Preheat oven to 350°F. Spray a 12-cup muffin pan with nonstick cooking spray and set aside.

**2.** To make the filling, beat together the goat cheese, egg, sugar, cinnamon, and vanilla extract in the bowl of a stand mixer, using the paddle attachment, until the filling is light and creamy. Transfer to a bowl and set aside until ready to use.

**3.** To make the muffin batter, whisk together the gluten-free all-purpose flour, baking powder, pumpkin pie spice, nutmeg, and salt in a mixing bowl. Set aside.

**4.** In the bowl of the stand mixer, using the paddle attachment, beat together the sugar, eggs, pumpkin purée, coconut oil, maple syrup, and vanilla extract.

**5.** Slowly add the dry ingredients into the wet ingredients, mixing well after each addition.

**6.** Fill each muffin cup about halfway with the muffin batter. You will not use all of the muffin batter in this step. Then, evenly distribute the creamy filling on top of the batter. Top the filling with remaining muffin batter.

**7.** Using a butter knife or kid's knife, gently swirl each muffin cup to artistically combine the filling and batter.

**8.** Bake for 30 to 35 minutes until a toothpick inserted into the center comes out clean. You may see some sticky filling on the toothpick, which is OK. Cool before serving.

 **Dr. Bear Fun Fact!** Pumpkins are a wonderful source of Vitamin A and beta-carotene. These nutrients keep your eyes healthy and your vision sharp!

# Flourless Chocolate Chip Sweet Potato Muffins

*These muffins come from my foodie friend Jackie Kestler. I'm totally obsessed with how easy they are to make and how much my kids love them. They get so excited to help me make them because they love to pierce the sweet potato with a fork, or as they say, "give the potato tattoos." For dairy-free muffins, use dairy-free mini chocolate chips.*

**YIELD: 12 MUFFINS**
Prep Time: 15 minutes
Total Time: 40 minutes

1 medium sweet potato
2 ripe bananas, peeled
2 eggs
1 cup creamy peanut butter
2 tablespoons maple syrup
1½ tablespoons vanilla extract
1 teaspoon baking soda
¼ teaspoon salt
½ cup mini chocolate chips

*Nutritional data reflects one muffin, based on a 12-muffin yield.*

**PER SERVING** Calories: 222; Total Fat: 14g; Saturated Fat: 4g; Cholesterol: 27mg; Sodium: 260mg; Total Carbohydrates: 21g; Dietary Fiber: 3g; Sugars: 12g; Protein: 6g

1. Preheat oven to 350°F. Line a muffin tin with cupcake liners or grease with nonstick spray. Set aside.

2. Place the sweet potato on a microwave-safe plate. Pierce the potato with a fork several times.

3. Microwave on high for 5 minutes. Remove from the microwave. If the potato is not soft, continue microwaving for 30 second increments until tender. Set aside and let cool completely.

4. In the bowl of a food processor, combine the bananas, eggs, peanut butter, maple syrup, vanilla extract, baking soda, and salt. Pulse until a smooth mixture forms.

5. Carefully peel the sweet potato and chop into pieces. Add the sweet potato into the food processor with the other ingredients and purée until smooth. Gently stir in the chocolate chips with a spatula.

6. Fill each of the prepared muffin tin cups about ¾ full with batter.

7. Bake for 20 to 22 minutes until the muffins are set and a toothpick inserted into the center comes out clean. Cool completely before serving.

 **Dr. Bear Fun Fact!** Baking soda has many uses, but when it's used in baking, it's as a leavening agent. This means it helps to make a product rise when cooked—a useful addition in a flourless baked good!

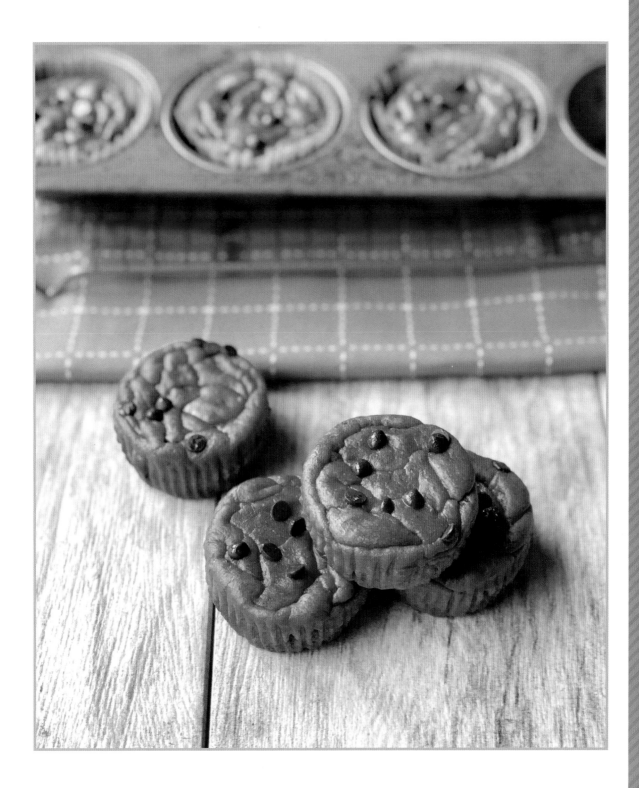

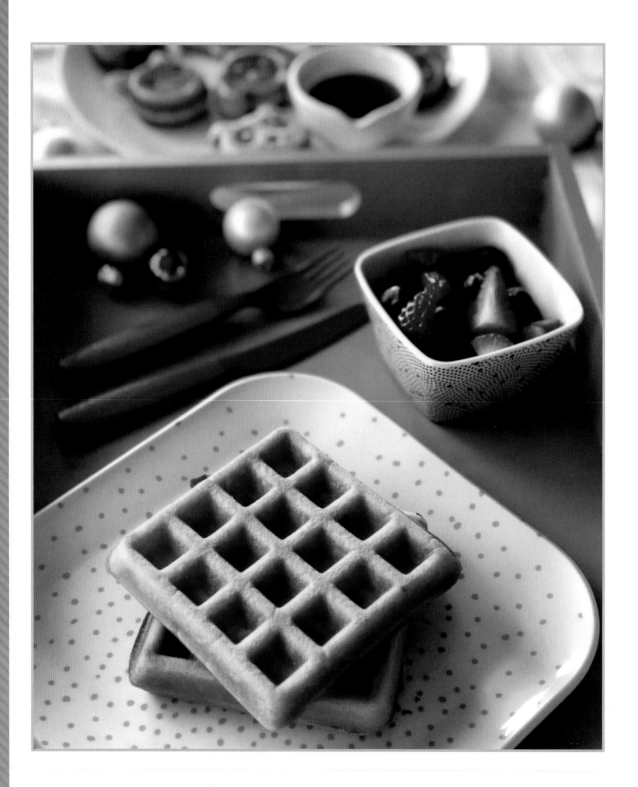

# Fluffy Waffles

*Waffles are a classic breakfast food that we make regularly in my house. My kids eat the normal square and round waffles just fine, but I couldn't resist getting an animal-shaped waffle maker when it was on sale at Bed Bath & Beyond. Not only do they taste great, but kids love having "animal talks" at the table with their little waffle friends.*

**YIELD: 4 SERVINGS**
Prep Time: 10 minutes
Total Time: 20 minutes

---

2 cups gluten-free all-purpose flour
2 tablespoons sugar
2 teaspoons baking powder
½ teaspoon salt
2½ cups milk
1 tablespoon lemon juice
1 egg yolk
2 tablespoons canola or vegetable oil
2 teaspoons vanilla extract
3 egg whites

1. Preheat waffle iron according to manufacturer instructions.

2. In a medium-sized mixing bowl, whisk together gluten-free all-purpose flour, sugar, baking powder, and salt.

3. In a separate large mixing bowl, whisk together milk, lemon juice, egg yolk, oil, and vanilla extract. Slowly mix the dry ingredients into the wet ingredients.

4. Using a handheld mixer, beat the egg whites until stiff peaks form.

5. Fold the egg whites into the batter.

6. Lightly grease the waffle iron with nonstick spray. Fill the waffle iron about ⅔ full with waffle batter and cook until golden brown on both sides. Repeat until all of the batter is cooked.

 **Dr. Bear Fun Fact!** The first waffles and waffle irons date back to the ninth century! They are a popular dish around the world but are mainly known as a famous Belgian treat.

*Nutritional data reflects one serving, based on a 4-serving yield.*

**PER SERVING** Calories: 411.4; Total Fat: 12.1g; Saturated Fat: 3g; Cholesterol: 57.2mg; Sodium: 658mg; Total Carbohydrates: 63.3g; Dietary Fiber: 1.9g; Sugars: 14.8g; Protein: 11.2g

# Sweet Potato Latke Waffles

*This is hands down my favorite recipe in the book. It came to life when I was craving sweet potato latkes, but didn't feel like going to the trouble of frying them. I really dislike that my kitchen smells for days and that there's oil all over the place. So, the sweet potato latke waffle was born! I now make them as a base for lox and cream cheese instead of a bagel. Grate the potatoes and onion using a food processor. This will save you lots of time and stress on your wrists.*

**YIELD: 10 WAFFLES** (when made in a 4-piece square waffle iron plate)
Prep Time: 15 minutes
Total Time: 45 minutes

---

4 eggs

1 cup cornstarch

2 tablespoons sugar

2 teaspoons ground cinnamon

1 teaspoon garlic powder

1 teaspoon salt

2 large sweet potatoes, peeled and shredded

2 large russet potatoes, peeled and shredded

1 sweet yellow onion, skin removed and shredded

Optional garnishes: (cream cheese + smoked salmon + cucumbers + chives), (avocado slices + sunny side up eggs), (butter + maple syrup)

*Nutritional data reflects one waffle, based on a 10-waffle yield. (Nutritional data does not include garnishes.)*

**PER SERVING** Calories: 168; Total Fat: 2g; Saturated Fat: 1g ; Cholesterol: 66mg; Sodium: 278mg; Total Carbohydrates: 34g; Dietary Fiber: 3g; Sugars: 5g; Protein: 4g

**1.** Preheat waffle iron over the highest heat setting.

**2.** In a large mixing bowl, whisk together the eggs, cornstarch, sugar, cinnamon, garlic powder, and salt until a smooth mixture forms.

**3.** Add the shredded potatoes and onion and toss to combine well.

**4.** Generously grease the waffle iron with nonstick spray. Stir the potato mixture again to make sure the liquid is evenly distributed just before adding to the hot waffle iron. If using a 4-piece waffle iron plate, add ½ cup of the potato mixture at a time to each section. Use a spoon to spread the mixture out evenly across the plate.

**5.** Close the waffle iron, and let the potato waffle cook for about 6 to 10 minutes, depending on the heat of your waffle iron. Check the waffles every few minutes to make sure they don't burn. You'll know they are done when the potato waffles are crispy and golden. Transfer to a serving plate and repeat with remaining potato mixture.

**6.** Serve hot and topped with garnishes of your choice. Store in an airtight container in the refrigerator. To reheat, place on foil in a toaster oven.

 **Dr. Bear Fun Fact!** Latkes are potato pancakes that Ashkenazi Jews created in the mid-nineteenth century to be served at Hanukkah. Latkes can also be made using cheese, vegetables, or legumes.

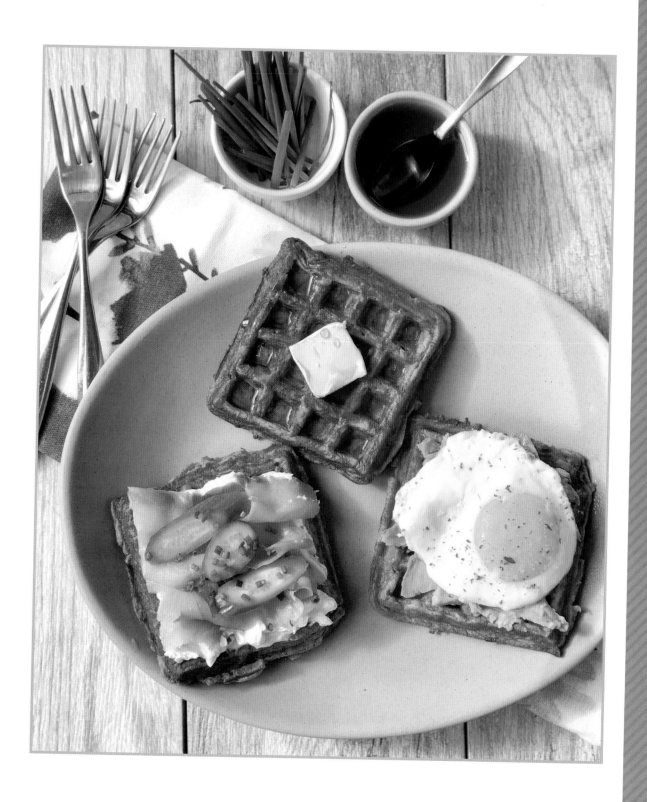

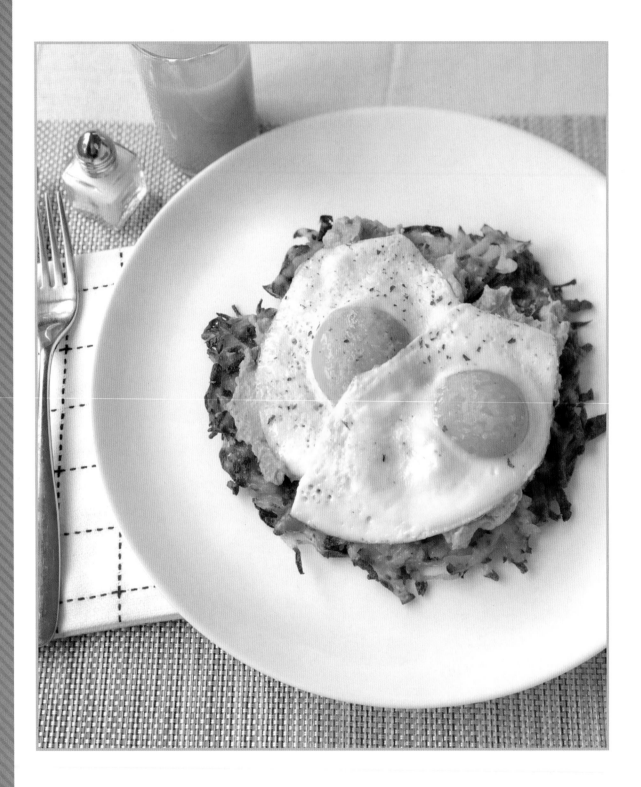

# Hash Brown Waffles with Avocado Purée and Eggs

*Hash brown waffles are the perfect gluten-free substitute for toast! If your family needs a dairy-free substitution, use vegetable oil or coconut oil in place of the butter.*

**YIELD: 6 WAFFLES** (made in a round 1-plate waffle iron)
Prep Time: 15 minutes
Total Time: 45 minutes

---

4 large russet potatoes, peeled and shredded

6 tablespoons butter, melted

1 teaspoon kosher salt

1 teaspoon freshly ground black pepper

2 avocados, skin and pit removed

½ cup crumbled goat cheese

Juice of 1 lemon

2 fresh mint leaves, rinsed and patted dry

12 eggs

 **Dr. Bear Fun Fact!** Hash browns are an American invention! They are very similar to the Swiss Rösti, as both are fritters made with shredded potatoes.

*Nutritional data reflects one waffle, based on a 6-waffle yield.*

**PER SERVING** Calories: 420.7; Total Fat: 30g; Saturated Fat: 13g; Cholesterol: 364mg; Sodium: 355mg; Total Carbohydrates: 23g; Dietary Fiber: 5g; Sugars: 2g; Protein: 16g

**1.** Preheat a waffle iron to its high setting and generously spray the plate with nonstick spray.

**2.** Wrap the shredded potatoes in a large paper towel and squeeze tightly to press out all of the liquid.

**3.** Transfer the potatoes to a large mixing bowl and add the melted butter, salt, and pepper. Toss to combine all of the ingredients well.

**4.** Press about 1¼ cups of the potato mixture into the greased waffle iron. Use a spoon to flatten the mixture.

**5.** Close the lid to the waffle maker and cook for about 10 to 12 minutes until the hash brown waffle is golden and crispy. Transfer the cooked hash brown waffle to a serving plate and repeat with remaining potato mixture.

**6.** While the waffles are cooking, make the avocado purée. In the bowl of a food processor, combine the avocados, goat cheese, lemon juice, and mint leaves. Pulse until a smooth mixture forms. Cover and refrigerate until ready to serve.

**7.** To make the eggs, grease a large skillet with nonstick spray and heat over medium-low heat. Add as many eggs as the skillet will hold, cover, and cook untouched for about 3 minutes. Remove from heat and season with salt. Repeat until all eggs are cooked.

**8.** To assemble the hash brown waffles, place a waffle on the serving plate. Spread a generous portion of the avocado purée on each hash brown waffle and then top with 2 sunny-side-up eggs.

# Pumpkin Oatmeal Banana Pancakes

*These pancakes are like eating pumpkin pie for breakfast. If your family can eat dairy, feel free to use regular milk and butter, but either way, they'll be delicious.*

**YIELD: 12 PANCAKES**
Prep Time: 10 minutes
Total Time: 30 minutes

———————

1½ cups coconut milk
1 cup pumpkin purée
1 egg
¼ cup sugar
¼ cup coconut oil, melted
1 cup gluten-free all-purpose flour
1 cup gluten-free oats
2 teaspoons baking powder
2 teaspoons pumpkin pie spice
½ teaspoon salt
2 bananas, peeled and thinly sliced
Maple syrup, for garnish

**1.** In a mixing bowl, whisk together the coconut milk, pumpkin purée, egg, sugar, and coconut oil. Set aside.

**2.** In a second mixing bowl, whisk together the gluten-free all-purpose flour, gluten-free oats, baking powder, pumpkin pie spice, and salt.

**3.** Slowly whisk the dry ingredients into the wet ingredients and mix until a smooth batter forms.

**4.** Spray a griddle pan with nonstick spray and heat over medium heat.

**5.** Pour ¼ cup of the pancake batter onto the griddle and place 4 slices of banana on top. Let the pancake sit for about 3 minutes until small bubbles begin forming on top of the pancake. Flip the pancake and cook an additional 3 minutes. Repeat with remaining batter.

**6.** Serve hot with maple syrup.

 **Dr. Bear Fact!** Did you know that pumpkin pie spice doesn't actually contain pumpkin? If you don't have this spice in your cabinet, simply mix together 4 parts cinnamon, 2 parts ground ginger, 1 part ground cloves, and ½ part ground nutmeg.

*Nutritional data reflects one pancake without syrup, based on a 12-pancake yield. (Nutritional data does not include maple syrup.)*

**PER SERVING** Calories: 155.1; Total Fat: 6.2g; Saturated Fat: 4.6g; Cholesterol: 13.7mg; Sodium: 186.8mg; Total Carbohydrates: 23.5g; Dietary Fiber: 2.2g; Sugars: 7.5g; Protein: 2.3g

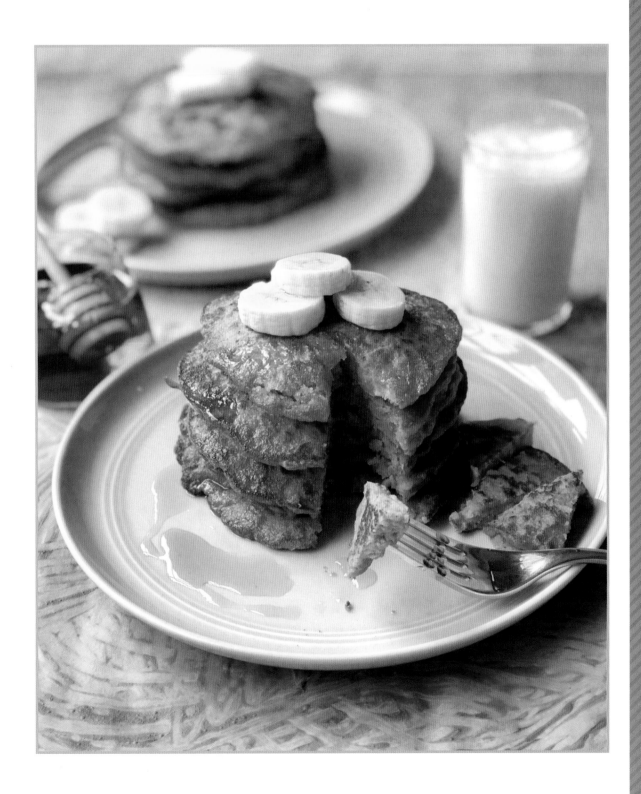

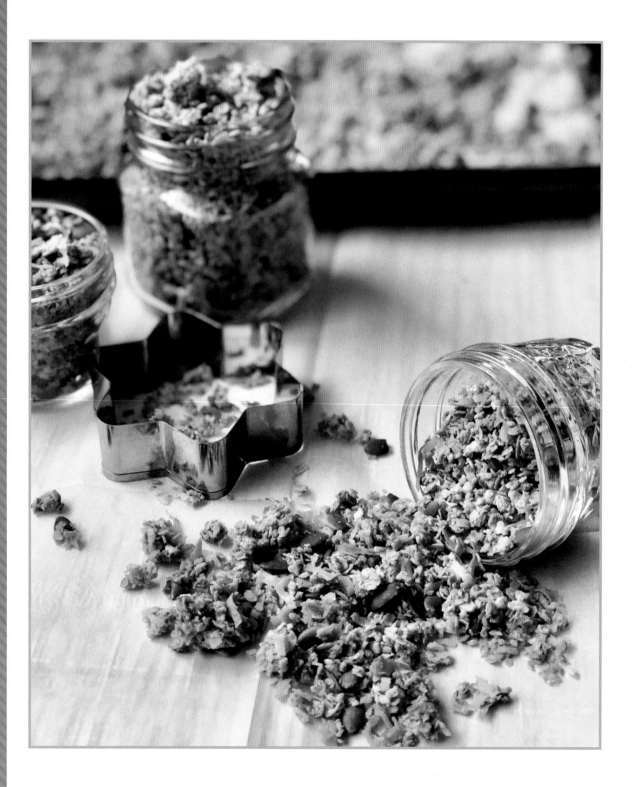

# Maple Coconut Granola with Pumpkin Seeds

*This is the best granola I've ever made, and now I'm scarred for buying packaged granola. My recommendation is to double the recipe and store the granola in the refrigerator so you always have it on hand.*

**YIELD: 10 (½ CUP) SERVINGS**
Prep Time: 10 minutes
Total Time: 40 minutes

———————

3 cups gluten-free rolled oats
1 cup coconut flakes
½ cup pumpkin seeds
½ cup maple syrup
¼ cup coconut oil
½ teaspoon sea salt
1 teaspoon vanilla extract

1. Preheat oven to 325°F. Line a baking sheet with parchment paper and set aside.

2. In a large mixing bowl, mix together gluten-free rolled oats, coconut flakes, and pumpkin seeds. Set aside.

3. In a small sauce pot set over medium-low heat, whisk together the maple syrup, coconut oil, and salt until the oil is melted and a smooth mixture forms. Remove from heat and whisk in the vanilla extract.

4. Pour the wet ingredients over the dry ingredients and mix until all of the dry ingredients are thoroughly coated with the maple-coconut mixture.

5. Spread the granola mixture out evenly onto the prepared baking sheet and bake for 25 to 30 minutes until golden. Stir the granola two times during baking to help the granola cook evenly.

6. Cool before serving. Store in an airtight container.

 **Dr. Bear Fun Fact!** Maple syrup provides more nutrients than white cane sugar. It's an excellent source of manganese, riboflavin, and zinc. Use it sparingly, though, as it's still high in sugar!

*Nutritional data reflects one serving, based on a 10-serving yield.*
**PER SERVING** Calories: 269.6; Total Fat: 15.1g; Saturated Fat: 9.9g; Cholesterol: 0mg; Sodium: 125.3mg; Total Carbohydrates: 29.8g; Dietary Fiber: 4.1g; Sugars: 10.5g; Protein: 5.5g

# Nutti-Licious Granola

*There are a handful of people with celiac disease who cannot tolerate oats. This is a great granola recipe for these individuals! It's packed with nuts and pumpkin seeds and just a hint of sweetness from the cocoa nibs and coconut chips.*

**YIELD: 16 (½ CUP) SERVINGS**
Prep Time: 5 minutes
Total Time: 10 minutes

---

2 cups roasted and salted almonds
2 cups roasted and salted cashews
2 cups dry roasted peanuts
1 cup roasted pumpkin seeds
⅓ cup cocoa nibs
1 (3-ounce) bag coconut chips

**1.** In the bowl of a food processor, combine the almonds, cashews, and peanuts. Pulse a few times until the nuts are crushed to your liking.

**2.** Transfer the nuts to a mixing bowl and stir in the pumpkin seeds, cocoa nibs, and coconut chips.

**3.** Transfer the granola to an airtight container and store in the refrigerator.

 **Dr. Bear Fun Fact!** Granola is also called "muesli" in many areas of the world!

*Nutritional data reflects one serving, based on a 16-serving yield.*

**PER SERVING**  Calories: 401.2; Total Fat: 32.7g; Saturated Fat: 7.1g; Cholesterol: 0mg; Sodium: 277mg; Total Carbohydrates: 19g; Dietary Fiber: 6.1g; Sugars: 4.5g; Protein: 14.3g

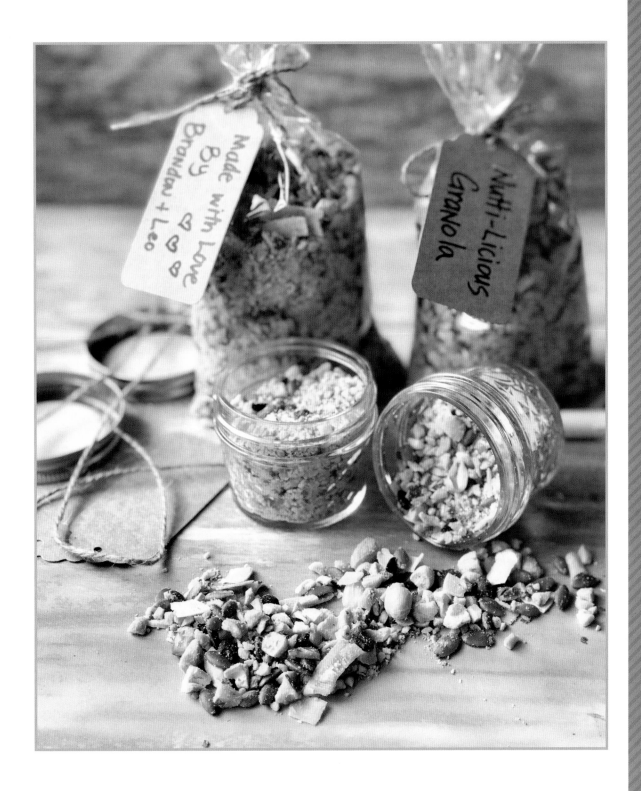

Made
By
with Love
Brandau + Leo ♡♡♡

Nutri-Licious
Granola

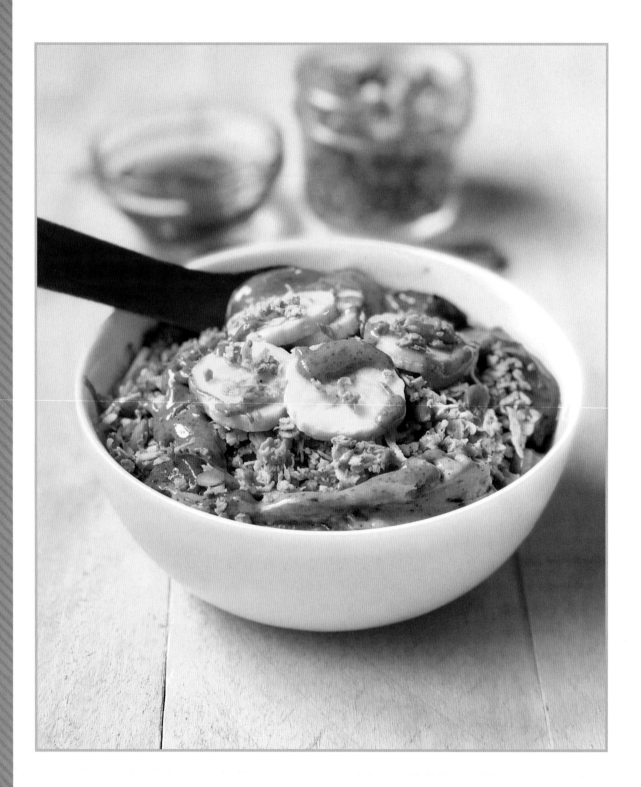

# Banana Blueberry Smoothie Bowl

*I always have a freezer full of frozen fruit, so if we're in the mood for these smoothie bowls, they are easy to toss together. If you're freezing bananas, take the skin off first for easier use later. Since the yogurt is pretty difficult to slice out of the container, I typically pour the yogurt into a Ziploc bag and press it out, flat, to about ½-inch thick. Freeze the bag flat so that when you're ready to use the frozen yogurt, it can easily be sliced with a sharp knife.*

**YIELD: 4 SERVINGS**
Prep Time: 20 minutes
Total Time: 30 minutes

---

3 frozen bananas, peeled

1½ cups frozen blueberries

1 cup Greek yogurt, frozen and cut into cubes

1 cup gluten-free granola

¼ cup almond butter, room temperature

Optional garnishes: sliced fruit, coconut shavings, mini chocolate chips

**1.** Remove the frozen fruit and yogurt from the freezer and let sit on the counter for about 20 minutes.

**2.** In the bowl of a food processor, combine the frozen bananas, blueberries, and yogurt cubes. Pulse for about 2 minutes until a smooth and creamy mixture forms. (If using a YoNana (or other machine), follow the manufacturer's instructions.)

 **Dr. Bear Fun Fact!** Frozen fruit is an underrated way of incorporating fruit into your diet! Because it stays frozen, the fruit is often picked when it's perfectly ripe. This means that the fruit tastes better and has more nutrients than fresh produce, which is often picked early and shipped unripe.

*Nutritional data reflects one serving without garnishes, based on a 4-serving yield.*

**PER SERVING** Calories: 395.4; Total Fat: 15.7g; Saturated Fat: 2g; Cholesterol: 4.6mg; Sodium: 28.1mg; Total Carbohydrates: 54g; Dietary Fiber: 8.2g; Sugars: 26.3g; Protein: 13.9g

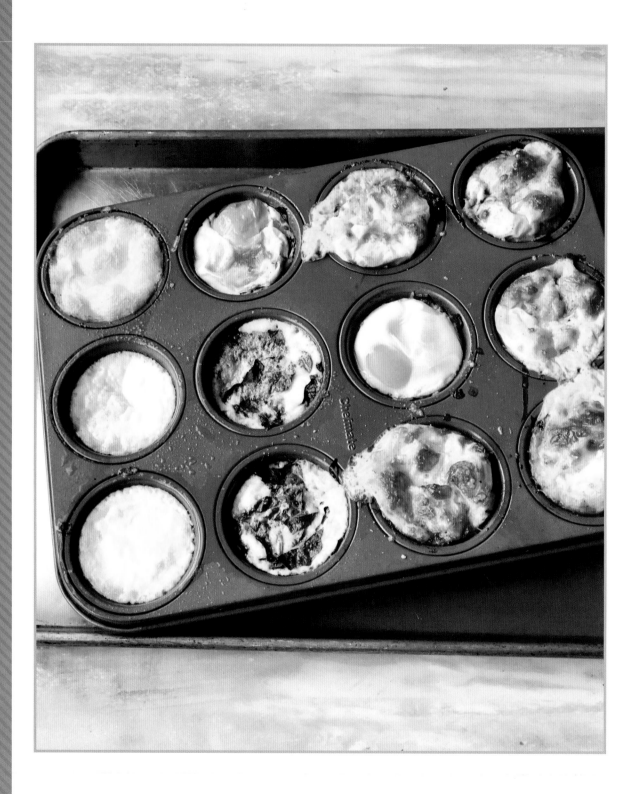

# Baked Egg Cups

*The possibilities for these eggs are endless. The recipe below is written as though you are going to make all of the eggs with the same egg base. But don't feel constrained. Like the photo shows, you can do some with whole eggs, some with beaten whole eggs, and some with just egg whites.*

**YIELD: 12 SERVINGS**
Prep Time: 5 minutes
Total Time: 25 minutes

6 eggs
½ cup milk
1 teaspoon salt
1 teaspoon garlic powder
4 cups mix-ins (such as chopped spinach, shredded cheese, chopped bacon or ham, sliced mushrooms)

**1.** Preheat oven to 375°F. Line a muffin pan with cupcake liners or spray heavily with nonstick spray. Set aside.

**2.** In a large mixing bowl, whisk together the eggs, milk, salt, and garlic powder.

**3.** Choose the mix-ins and evenly distribute in the muffin cups.

**4.** Pour the egg mixture evenly into the 12 muffin cups and bake for 15 to 18 minutes until the eggs are fully set. Serve immediately.

 **Dr. Bear Fun Fact!** Eggs provide an excellent source of protein, Vitamin $B_{12}$, choline, riboflavin, and phosphorus. The color of eggs just depends on the breed of the hen and has no influence on how nutritious the egg is.

*Nutritional data reflects one serving without optional add-ins, based on a 12-serving yield.*

**PER SERVING** Calories: 40.1; Total Fat: 2.5g; Saturated Fat: 0.9g; Cholesterol: 82.9mg; Sodium: 228.7mg; Total Carbohydrates: 0.9g; Dietary Fiber: 0g; Sugars: 0.8g; Protein: 3.2g

# Velvety Gruyère Sous Vide Egg Jars

*Why sous vide? It's easy…I could tell you about all of the health benefits of cooking with less butter and oil (there are many), but the truth is that I like sous vide eggs because I'm guaranteed to have no brown spots, which means my kids will eat them 100 percent of the time. With sous vide eggs, you'll get perfectly bright yellow eggs with no browning on them whatsoever. It's a mom's dream to put a plate down and not be asked fifteen times to remove every last piece of crust or brown spots. Phew!*

*These recipes are inspired by Starbucks egg bites. After I had that first bite of the Bacon and Gruyère Egg Bite, I knew I had to figure it out at home. If you don't have mason jars to make these in, don't worry. Use a small Ziploc bag, and you'll get equally as tasty eggs in the shape of an omelet (see photo). The eggs made in baggies are used on the sandwiches using croissants from Rise Bakery in Washington, DC.*

**YIELD: 12 (4-OUNCE) EGG JARS**
Prep Time: 20 minutes
Total Time: 80 minutes

————————

12 eggs
½ cup cream cheese
½ cup cottage cheese
½ cup grated Gruyère cheese
1 teaspoon salt
12 (4-ounce) canning jars

**Mix-in Ideas**
Spinach and basil
Sautéed mushrooms and rosemary
Cooked bacon and chives

**1.** Set up a large, high-sided roasting pan on a heat-safe surface (I set mine on top of the stove). Fill the pan about halfway with water. Place your sous vide device in the water and heat to 175°F.

**2.** To make the egg batter, combine the eggs, cream cheese, cottage cheese, grated Gruyère, and salt in the bowl of a food processor or blender. Pulse until the mixture is very smooth.

**3.** Spray each of the 4-ounce jars with nonstick spray. Fill the jars with a spoonful of your desired mix-ins.

**4.** Pour the egg mixture evenly into the jars. You want them to be about ¾ full.

**5.** Screw the lids on gently. Do not seal the jars tightly. You want some air to be able to escape.

**6.** Place the jars in the water bath and cook for 1 hour.

**7.** Carefully remove the jars from the water and enjoy immediately. You can eat the eggs right out of the jars, or slide a butter knife around the sides and transfer them to a plate. If you're making ahead for later in the week, let the jars cool completely, then refrigerate until ready to eat.

### Mix-in Directions

- **Spinach and basil:** Sauté 1 tablespoon olive oil with 3 cups baby spinach leaves and a pinch of salt. When the spinach is wilted, remove from heat and toss in 10 thinly-sliced basil leaves. Divide mixture evenly amongst the egg jars.

- **Sautéed mushrooms and rosemary:** Sauté 2 tablespoons olive oil with 2 cups thinly sliced wild mushrooms and 1 teaspoon finely chopped rosemary until the mushrooms begin to brown. Divide the mixture evenly amongst the egg jars.

- **Cooked bacon and chives:** Preheat oven to 400°F. Arrange bacon on a parchment-lined baking sheet and bake for 15 to 18 minutes until crispy. Chop the bacon and place in a small bowl. Mix in ¼ cup chopped chives and then divide the mixture evenly amongst the egg jars.

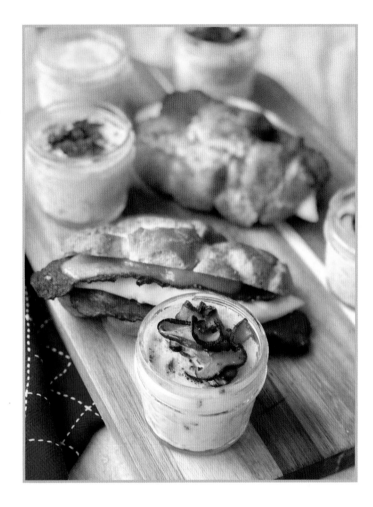

 **Dr. Bear Fun Fact!** "Sous vide" is French for "under vacuum." Food that is cooked using this method is cooked at lower temperatures for longer periods of time, making the food evenly cooked and moist.

*Nutritional data reflects one serving without optional add-ins, based on a 12-serving yield.*

**PER SERVING** Calories: 147.6; Total Fat: 11g; Saturated Fat: 5.1g; Cholesterol: 185mg; Sodium: 389.2mg; Total Carbohydrates: 1.7g; Dietary Fiber: 0g; Sugars: 1.4g; Protein: 10.1g

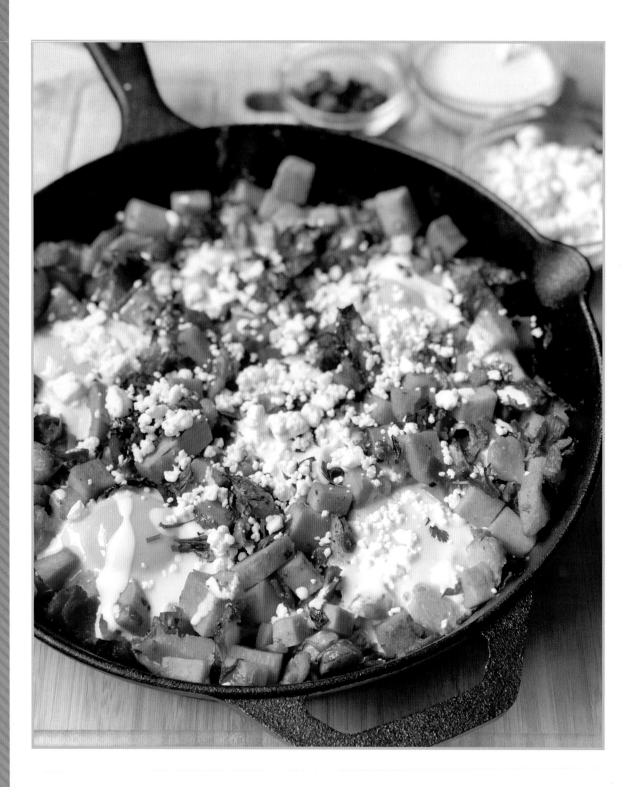

# Sweet Potato, Brussels Sprouts, & Bacon Hash with Baked Eggs

*You would have thought I was pregnant when I created this recipe, but really, I just had cravings for Mexican-themed breakfast food. The lime sour cream and chopped cilantro are the perfect cut for the salty bacon. I typically prepare all of the ingredients for this dish the night before, so when it's breakfast time, all I have to do is cook the ingredients.*

**YIELD: 6 SERVINGS**
Prep Time: 15 minutes
Total Time: 35 minutes

---

2 tablespoons butter

2 tablespoons olive oil

2 large sweet potatoes, peeled and chopped into 1-inch cubes

1 (8-ounce) package bacon, chopped into bite-sized pieces

1 (12-ounce) package shredded Brussels sprouts

1 teaspoon garlic powder

1 teaspoon ground cumin

¼ teaspoon salt

6 eggs

¼ cup sour cream

Juice of 1 lime

½ cup goat cheese

¼ cup chopped fresh cilantro leaves, rinsed and patted dry

**1.** Preheat oven to 400°F.

**2.** In a large cast-iron skillet, heat the butter and olive oil over medium-high heat on the stove. Add the sweet potatoes and cook, stirring frequently, until they begin to soften, about 7 minutes.

**3.** Add the bacon and cook, stirring occasionally, until it begins to brown, about 5 minutes. Add the Brussels sprouts, garlic powder, cumin, and salt and toss to combine. Cook, stirring occasionally, for an additional 3 minutes.

**4.** Push the vegetables around to form 6 wells in the pan. Crack an egg into each of the wells and bake for 10 to 12 minutes, just until the whites of the eggs have set.

**5.** While the hash and eggs are baking, whisk together the sour cream and the lime juice in a small mixing bowl. Set aside.

**6.** To garnish, drizzle the lime cream on top of the eggs and vegetables. Evenly distribute the goat cheese and cilantro across the top of the hash before serving.

 **Dr. Bear Fun Fact!** Bacon is one of the world's oldest preserved meats! The Chinese began salting and cooking pork bellies around 1,500 BC.

*Nutritional data reflects one serving, based on a 6-serving yield.*

**PER SERVING** Calories: 490.2; Total Fat: 34.8g; Saturated Fat: 14.4g; Cholesterol: 231.2mg; Sodium: 974.4mg; Total Carbohydrates: 18g; Dietary Fiber: 3.8g; Sugars: 4.7g; Protein: 27g

# Butternut Squash & Goat Cheese Quiche

*Make the butternut squash mash the night before for easy morning assembly. Perfect for a Sunday brunch. The puff pastry comes with two pieces, so if kids want a more basic version, make a second quiche with just eggs and grated cheddar cheese.*

**YIELD: 8 SERVINGS**
Prep Time: 20 minutes
Total Time: 50 minutes

---

1 sheet gluten-free puff pastry (pictured is GeeFree Gluten-Free Puff Pastry sheets)

1 cup Butternut Squash & Caramelized Onion Mash (see page 226)

1 cup crumbled goat cheese

6 eggs

1 cup heavy cream

½ cup skim milk

½ teaspoon salt

**1.** Preheat oven to 375°F. Spray a 9-inch tart or pie dish with nonstick spray and place on a baking sheet. The baking sheet will make it easier to transport the quiche in and out of the oven.

**2.** Sprinkle gluten-free all-purpose flour or cornstarch on a clean work surface, and lay out the gluten-free puff pastry. Sprinkle a small amount of gluten-free flour on top of the puff pastry. Using a rolling pin, roll the pastry dough out to about a 10-inch square. Carefully pick up the puff pastry and place it inside of the prepared baking dish. Press the dough down to fit snugly in the baking dish. If using a tart pan, press the dough gently into the grooves.

**3.** Using a spoon, spread the Butternut Squash & Caramelized Onion Mash mixture across the bottom of the dough.

**4.** Sprinkle the goat cheese crumbles on top of the mash.

**5.** In a mixing bowl, whisk together the eggs, heavy cream, milk, and salt until a smooth mixture forms. Pour this liquid mixture over the mash and goat cheese.

**6.** Bake for 35 to 40 minutes until the egg mixture is set. Cool slightly before slicing.

 **Dr. Bear Fun Fact!** What makes puff pastry so flaky? During the baking process, steam from water makes the fat in the dough push the thin layers apart and rise up.

*Nutritional data reflects one serving, based on an 8-serving yield.*

**PER SERVING** Calories: 277.3; Total Fat: 21.9g; Saturated Fat: 11.5g; Cholesterol 168.2mg; Sodium: 469.2mg; Total Carbohydrates: 11.8g; Dietary Fiber: 1.4g; Sugars: 5.8g; Protein: 9.2g

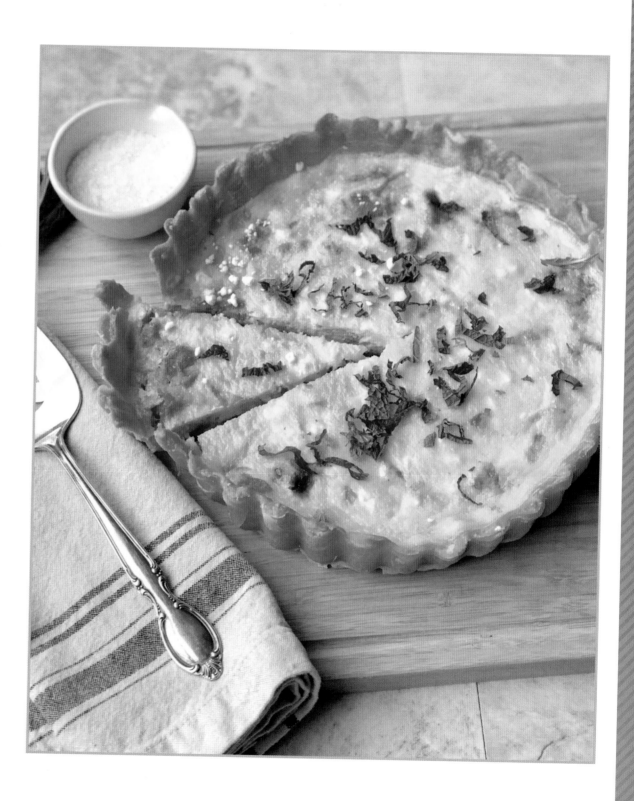

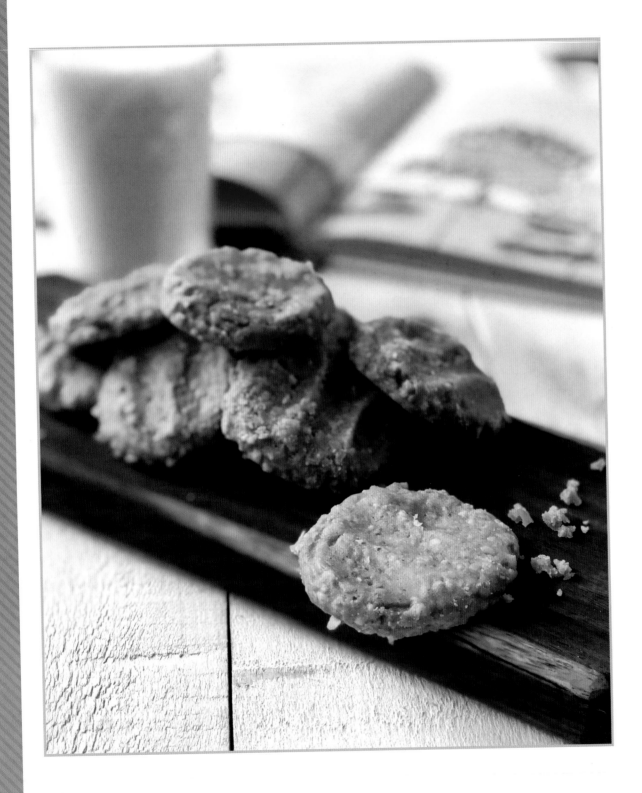

# Peanut Butter Coconut Breakfast Cookies

*My kids are known for begging for cookies for breakfast. So, I finally gave in and came up with a recipe that I'm OK letting them eat for breakfast! Serve these with a bowl of fruit and a glass of milk. The kids will be begging for seconds and thirds!*

**YIELD: 24 COOKIES**
Prep Time: 10 minutes
Total Time: 20 minutes

---

20 pitted dates

½ cup hot water

⅓ cup coconut oil, warmed

1 teaspoon vanilla extract

½ teaspoon salt

1 cup peanut butter

1 egg

½ cup gluten-free rolled oats

½ cup shredded coconut

½ cup gluten-free all-purpose flour

**1.** Preheat oven to 350°F. Line two baking sheets with parchment paper and set aside.

**2.** In a food processor, combine dates and hot water, and let sit for 5 minutes to soften. Add in the warmed coconut oil, vanilla extract, and salt. Pulse until a very smooth mixture forms.

**3.** Add the peanut butter and egg and pulse until combined.

**4.** Add the gluten-free oats, shredded coconut, and gluten-free all-purpose flour, and pulse for about 30 seconds until the dough pulls together.

**5.** Scoop the dough by rounded tablespoonfuls onto the prepared baking sheets and bake for 10 minutes. Cool before serving.

*Optional variation:* Line an 8-by-8-inch glass baking dish with parchment paper. Press the batter into the lined baking dish and spread out evenly. Bake for 20 minutes. Cool completely before slicing into bars.

 **Dr. Bear Fun Fact!** Why do we add hot water to this recipe? Dates can be a little tough right out of the package. Letting them sit in warm water softens them and will make them easier to purée.

*Nutritional data reflects one cookie, based on a 24-cookie yield.*

**PER SERVING** Calories: 137.7; Total Fat: 10g; Saturated Fat: 4.7g; Cholesterol: 6.8mg; Sodium: 52.2mg; Total Carbohydrates: 10.4g; Dietary Fiber: 1.5g; Sugars: 5.1g; Protein: 3.2g

# Baked Oatmeal with Apples, Chia, & Brown Sugar

*I promised our Children's National Community Education Specialist Kate that I would come up with a baked oatmeal recipe for her that used chia seeds, and this is the result. I typically make the oatmeal mixture the day before, refrigerate overnight, and bake it first thing in the morning. While I'm getting the kids dressed and brushing their teeth, the oatmeal is baking and ready by the time we get downstairs.*

**YIELD: 12 SERVINGS**
Prep Time: 15 minutes
Total Time: 45 minutes

---

2 eggs
1½ cups coconut milk
¼ cup coconut oil, melted
¼ cup maple syrup
1 teaspoon vanilla extract
2 cups gluten-free rolled oats
1 cup chopped apples, core removed
1 cup chopped pitted dates
½ cup chopped pecans
2 tablespoons chia seeds
2 teaspoons ground cinnamon, divided
½ teaspoon salt
½ cup brown sugar

**1.** Preheat oven to 350°F. Spray an 8-by-8-inch glass baking dish with nonstick spray and set aside.

**2.** In a large mixing bowl, whisk together the eggs, coconut milk, coconut oil, maple syrup, and vanilla extract.

**3.** Stir in the gluten-free oats, apples, dates, pecans, chia seeds, 1 teaspoon cinnamon, and salt, and mix until well combined. Pour this mixture in the prepared baking dish.

**4.** In a small mixing bowl, mix together the brown sugar, remaining cinnamon, and a pinch of salt.

**5.** Sprinkle the cinnamon sugar mixture over the top of the oatmeal and bake for 30 to 35 minutes until set. Let cool slightly before serving.

**Dr. Bear Fun Fact!** Chia seeds are a great addition to oatmeal or any baked good to add texture! They are also a great source of nutrients and energy. In fact, "chia" means "strength" in the ancient Mayan language!

*Nutritional data reflects one serving, based on a 12-serving yield.*

**PER SERVING** Calories: 230; Total Fat: 10.6g; Saturated Fat: 5g; Cholesterol: 27.4mg; Sodium: 111.6mg; Total Carbohydrates: 32g; Dietary Fiber: 3.9g; Sugars: 19.2g; Protein: 3.8g

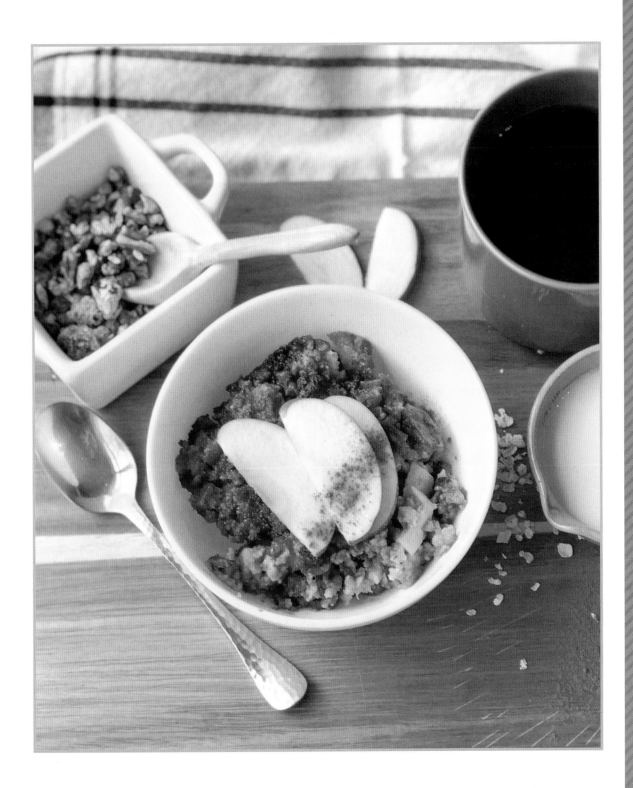

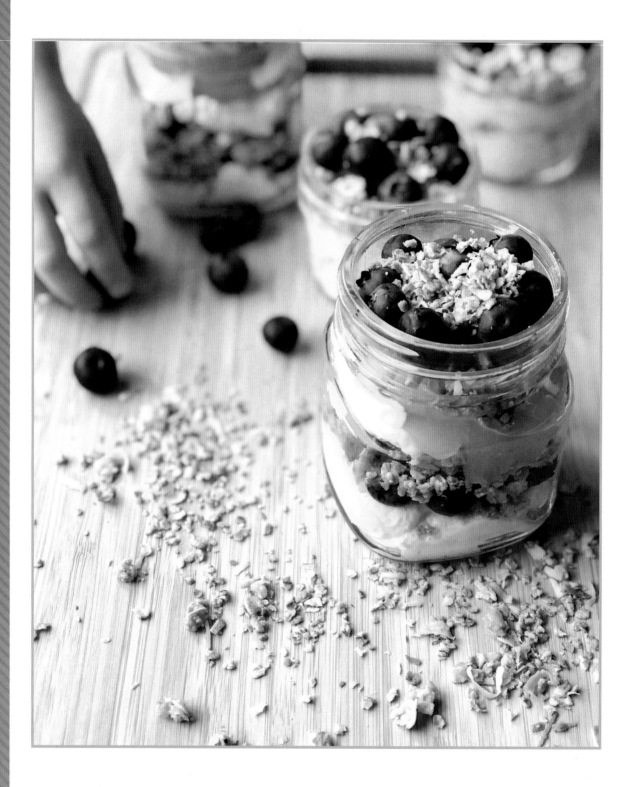

# Granola Parfaits with Lemon Curd & Blueberries

*The sweet lemon curd is the perfect combination for the tart yogurt. I added blueberries, but these parfaits are excellent with strawberries as well.*

**YIELD: 4 SERVINGS**
Prep Time: 5 minutes
Total Time: 10 minutes

---

2 cups Greek yogurt, divided

1 pint blueberries, rinsed, patted dry, and divided

1½ cups gluten-free granola, divided (pictured is Maple Coconut Granola on page 59)

4 tablespoons lemon curd, divided

**1.** To assemble the parfaits, place 2 tablespoons Greek yogurt in the bottom of each parfait dish. Layer with a sprinkling of blueberries and 1 tablespoon of gluten-free granola.

**2.** Continue by adding 2 more tablespoons yogurt to each parfait and then 1 tablespoon lemon curd, followed by 1 tablespoon of granola.

**3.** Continue layering by adding 2 additional tablespoons of Greek yogurt and a few more blueberries. Garnish the top of parfaits with a spoonful of granola.

 **Dr. Bear Fun Fact!** Curd is usually made from sour milk! Fruit curds are different, though—it's usually a mixture of egg yolks, fruit juice, sugar, and zest, combined and cooked in a saucepan.

*Nutritional data reflects one serving using the Maple Coconut Granola recipe, based on a 4-serving yield.*

**PER SERVING** Calories: 415.1; Total Fat: 15.2g; Saturated Fat: 9.3g; Cholesterol: 24.2mg; Sodium: 156mg; Total Carbohydrates: 54.7g; Dietary Fiber: 5.8g; Sugars: 35.1g; Protein: 18.1g

# Apple Slices with Peanut Butter & Granola

*Quickest and easiest breakfast ever. For those days when it takes too long to get out of bed, this breakfast ensures an energizing meal for your little kiddos.*

**YIELD: 4 SERVINGS**
Prep Time: 5 minutes
Total Time: 10 minutes

---

2 apples, core removed,
   sliced into thin rounds
½ cup peanut butter
1 cup granola

**1.** Place apple slices on a serving platter. Spread a thin layer of peanut butter, about 2 teaspoons, onto each slice.

**2.** Top each slice of apple with a sprinkle of granola. Serve immediately.

 **Dr. Bear Fun Fact!** Granny Smith apples are named after the woman who began cultivating them in the nineteenth century—Maria Ann "Granny" Smith!

*Nutritional data reflects one serving, based on a 4-serving yield.*

**PER SERVING**  Calories: 367.3; Total Fat: 21.2g; Saturated Fat: 3g; Cholesterol: 0mg; Sodium: 135.9mg; Total Carbohydrates: 38.6g; Dietary Fiber: 6.2g; Sugars: 17.5g; Protein: 10.2g

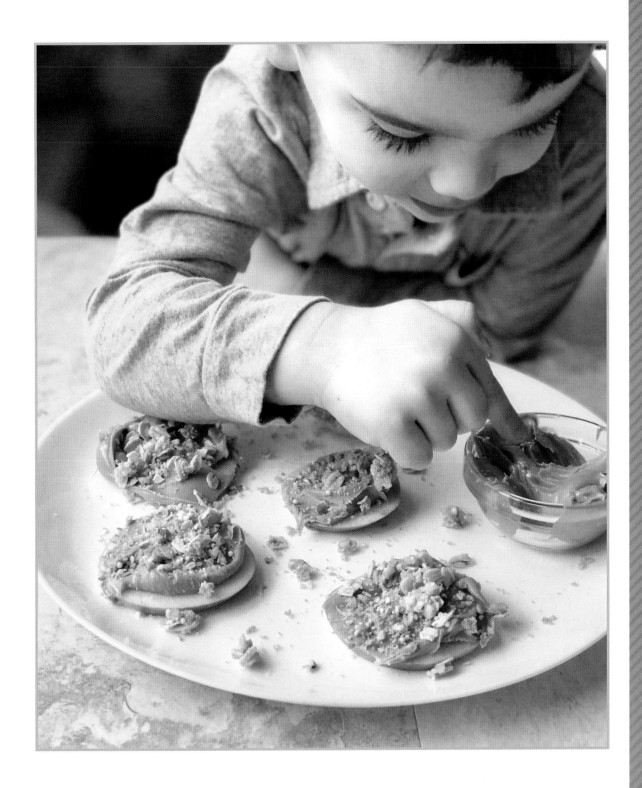

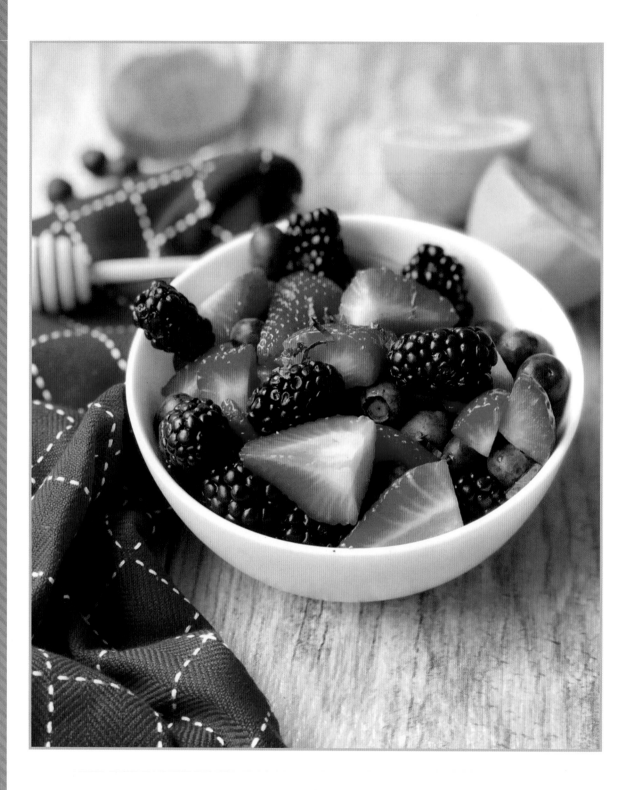

# Lemon Mint Berry Fruit Salad

*Fruit salad is something I make all the time when my family comes to visit, and I also regularly take one to brunches at friends' houses. This berry fruit salad is simple to make, and the addition of lemon, honey, and mint takes it from a good salad to a great one.*

**YIELD: 8 SERVINGS**
Prep Time: 10 minutes
Total Time: 10 minutes

---

1 pint strawberries, rinsed, stems removed and cut into quarters

1 pint blueberries, rinsed and patted dry

1 pint blackberries, rinsed and patted dry

Juice of 1 lemon

1 teaspoon honey

¼ cup finely chopped fresh mint leaves, rinsed and patted dry

**1.** In a serving bowl, toss together the strawberries, blueberries, and blackberries.

**2.** In a small bowl, whisk together the lemon juice and honey. Drizzle the mixture over the top of the berries and toss to combine.

**3.** Sprinkle the mint on top of the fruit salad and toss gently to combine.

**4.** Cover and refrigerate until ready to serve.

 **Dr. Bear Fun Fact!** Blackberries are packed with antioxidants!

*Nutritional data reflects one serving, based on an 8-serving yield.*

**PER SERVING** Calories: 60.7; Total Fat: 0.5g; Saturated Fat: 0g; Cholesterol: 0mg; Sodium: 1.6g; Total Carbohydrates: 14.8g; Dietary Fiber: 4.1g; Sugars: 9.3g; Protein: 1.2g

# Tropical Fruit Salad with Honey & Lime

*I learned about squeezing lime juice over papaya when my husband and I were on our honeymoon in Thailand. And, after experimenting, I learned that lime juice is great on lots of other fruits too!*

**YIELD: 8 SERVINGS**
Prep Time: 15 minutes
Total Time: 15 minutes

---

1 mango, skin and pit removed, cut into bite-sized pieces

1 pineapple, skin and top removed, cut into bite-sized pieces

1 papaya, skin and seeds removed, cut into bite-sized pieces

1 kiwi, skin removed, sliced in half and cut into bite-sized pieces

Juice of 2 limes

1 tablespoon honey

**1.** In a serving bowl, toss together the mango, pineapple, papaya, and kiwi.

**2.** In a small bowl, whisk together the lime juice and honey. Drizzle this mixture over the fruit and gently toss together.

**3.** Cover and refrigerate until ready to serve.

 **Dr. Bear Fun Fact!** Papayas are a good source of Vitamin C and folate!

*Nutritional data reflects one serving, based on an 8-serving yield.*

**PER SERVING** Calories: 118.3; Total Fat: 0.5g; Saturated Fat: 0.1g; Cholesterol: 0mg; Sodium: 5.9mg; Total Carbohydrates: 30.7g; Dietary Fiber: 3.4g; Sugars: 23.7g; Protein: 1.3g

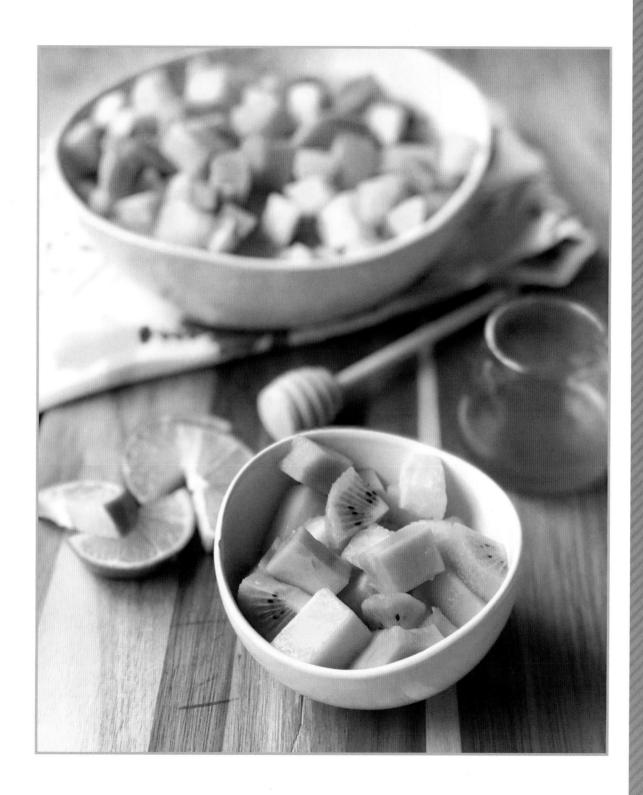

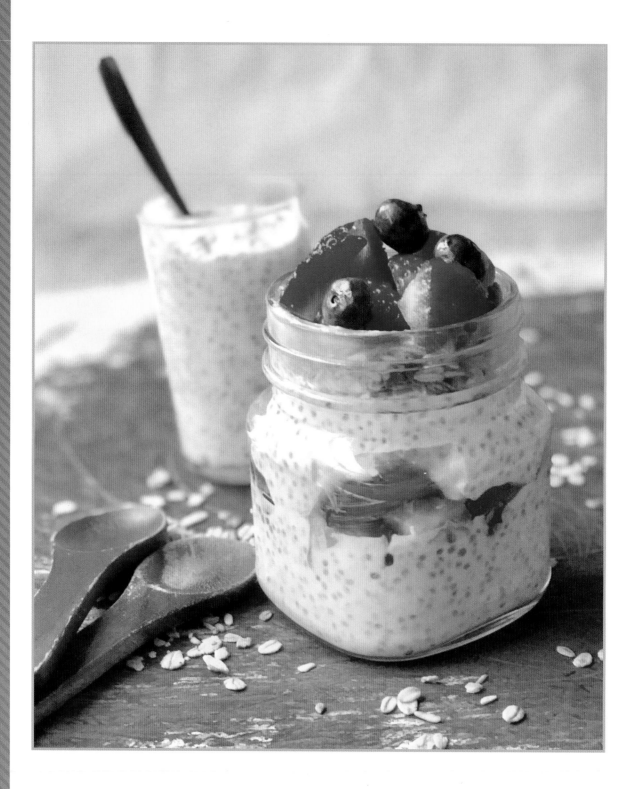

# Coconut Chia Yogurt

*This recipe can be made using full-fat Greek Yogurt or any dairy-free yogurt as well. Don't be alarmed if the chia seeds look spread out and gelled when you go to eat the yogurt. This is normal! For an easy breakfast, make this before bed and pull it out of the refrigerator the next morning.*

**YIELD: 4 SERVINGS**
Prep Time: 5 minutes
Total Time: 8 hours (includes chilling)

———————

1 cup coconut milk

1 cup full-fat plain yogurt

2 tablespoons honey

½ tablespoon vanilla extract

¼ cup chia seeds

Fruit, for garnish (pictured with Lemon Mint Berry Fruit Salad, page 81)

Granola, for garnish

1. In a glass mixing bowl, whisk together the coconut milk, yogurt, honey, and vanilla extract until a smooth mixture forms. Gently stir in the chia seeds.

2. Cover and refrigerate for at least 6 to 8 hours.

3. Serve with fresh fruit and granola.

 **Dr. Bear Fun Fact!** Chia seeds are a fantastic source of fiber!

*Nutritional data reflects one serving without garnish, based on a 4-serving yield.*

**PER SERVING** Calories: 130.5; Total Fat: 6.2g; Saturated Fat: 2.7g; Cholesterol: 8mg; Sodium: 30.7mg; Total Carbohydrates: 16.1g; Dietary Fiber: 3.5g; Sugars: 11.9g; Protein: 3.9g

# Braided Challah

*This is one of the more complicated recipes in the book, so I make it large enough to come out with two loaves. This way you can freeze one to have on hand for your next Shabbat dinner.*

**YIELD: 2 LARGE, BRAIDED LOAVES
(32 SERVINGS)**
Prep Time: 30 minutes
Total Time: 80 minutes

---

⅓ cup very warm water

1 package rapid rise yeast

4 cups gluten-free all-purpose flour

¼ cup granulated sugar

3 teaspoons baking powder

1 teaspoon salt

5 egg yolks

1 cup plain yogurt

⅓ cup vegetable oil

¼ cup honey

1 teaspoon apple cider vinegar

½ teaspoon vanilla extract

1 whole egg

1 teaspoon water

**1.** Cut two pieces of parchment paper the length of a baking sheet. Set each piece of parchment paper in front of a baking sheet on the counter. Being prepared and having the parchment close to the baking sheets is very important for this recipe!

**2.** In a small bowl, combine the warm water and yeast. Let sit for about 5 minutes until foamy.

**3.** In a mixing bowl, whisk together the gluten-free all-purpose flour, sugar, baking powder, and salt. Set aside.

**4.** In the bowl of a stand mixer, using the paddle attachment, beat together the yeast mixture, egg yolks, yogurt, oil, honey, apple cider vinegar, and vanilla extract.

**5.** Slowly add the dry ingredients into the wet ingredients, mixing well after each addition.

**6.** Oil your hands well, and transfer the dough to one piece of parchment paper. Divide the dough into six equally-sized pieces. Place three pieces on one piece of parchment paper and three on the other.

**7.** Roll each piece of dough into a ball and then roll out into a rope about 15 inches long. Pinch together one end of each rope and then gently braid the dough ropes together. Pinch together at the opposite end. Repeat with the other three pieces of dough.

**8.** In a small bowl, whisk together the whole egg and water to make the egg wash.

**9.** Brush the egg wash mixture over the surface of each braided loaf, then cover and place in a warm place to rise for about 20 minutes.

**10.** While the dough is rising, preheat oven to 350°F. Bake the braided loaves for 30 minutes. Remove from oven and cool before slicing.

**11.** If you don't plan to eat both loaves right away, wrap the loaves in foil, then place in a plastic zip-lock bag before freezing.

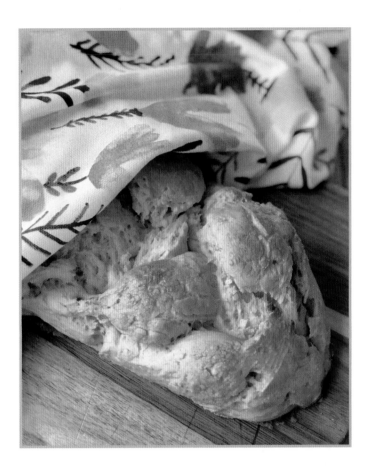

 **Dr. Bear Fun Fact!** Challah bread is a special bread made in Jewish cuisine around the world. It is typically eaten on major Jewish holidays (with the exception of Passover) and on the Sabbath.

*Nutritional data reflects one serving, based on a 32-serving yield.*

**PER SERVING** Calories: 104.5; Total Fat: 3.6g; Saturated Fat: 0.9g; Cholesterol: 34.3mg; Sodium: 127.1mg; Total Carbohydrates: 16.5g; Dietary Fiber: 0.5g; Sugars: 4.2g; Protein: 1.6g

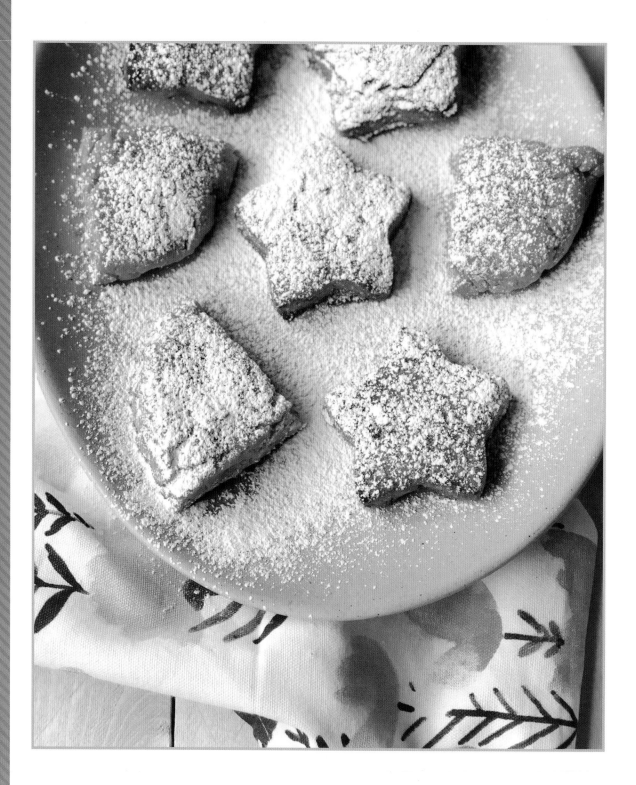

# Sweet Potato Scones

*These mildly flavored scones are delicious toasted with peanut butter. If your household is OK with dairy, you can replace the coconut oil with butter.*

**YIELD: 14–16 SCONES**
(depending on cookie cutter size)
Prep Time: 20 minutes
Total Time: 50 minutes

---

1 large sweet potato
1½ cups gluten-free all-purpose flour
¼ cup gluten-free quick cook oats
½ cup sugar
1 tablespoon baking powder
1 teaspoon ground cinnamon
1 teaspoon salt
½ cup solid coconut oil
¼ cup coconut milk
Powdered sugar, for dusting

*Nutritional data reflects one scone, based on a 15-scone yield.*

**PER SERVING** Calories: 155; Total Fat: 8g; Saturated Fat: 6g; Cholesterol: 0mg; Sodium: 261mg; Total Carbohydrates: 21g; Dietary Fiber: 1g; Sugars: 9g; Protein: 1g

1. Preheat oven to 400°F. Line a baking sheet with parchment paper and set aside.

2. Place the sweet potato on a paper towel and, using a fork, pierce the potato all over its surface. Cook the sweet potato in the microwave for 5 to 7 minutes, until soft to the touch. Remove from microwave, cool, peel, and mash the potato flesh.

3. In a large mixing bowl, whisk together the gluten-free all-purpose flour, gluten-free oats, sugar, baking powder, ground cinnamon, and salt.

4. Using a fork or pastry cutter, cut in the solid coconut oil until the mixture resembles pea-like crumbles.

5. Add the coconut milk and cooled, mashed sweet potato, and mix until well combined. (I find this step is easiest by mixing with a fork, and once the coconut milk is mixed in, transfer the dough to your clean countertop and knead it with your hands.)

6. Using your hands, press the dough out to a 1-inch thick round.

7. Cut out the dough using your cookie cutter of choice, or simply slice into rectangles or triangles.

8. Place the pieces of dough on the prepared baking sheet and bake for 18 to 22 minutes until golden. Dust with powdered sugar before serving.

 **Dr. Bear Fun Fact!** Sweet potatoes are a rich source of complex carbohydrates, fiber, and beta-carotene (which turns into Vitamin A in the body)!

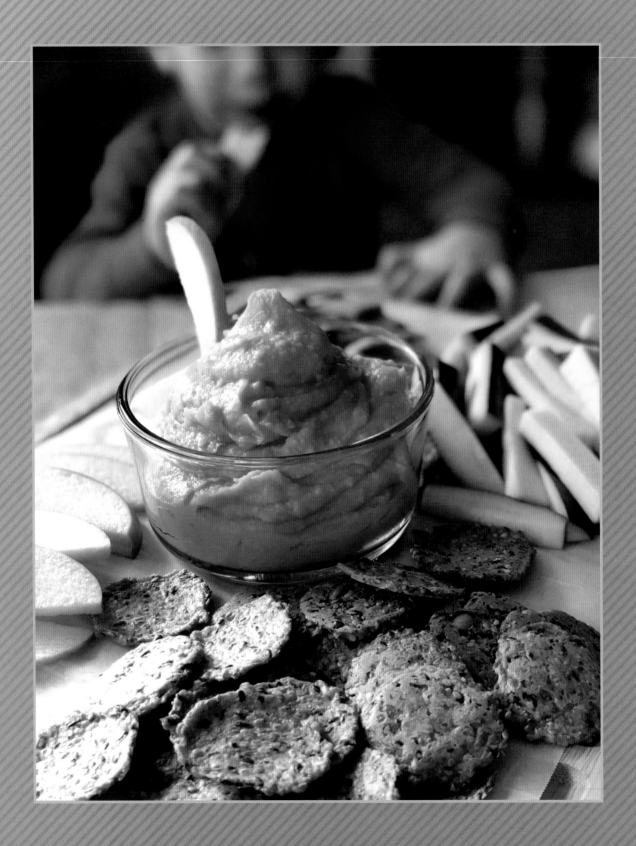

# 6

# Everyday Snacks

Kid-friendly participation steps are printed in **ORANGE**

# Almond Butter Chocolate Chip Granola Bars

*These no-bake granola bars are super easy to make, and my kids adore them. If nuts are a concern, swap out the almond butter, and use Sunbutter instead.*

**YIELD: 10 BARS**
Prep Time: 20 minutes
Total Time: 80 minutes

---

2 cups gluten-free oats

1 cup pitted dates, packed

¼ cup hot water

½ cup almond butter

½ cup honey

2 tablespoons coconut oil

1 cup gluten-free honey-oat O's cereal, slightly crushed

¼ cup mini dairy-free chocolate chips

 **Dr. Bear Fun Fact!** Almonds are a great source of potassium, fiber, iron, magnesium, calcium, and good fat!

*Nutritional data reflects one bar, based on a 10-bar yield.*

**PER SERVING** Calories: 286; Total Fat: 13g; Saturated Fat: 4g; Cholesterol: 0mg; Sodium: 21mg; Total Carbohydrates: 42g; Dietary Fiber: 5g; Sugars: 23g; Protein: 6g

**1.** Preheat oven to 350°F. Line an 8-by-8-inch baking dish with parchment paper and spray lightly with nonstick spray. Set aside.

**2.** Line a separate baking sheet with parchment paper, and spread the gluten-free oats across the baking sheet. Toast the oats for 15 to 18 minutes until lightly golden, stirring about halfway through baking.

**3.** While the oats are toasting, combine the dates and hot water in a small food processor or blender. Let sit for about 5 minutes. Once the dates have softened, purée until nearly smooth. It's OK for the date purée to have little chunks. Set aside.

**4.** In a small pot, combine the almond butter, honey, date purée, and coconut oil over medium heat. Cook, stirring frequently, until the almond butter is melted and the mixture is well combined. Remove from heat.

**5.** In a large mixing bowl, toss together the honey-oat O's cereal and chocolate chips. Stir in the toasted oats and mix well.

**6.** Pour the almond butter mixture over the dry ingredients in the bowl and stir together well.

**7.** Using a rubber spatula or damp hands, press the mixture evenly into the prepared baking dish.

**8.** Cover and refrigerate the bars for about 1 hour before slicing. To slice, lift the bars out of the pan in one piece using the edges of the parchment paper. Cut into 10 rectangular-shaped pieces. Store in an airtight container.

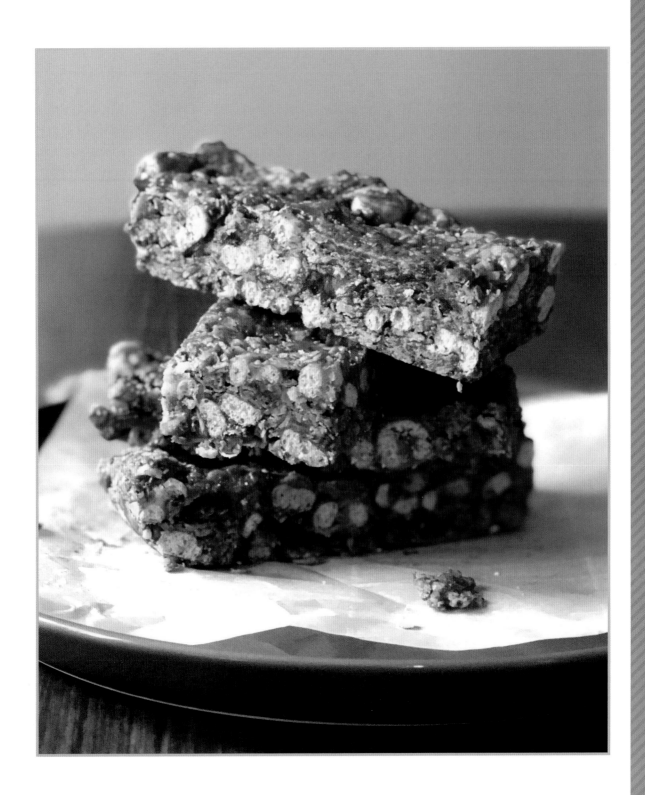

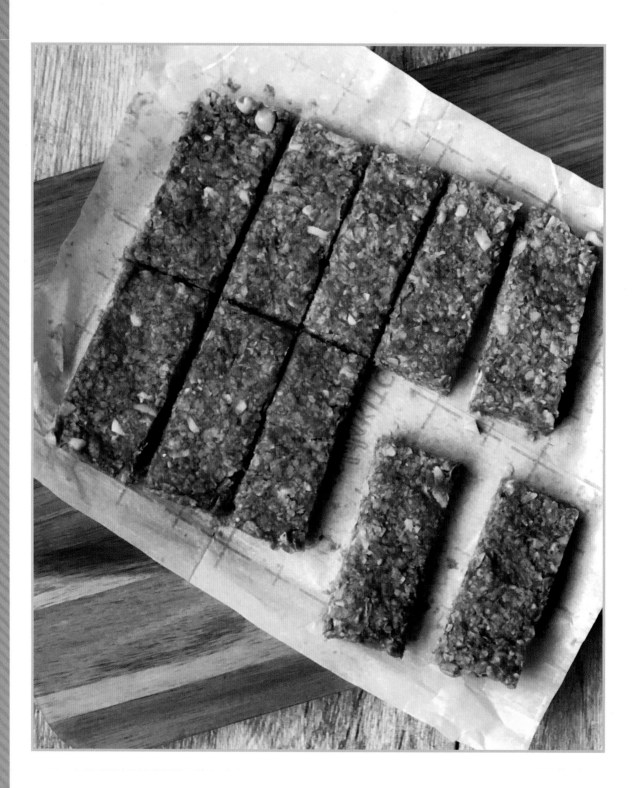

# Peanut Butter Coconut Granola Bars

*We go through peanut butter like water in my house, so of course I have a recipe for peanut butter granola bars. These no-bake bars are soft, sweet, and perfect for a quick morning bite.*

**YIELD: 10 BARS**
Prep Time: 20 minutes
Total Time: 80 minutes

---

2 cups gluten-free oats
1 cup pitted dates, packed
¼ cup hot water
½ cup peanut butter
½ cup honey
2 tablespoons coconut oil
1 cup gluten-free puffed rice cereal
1 cup shredded coconut
½ cup finely chopped peanuts

 **Dr. Bear Fun Fact!** Many puffed rice cereals use malt or malt flavoring in the ingredients. Always make sure the box says "gluten-free" on it!

*Nutritional data reflects one bar, based on a 10-bar yield.*

**PER SERVING**  Calories: 371; Total Fat: 20g; Saturated Fat: 9g; Cholesterol: 0mg; Sodium: 88mg; Total Carbohydrates: 46g; Dietary Fiber: 6g; Sugars: 26g; Protein: 8g

**1.** Preheat oven to 350°F. Line an 8-by-8-inch baking dish with parchment paper and spray lightly with nonstick spray. Set aside.

**2.** Line a separate baking sheet with parchment paper, and spread the gluten-free oats across the baking sheet. Toast the oats for 15 to 18 minutes until lightly golden.

**3.** While the oats are toasting, combine the dates and hot water in a small food processor or blender. Let sit for about 5 minutes. Once the dates have softened, purée until nearly smooth. It's OK for the date purée to have little chunks. Set aside.

**4.** In a small pot, combine the peanut butter, honey, date purée, and coconut oil over medium heat. Cook, stirring frequently, until the peanut butter is melted and the mixture is well combined, about 5 minutes. Remove from heat.

**5.** In a large mixing bowl, toss together the puffed rice cereal, shredded coconut, and chopped peanuts. Stir in the toasted oats and toss well.

**6.** Pour the peanut butter mixture over the dry ingredients in the bowl and stir until well combined.

**7.** Using a rubber spatula or damp hands, press the mixture evenly into the prepared baking dish.

**8.** Cover and refrigerate the bars for about 1 hour before slicing. To slice, lift the bars out of the pan in one piece using the edges of the parchment paper. Cut into 10 rectangular-shaped pieces. Store in an airtight container.

# Bright Beet Hummus

*All kids love bright colors, and this hummus certainly brings the brightness! It's loaded with good-for-you ingredients and tastes great with gluten-free crackers and veggies.*

**YIELD: 2 CUPS (8 SERVINGS)**
Prep Time: 50 minutes
Total Time: 75 minutes

---

1 large beet (or 3 small), scrubbed, ends removed, and peeled

3 tablespoons olive oil, divided

1 (15-ounce) can garbanzo beans, drained and rinsed

Juice of 1 lemon

1 teaspoon salt

Gluten-free crackers and vegetables for dipping

**1.** Preheat oven to 400°F. Place the beet(s) on a piece of foil, drizzle with olive oil and rub in. Wrap the beet(s) in foil, and place on a baking sheet. Roast for 20 to 50 minutes (depending on their size) until the beet is soft. Remove from oven and cool completely.

**2.** Once the beet is cool enough to handle, cut into chunks.

**3.** In the bowl of a food processor, combine the chopped beets, garbanzo beans, lemon juice, and salt. Purée until a smooth mixture forms.

**4.** Serve with gluten-free crackers and veggies.

 **Dr. Bear Fun Fact!** Beets have an earthy flavor, but they are also quite sweet! Beet juice also serves as a great natural food coloring.

*Nutritional data reflects one serving without crackers, based on an 8-serving yield.*

**PER SERVING** Calories: 128; Total Fat: 6.6g; Saturated Fat: 0.8g; Cholesterol: 0mg; Sodium: 422mg; Total Carbohydrates: 14.3g; Dietary Fiber: 3.8g; Sugars: 3.8g; Protein: 4.1g

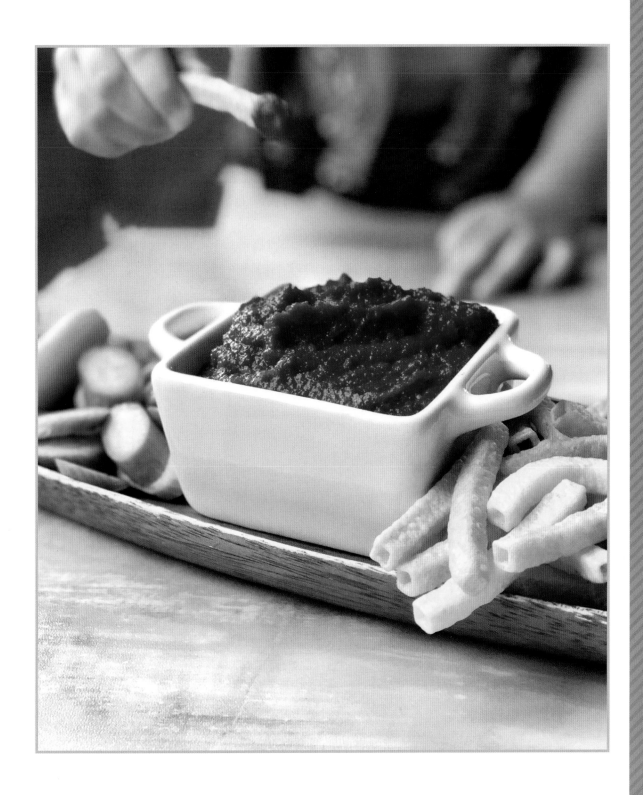

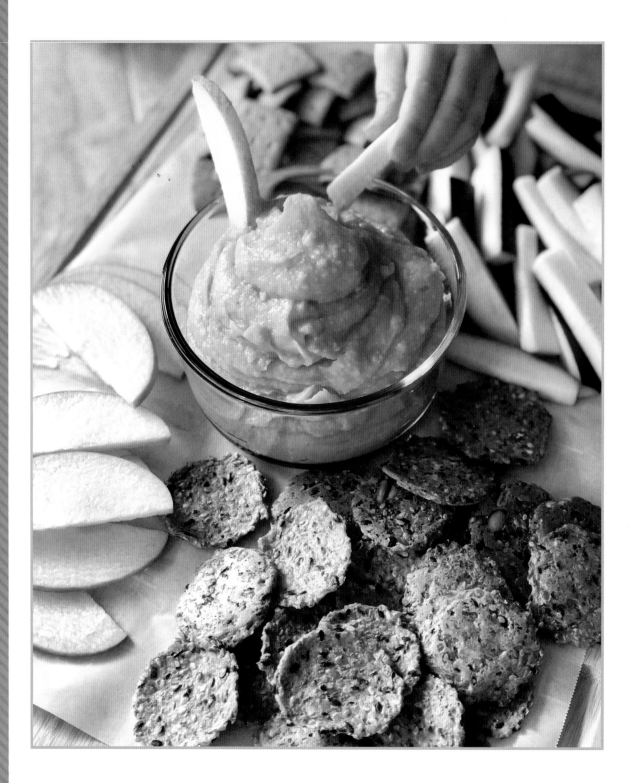

# Sweet Potato & White Bean Dip

*I developed this recipe on a whim when I intended to make hummus but didn't have any garbanzo beans in my pantry. I learned a very valuable lesson. You can make a hummus-like dip with lots of things! It's a little sweet, a little savory, and a whole lot delicious.*

**YIELD: 2 CUPS (8 SERVINGS)**
Prep Time: 35 minutes
Total Time: 40 minutes

---

1 large sweet potato

1 (15-ounce) can white beans, drained and rinsed

10 fresh basil leaves, rinsed and patted dry

1 teaspoon minced fresh ginger, peeled

1 garlic clove, peeled

Zest of 1 lemon

Juice of 1 lemon

3 tablespoons olive oil

Gluten-free crackers, bread, or vegetables for serving

1. Preheat oven to 400°F. Line a baking sheet with foil.

2. Place the sweet potato on the baking sheet and roast for 30 minutes, or until the sweet potato is soft and easily pierced with a fork. Remove from oven and cool completely.

3. Once cool, peel the skin off of the sweet potato and cut into chunks.

4. In the bowl of a food processor, combine white beans, basil, ginger, garlic, lemon zest, lemon juice, olive oil, and cooled sweet potato. Pulse until a smooth mixture forms.

5. Serve with gluten-free crackers, bread, or vegetables.

 **Dr. Bear Fun Fact!** White beans can refer to many different types of beans, like navy beans, cannellini, or Great Northern beans. Try variations of this recipe with different white beans to see which one you like best!

*Nutritional data reflects one serving without crackers or bread, based on an 8-serving yield.*

**PER SERVING** Calories: 120.7; Total Fat: 5.3g; Saturated Fat: 0.8g; Cholesterol 0mg; Sodium: 186.2mg; Total Carbohydrates: 14.9g; Dietary Fiber: 3.1g; Sugars: 1.2g; Protein: 4.2g

# Herby Hummus with Veggie Chips

*My kids are obsessed with veggie chips, so instead of always buying them, I figured out a way to make them at home. With the help of my friend Jackie, I came up with this recipe, which has three types of crispy chips to go along with the herby hummus.*

**YIELD: 2 CUPS (8 SERVINGS)**
Prep Time: 20 minutes
Total Time: 45 minutes

---

**For the Veggie Chips**

2 large parsnips, peeled

2 large sweet potatoes, peeled

2 large purple beets, scrubbed, ends removed, and peeled

Fine sea salt

Olive oil cooking spray

**For the Hummus**

1 (15-ounce) can garbanzo beans, drained and rinsed

½ cup roughly chopped fresh parsley, rinsed and patted dry

¼ cup roughly chopped fresh basil leaves, rinsed and patted dry

¼ cup roughly chopped fresh chives

¼ cup tahini

2 tablespoons lemon juice

2 tablespoons olive oil

1 garlic clove, peeled and minced

¾ teaspoon sea salt, divided

Optional: 1 tablespoon warm water

*Nutritional data reflects one serving, based on an 8-serving yield.*

**PER SERVING** Calories: 222; Total Fat: 9g; Saturated Fat: 1g; Cholesterol: 0mg; Sodium: 405mg; Total Carbohydrates: 31g; Dietary Fiber: 8g; Sugars: 7g; Protein: 7g

1. Position racks in the upper and lower thirds of the oven and preheat to 375°F. Line two baking sheets with parchment paper and set aside.

2. Using a mandolin or handheld slicer, carefully slice the vegetables to approximately ⅛-inch thick.

3. Place the sliced vegetables on paper towels in a single layer and sprinkle with half of the sea salt. Let sit for 15 minutes, then blot dry to remove excess water. This will help the chips get crispier in the oven.

4. Place the vegetable slices in a single layer on the baking sheets, and spray with a light coating of nonstick cooking spray. Bake for about 10 minutes. Toss and then bake an additional 10 to 12 minutes until crispy.

5. Remove veggie chips from the oven and sprinkle with remaining sea salt. Cool while making the hummus.

6. To make the hummus, combine the garbanzo beans, parsley, basil, chives, tahini, lemon juice, olive oil, garlic, and salt in the bowl of a food processor. Pulse until the hummus is thick, smooth, and creamy. Pause every few seconds to scrape down the sides of the bowl. If the hummus feels too thick, add 1 tablespoon warm water to thin it out slightly.

7. Serve hummus with the veggie chips.

**Dr. Bear Fun Fact!** The word "hummus" comes from the Arabic word for "chickpeas!" So, why do we use garbanzo beans in the recipe instead of chickpeas? While these two ingredients seem unrelated, they are actually the same bean. Use them interchangeably in recipes, but keep in mind that you're more likely to find a can labeled as garbanzo beans than chickpeas.

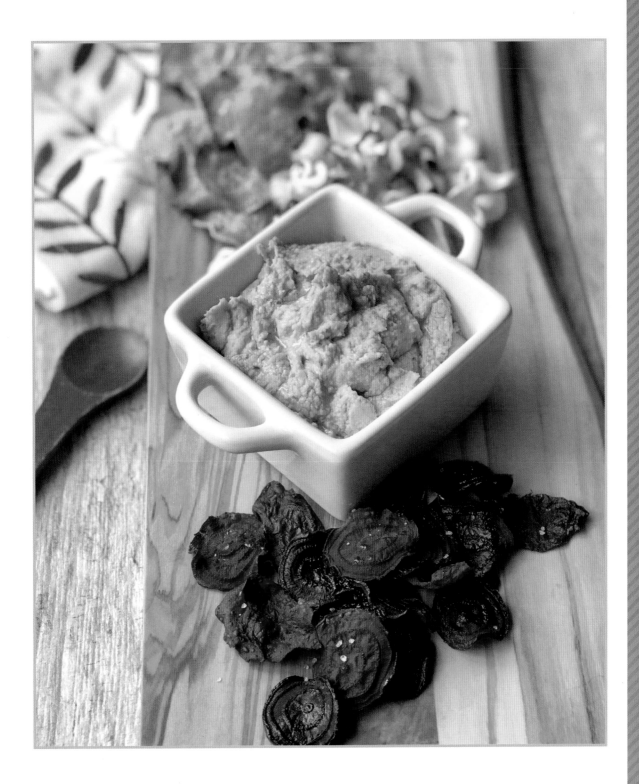

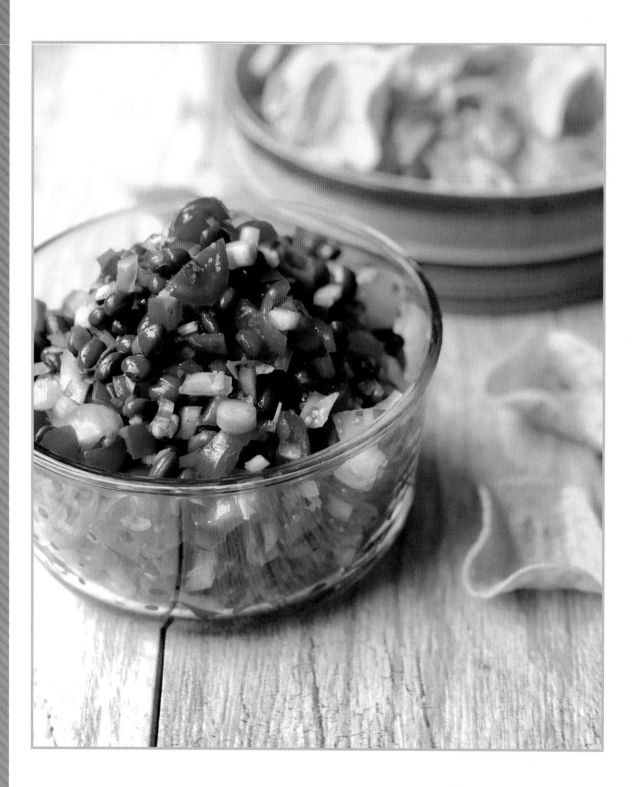

# Chunky Black Bean & Tomato Dip

*Dip or salsa? It really could be called either one, but regardless of its name, this chunky, flavor-packed dip is great on its own or served with corn chips.*

**YIELD: 8 SERVINGS**
Prep Time: 10 minutes
Total Time: 70 minutes
　(including chill time)

2 (15-ounce) cans black beans,
　drained and rinsed

2 cups chopped tomatoes

½ cup chopped fresh cilantro leaves,
　rinsed and patted dry

6 scallions, ends removed and
　finely chopped

½ cup finely chopped red onion,
　skin removed

2 teaspoons finely chopped jalapeño,
　stem and seeds removed

Juice of 1 lime

Corn chips, for serving

1. **In a large** glass mixing bowl, toss together the black beans, tomatoes, cilantro, scallions, red onion, jalapeño, and lime juice.

2. Cover and refrigerate for 1 hour before serving.

3. Serve black bean dip with corn chips.

 **Dr. Bear Fun Fact!** Black beans are one of the superheroes of the legume group! They have been shown to help lower blood pressure, manage insulin levels, maintain healthy bones, and boost brain function.

*Nutritional data reflects one serving without corn chips, based on an 8-serving yield.*

**PER SERVING** Calories: 166; Total Fat: 0.8g; Saturated Fat: 0.1g; Cholesterol: 0mg; Sodium: 414mg; Total Carbohydrates: 31.6g; Dietary Fiber: 12.1g; Sugars: 2.6g; Protein: 9.4g

# Mango Guacamole

*I could eat this guacamole every single day and never get tired of it. It is great served on its own with corn chips, or as a topping for tacos, grilled fish, or chicken.*

**YIELD: 6–8 SERVINGS**
Prep Time: 10 minutes
Total Time: 15 minutes

———————

2 ripe avocados, skin and
    pit removed

½ cup finely chopped white onion,
    skin removed

½ cup chopped fresh cilantro leaves,
    rinsed and patted dry

1 teaspoon finely chopped jalapeño,
    stem and seeds removed

Zest of 1 lime

Juice of 1 lime

1 teaspoon sugar

1 cup chopped mango, skin and
    pit removed

1 cup chopped tomatoes

Corn chips, for serving

**1.** In a glass mixing bowl, mash together the avocado, onion, cilantro, jalapeño, lime zest, lime juice, and sugar until you're happy with the texture.

**2.** Gently stir in the mango and tomatoes. Cover and refrigerate until ready to serve with chips or on top of your favorite tacos.

 **Dr. Bear Fun Fact!** Mangoes and cashews are in the same family; however, having an allergy to one does not mean you're necessarily allergic to both.

*Nutritional data reflects one serving without corn chips, based on an 8-serving yield.*

**PER SERVING** Calories: 83; Total Fat: 5.4g; Saturated Fat: 0.8g; Cholesterol: 0mg; Sodium: 38.5mg; Total Carbohydrates: 9.3g; Dietary Fiber: 3.5g; Sugars: 4.8g; Protein: 1.3g

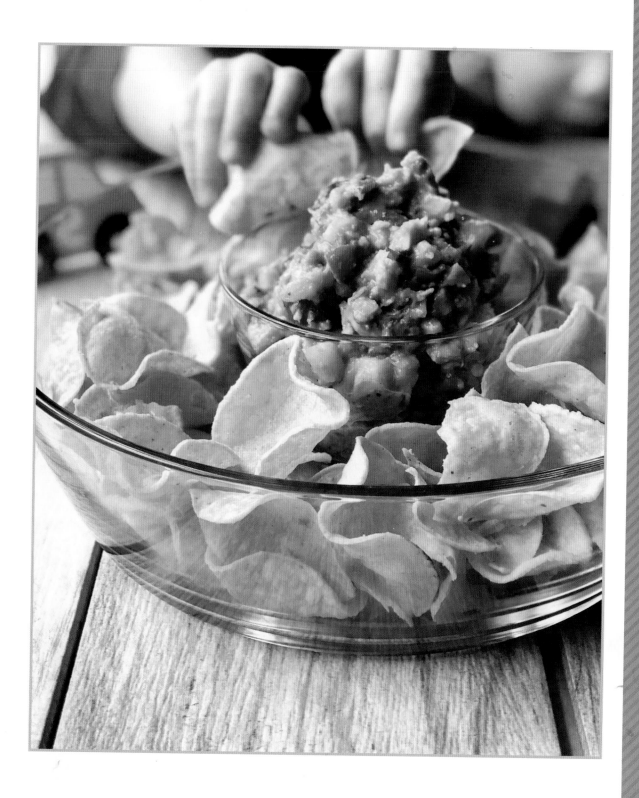

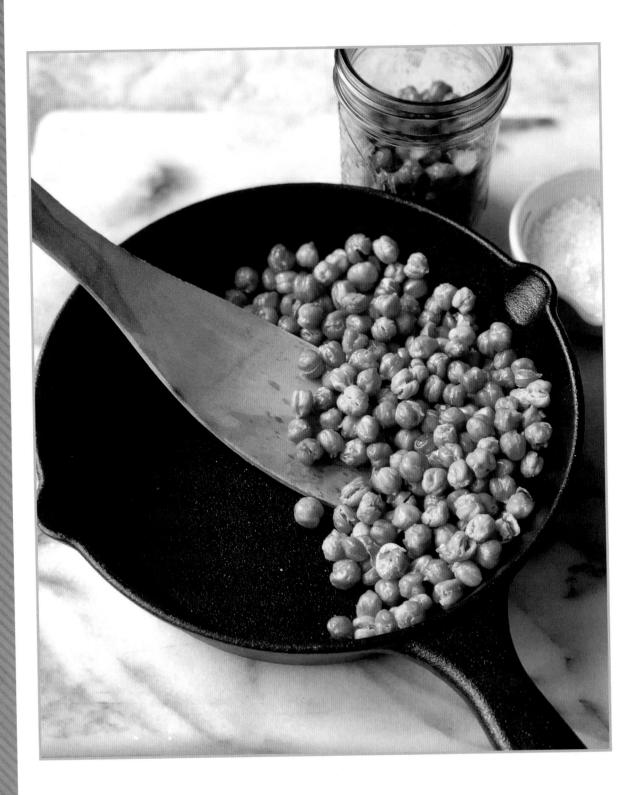

# Rosemary Sea Salt Roasted Chickpeas

*These crunchy bites are great as an on-the-go snack. I make large batches before a trip and snack on them on the train or airplane. Rosemary and sea salt are just one option for seasoning, but the sky's the limit. Try Old Bay, chili powder, or lime zest.*

**YIELD: 4 SERVINGS**
Prep Time: 5 minutes
Total Time: 75 minutes

---

2 (15-ounce) cans chickpeas, rinsed and drained

1 tablespoon olive oil

2 teaspoons finely chopped fresh rosemary, rinsed and patted dry

1 teaspoon sea salt

1. Preheat oven to 300°F. Line a baking sheet with parchment and set aside.

2. Arrange chickpeas in a single layer on the parchment paper and dry with a paper towel to remove any excess moisture.

3. Roast the chickpeas for 60 minutes, stirring every 10 to 15 minutes to help them roast evenly.

4. Remove from oven and place the chickpeas in a mixing bowl. Drizzle the olive oil, rosemary, and salt over the chickpeas and toss to combine. Transfer the chickpeas back to the lined baking pan. Increase oven temperature to 375°F and bake for another 10 minutes.

5. Remove from oven and let chickpeas cool completely before serving.

 **Dr. Bear Fun Fact!** Chickpeas are very high in fiber, which means they keep you fuller longer. A great choice for a snack!

*Nutritional data reflects one serving, based on a 4-serving yield.*

**PER SERVING** Calories: 327; Total Fat: 9.4g; Saturated Fat: 1g; Cholesterol: 0mg; Sodium: 1035.7mg; Total Carbohydrates: 48.3g; Dietary Fiber: 13.8g; Sugars: 8.5g; Protein: 15g

# Sweet & Crunchy Snack Mix

*My kids call this snack mix "mommy's yummy in my tummy mix" because it includes all of their favorite snack foods. Make as directed below or toss in whatever nuts you have in your pantry.*

**YIELD: 5 CUPS (10 SERVINGS)**
Prep Time: 5 minutes
Total Time: 5 minutes

---

2 cups gluten-free pretzels

1 cup roasted and salted peanuts

1 cup raisins

½ cup chopped dark chocolate pieces

¼ cup roasted and salted
   pumpkin seeds

1. Toss all ingredients together in a large mixing bowl.

2. Spoon into a serving dish or store in an airtight container.

**Dr. Bear Fun Fact!** The history of the pretzel is unknown, but it is mostly associated with Germany!

*Nutritional data reflects one serving, based on a 10-serving yield.*

**PER SERVING** Calories: 292; Total Fat: 12.5g; Saturated Fat: 3.5g; Cholesterol: 0.6mg; Sodium: 309.6mg; Total Carbohydrates: 42.5g; Dietary Fiber: 3.1g; Sugars: 13.5g; Protein: 5.3g

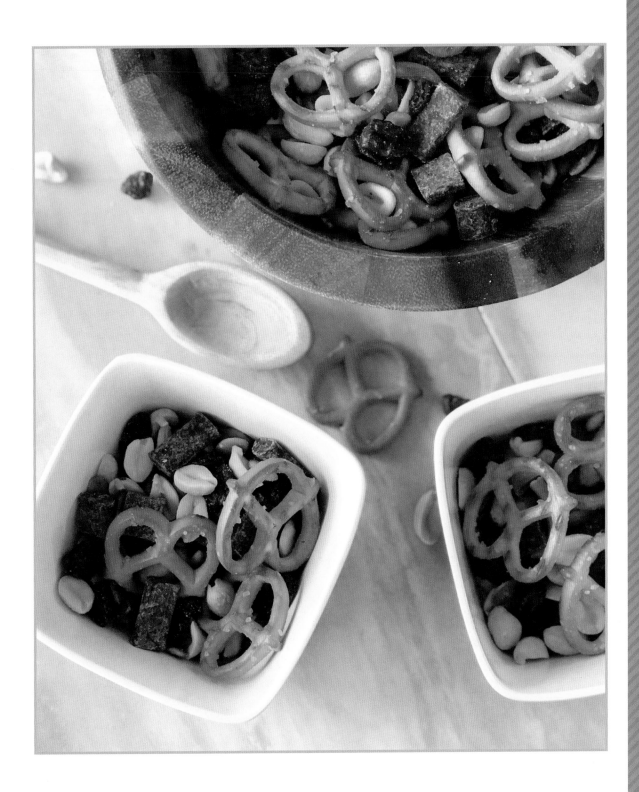

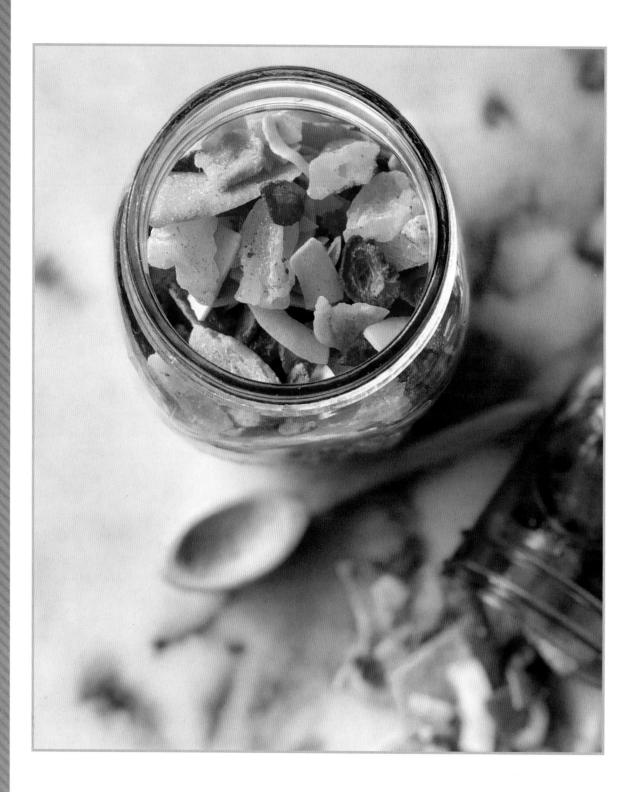

# Caribbean Crunch Snack Mix

*As we were getting ready to travel to Jamaica, my kids went grocery shopping with me to pick out a bunch of snacks for the airplane ride. They picked a bunch of different dried fruits, so when we got home we tossed them all together and voila! The Caribbean Crunch Snack Mix came to life. Its flavors will certainly remind you of vacation on a tropical beach.*

**YIELD: 6 CUPS (12 SERVINGS)**
Prep Time: 5 minutes
Total Time: 5 minutes

---

1 (1-ounce) package dried strawberries

1 (6-ounce) package dried pineapple

1 (6-ounce) package dried mango pieces, chopped

1 (3-ounce) package coconut chips

**1.** Toss all ingredients together in a large mixing bowl.

**2.** Spoon into serving dish or store in an airtight container.

 **Dr. Bear Fun Fact!** Ancient Egyptians included dried fruit in tombs of Pharaohs as food for the afterlife!

*Nutritional data reflects one serving, based on a 12-serving yield.*

**PER SERVING** Calories: 130; Total Fat: 2.7g; Saturated Fat: 2.2g; Cholesterol: 0mg; Sodium: 27.1mg; Total Carbohydrates: 26.8g; Dietary Fiber: 2.7g; Sugars: 21.6g; Protein: 2g

# Salty, Sweet, & Crunchy Popcorn

*I have this ongoing problem of forgetting when I'm snack mom for the week. Thankfully, I always have popcorn and gluten-free pretzels in my pantry, so I can whip up a batch of trail mix. One day I also happened to have dried pineapple, so I tossed it in and the feedback was amazing! At least three parents sent me a message to tell me their child came home raving about the snack mix and they needed the recipe. Who knew cleaning out the cupboards would lead to such success with a group of five-year-olds!*

**YIELD: 18 CUPS (18 SERVINGS)**
Prep Time: 5 minutes
Total Time: 5 minutes

1 (4.75-ounce) bag lightly salted popcorn
1 (8-ounce) bag gluten-free pretzels
1 (9.6-ounce) bag M&Ms
1 cup raisins
1 (6-ounce) package dried pineapple

**1.** Toss all ingredients together in a large mixing bowl.

**2.** Spoon into a serving dish or store in an airtight container.

**Dr. Bear Fun Fact!** Popcorn has always been a popular snack—ancient popcorn was found in a cave in Mexico dating back to 3,600 BC!

*Nutritional data reflects one serving, based on an 18-serving yield.*

**PER SERVING** Calories: 448; Total Fat: 15.9g; Saturated Fat: 8.2g; Cholesterol: 0mg; Sodium: 212.2mg; Total Carbohydrates: 75.2g; Dietary Fiber: 3.5g; Sugars: 53.3g; Protein: 4.3g

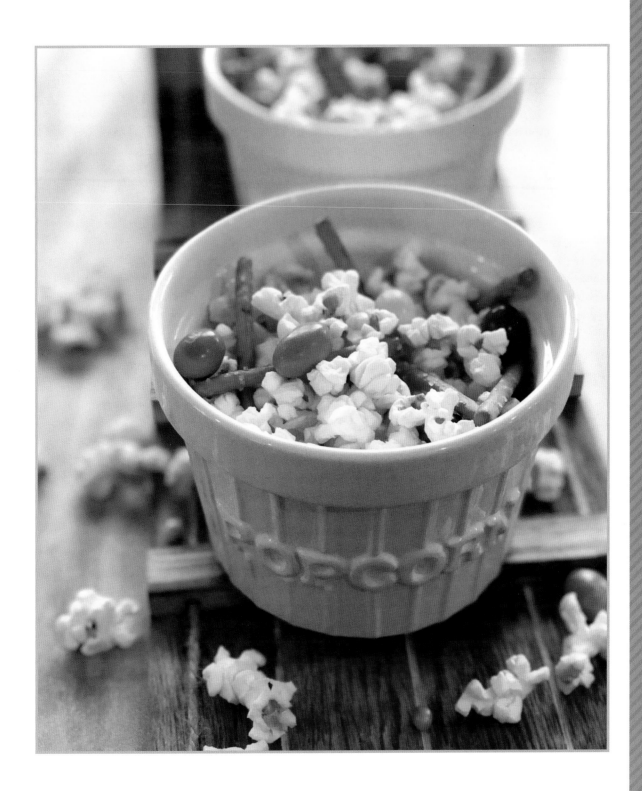

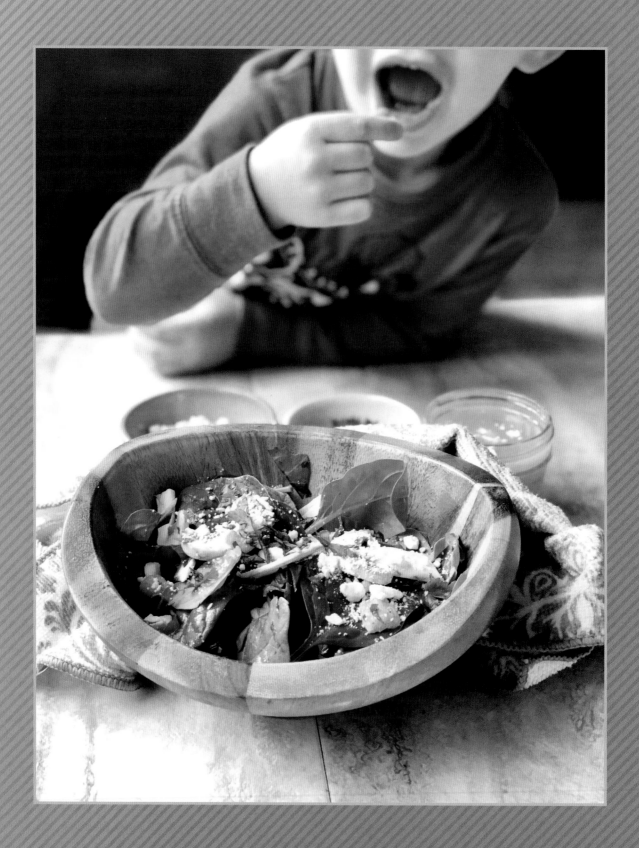

# 7

# Salads & Soups

Kid-friendly participation steps are printed in **ORANGE**

# Quinoa Salad with Black Beans & Herbs

*This salad comes together quite quickly and is the perfect side dish for grilled fish or steaks. My kids won't eat it all combined in the salad form, but if I plate each of the ingredients separately, they'll joyfully eat it all up.*

**YIELD: 4 SERVINGS**
Prep Time: 10 minutes
Total Time: 30 minutes

———————

3 cups water

1½ cups quinoa

¼ cup avocado or olive oil

¼ cup lemon juice

2 tablespoons white wine vinegar

2 teaspoons lemon zest

½ teaspoon salt

1 cup chopped tomatoes

¾ cup chopped fresh basil leaves, rinsed and patted dry

¼ cup chopped fresh Italian parsley leaves, rinsed and patted dry

¼ cup chopped fresh cilantro leaves, rinsed and patted dry

1 (14.5-ounce) can black beans, drained and rinsed

**1.** In a medium sauce pot, add the water and quinoa. Bring to a boil over medium-high heat. Reduce the heat to a simmer, cover, and cook for about 12 to 15 minutes until all of the liquid is absorbed. Remove from heat and cool completely.

**2.** To make the dressing, whisk together the avocado or olive oil, lemon juice, white wine vinegar, lemon zest, and salt in a small bowl. Set aside.

**3.** In a large mixing bowl, toss together the cooled quinoa, tomatoes, basil, parsley, cilantro, black beans, and dressing. Chill until ready to serve.

 **Dr. Bear Fun Fact!** Quinoa is a naturally gluten-free superfood that contains all nine essential amino acids. Technically, it's a seed that's eaten like a grain, and it comes in a variety of colors like red, white, and black. In this recipe we've tossed it with fresh herbs, black beans, and tomatoes for a light lunchtime salad! Or serve it as a side dish with your favorite protein.

*Nutritional data reflects one serving, based on a 4-serving yield.*

**PER SERVING** Calories: 427; Total Fat: 6.8g; Saturated Fat: 1g; Cholesterol: 0mg; Sodium: 710.1mg; Total Carbohydrates: 73g; Dietary Fiber: 17.5g; Sugars: 6.8g; Protein: 19.2g

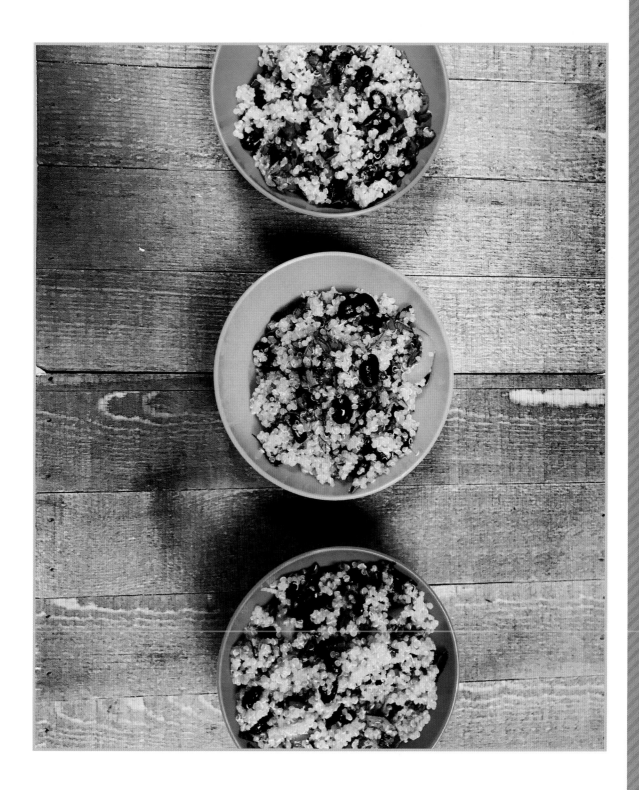

# Shaved Apple & Spinach Salad with Honey Dijon Vinaigrette

*The founder of our Celiac Program at Children's National, Blair Raber, made this amazing salad for dinner when we had an out-of-town visitor from Uganda. It's a long story of how this dinner came to be, but the patient had a lot of difficulty getting tested for celiac disease in her home country and was able to get a visa to visit us in the United States for testing. It all worked out well, and I was still thinking about this salad days later. The highlights of the salad were the shaved apples and white cheddar cheese, so I had to figure it out at home. Here's what I came up with.*

**YIELD: 4–6 SERVINGS**
Prep Time: 15 minutes
Total Time: 45 minutes

---

1 pound shredded Brussels sprouts

½ cup, plus 2 tablespoons olive oil, divided

1 teaspoon salt, divided

1 teaspoon garlic powder

10 slices turkey bacon

3 tablespoons apple cider vinegar

1 shallot, skin removed and finely chopped

1 tablespoon Dijon mustard

2 teaspoons honey

Juice of 1 lemon

1 (5-ounce) package baby arugula, rinsed and patted dry

4 cups baby spinach, rinsed and patted dry

1 cup grated sharp white cheddar cheese

1 cold Honeycrisp apple, grated using a box grater

Optional add-Ins: Rotisserie chicken, hard-boiled eggs, and chopped avocado

**1.** Preheat oven to 375°F. Line two baking sheets with foil and set aside.

**2.** Place the shredded Brussels sprouts on one prepared baking sheet and toss with 2 tablespoons olive oil, ½ teaspoon salt, and garlic powder. Roast for 25 to 30 minutes until golden brown, tossing at least twice during roasting to brown evenly.

**3.** Arrange turkey bacon on the second prepared sheet pan and roast alongside the Brussels sprouts for 15 to 20 minutes until crispy and starting to brown. Remove from oven and cool. Once cool, chop into bite-sized pieces.

**4.** To make the salad dressing, whisk together the remaining ½ cup olive oil, apple cider vinegar, chopped shallot, Dijon mustard, honey, juice of one lemon, and remaining ½ teaspoon salt in a glass mixing bowl or mason jar. Cover and refrigerate until ready to serve.

**5.** To assemble the salad, in a large salad bowl, toss together the baby arugula, spinach, roasted Brussels sprouts, chopped turkey bacon, grated white cheddar cheese, and grated apple.

**6.** Pour the dressing over the salad and toss to combine. Add any desired garnishes and serve immediately.

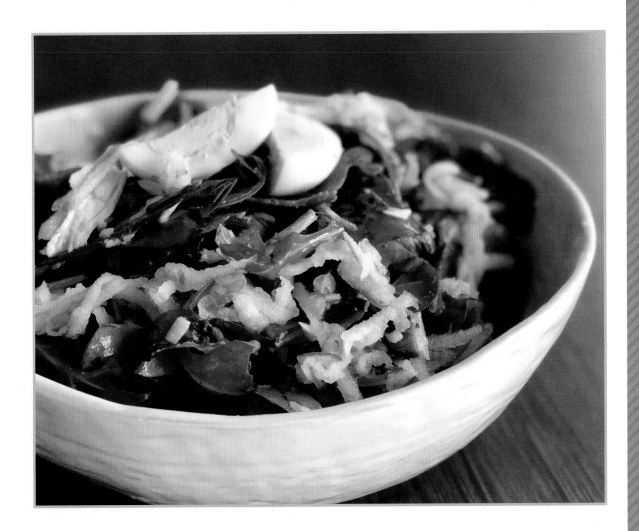

 **Dr. Bear Fun Fact!** Spinach is considered a super-food. It's jam-packed with Vitamins A, C, and K, as well as folate, iron, manganese, and magnesium. We can see why Popeye the Sailor Man is spinach's biggest fan!

*Nutritional data reflects one serving without optional add-ins, based on a 6-serving yield.*

**PER SERVING** Calories: 436.9; Total Fat: 35g; Saturated Fat: 8.4g; Cholesterol 54mg; Sodium: 1108.4mg; Total Carbohydrates: 18.3g; Dietary Fiber: 4.8g; Sugars: 9g; Protein: 15.9g

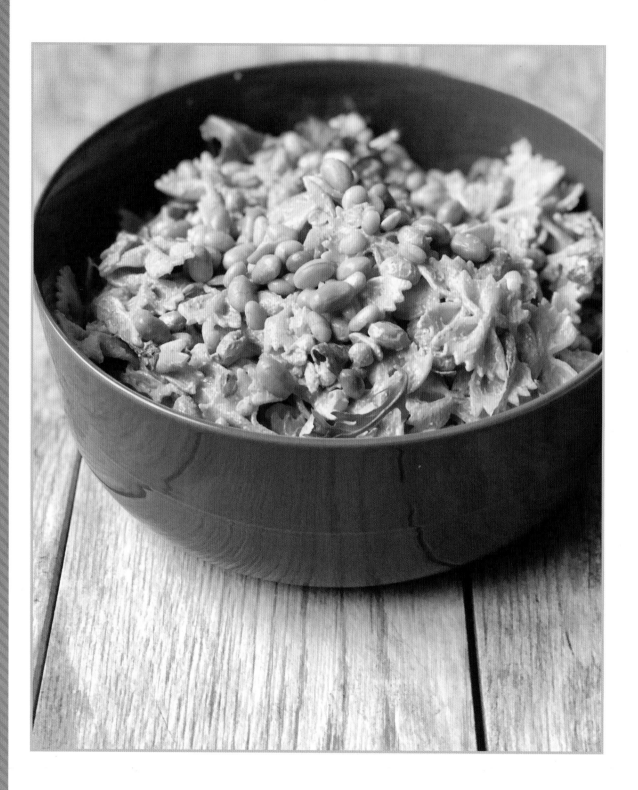

# Pasta Salad with Edamame & White Beans

*This pasta salad can be made with any gluten-free pasta shape. If your kids aren't a fan of green leaves, toss in the arugula after serving them.*

**YIELD: 4–6 SERVINGS**
Prep Time: 20 minutes
Total Time: 30 minutes

---

1 (12-ounce) package gluten-free
    farfalle pasta

2 cups frozen shelled edamame

½ cup sour cream

¼ cup mayonnaise

3 teaspoons lemon juice

1 teaspoon water

2 teaspoons paprika

1 teaspoon garlic powder

1 teaspoon salt

½ teaspoon dry mustard

1 cup small white beans, drained
    and rinsed

2 cups baby arugula, rinsed
    and patted dry

Optional add-ins: shredded rotisserie
    chicken, chopped crispy bacon,
    chopped spinach, avocado, etc.

**1.** Fill a large pot with water and bring to a boil over high heat. Add the gluten-free farfalle pasta and cook according to package instructions. Drain, rinse with cold water, and set aside.

**2.** Cook the edamame according to package instructions. Cool completely.

**3.** In a large mixing bowl, whisk together the sour cream, mayonnaise, lemon juice, water, paprika, garlic powder, salt, and dry mustard until a smooth mixture forms.

**4.** Add the pasta into the mixing bowl with the dressing and toss to coat well. Add the edamame, white beans, and arugula and toss to combine.

**5.** Toss in any extra ingredients that sound good to you!

**6.** Cover and refrigerate until ready to serve.

 **Dr. Bear Fun Fact!** Edamame is actually just un-ripened soybeans! They have a subtle sweet flavor and pack a nutritional punch with protein, fiber, and micronutrients.

*Nutritional data reflects one serving without optional add-ins, based on a 6-serving yield.*

**PER SERVING** Calories: 431; Total Fat: 15.6g; Saturated Fat: 3.4g; Cholesterol: 15.2mg; Sodium: 613.7mg; Total Carbohydrates: 59.2g; Dietary Fiber: 7.3g; Sugars: 2.4g; Protein: 15.5g

# Italian Salad with Gluten-Free Orzo

*I was thrilled to find the gluten-free orzo from Delallo on my grocery store shelf. It's a great side dish but also a wonderful addition to a salad.*

**YIELD: 4–6 SERVINGS**
Prep Time: 25 minutes
Total Time: 35 minutes

---

### For the Italian Dressing
2 tablespoons red wine vinegar

Juice of 1 lemon

1 teaspoon Dijon mustard

2 tablespoons grated Romano cheese

1 teaspoon sugar

1 teaspoon Italian seasoning blend

¼ teaspoon garlic powder

¼ teaspoon salt

¼ cup olive oil

### For the Salad
1 (12-ounce) package gluten-free orzo

1 (15-ounce) can small white beans, drained and rinsed

4 cups baby spinach, rinsed and patted dry

1 cup chopped Italian salami

1 cup chopped tomatoes

½ cup chopped cucumbers, rinsed, patted dry, and ends removed

½ cup chopped provolone cheese

1. To make the dressing, whisk together the red wine vinegar, lemon juice, Dijon mustard, Romano cheese, sugar, Italian seasoning, garlic powder, and salt in a small glass mixing bowl. Add the olive oil, and whisk until an emulsified mixture forms. Cover and refrigerate until ready to use.

2. In a pot of boiling water, cook the gluten-free orzo according to package instructions. Drain and cool completely.

3. To make the salad, toss together the cooked gluten-free orzo, white beans, spinach, Italian salami, tomatoes, cucumbers, and provolone cheese in a large mixing bowl.

4. Drizzle the salad dressing over the salad and toss to coat all of the ingredients.

5. Cover and refrigerate until ready to serve.

 **Dr. Bear Fun Fact!** Orzo is a type of pasta that's shaped like a large grain of rice. It can be tricky to tell the difference between orzo and rice at a restaurant, so always be sure to double-check its gluten-free status!

*Nutritional data reflects one serving, based on a 6-serving yield.*

**PER SERVING** Calories: 553.6; Total Fat: 23.5g; Saturated Fat: 6.8g; Cholesterol 29.2mg; Sodium: 748.3mg; Total Carbohydrates: 67.1g; Dietary Fiber: 7.2g; Sugars: 2g; Protein: 19.9g

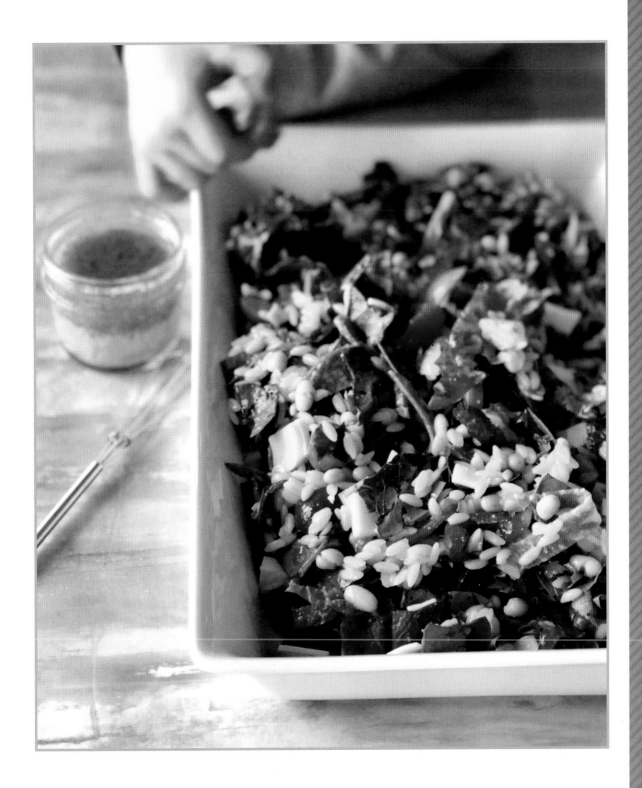

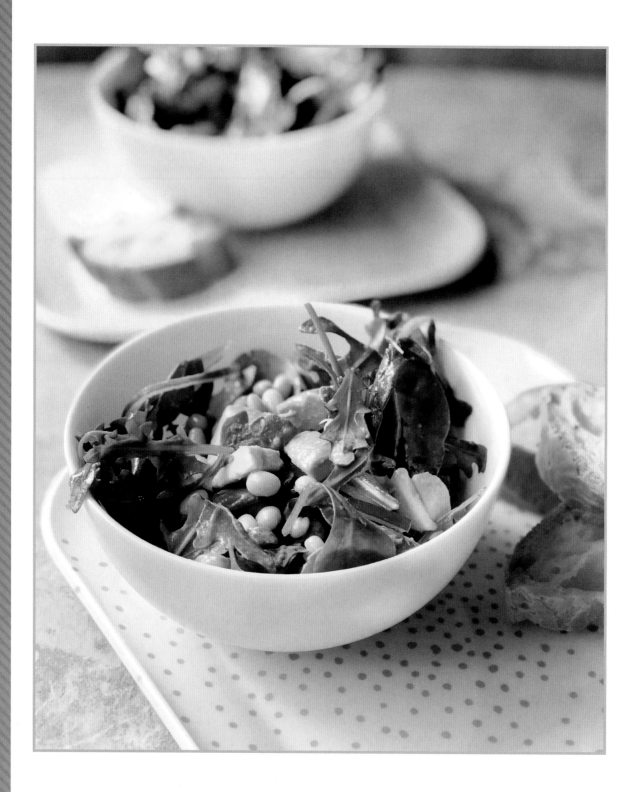

# Tossed Arugula Salad with Sweet Lemon Vinaigrette

*This is a bright and fresh salad with tangy and sweet flavors. It's excellent for a Sunday brunch or served alongside grilled fish.*

**YIELD: 6–8 SERVINGS**

Prep Time: 10 minutes
Total Time: 15 minutes

---

¼ cup olive oil

Zest of 1 lemon

¼ cup lemon juice

2 teaspoons sugar

2 teaspoons Dijon mustard

¼ teaspoon sea salt

4 cups baby arugula, rinsed and patted dry

2 cups baby spinach, rinsed and patted dry

1 (15-ounce) can small white beans, drained and rinsed

¼ cup thinly sliced red onions, skin removed

1 avocado, skin and pit removed and finely chopped

**1.** To make the salad dressing, whisk together the olive oil, lemon zest, lemon juice, sugar, Dijon mustard, and salt in a glass mixing bowl or mason jar. Cover and refrigerate until ready to serve.

**2.** In a large salad or mixing bowl, toss together the arugula, spinach, white beans, red onions, and avocado. Drizzle the dressing over the salad and toss together until well coated.

**3.** Serve immediately!

 **Dr. Bear Fun Fact!** Arugula is often called "rocket" in other parts of the world. It has a slightly peppery taste and is usually added to lettuce blends. It's a great source of calcium too!

*Nutritional data reflects one serving, based on a 6-serving yield.*

**PER SERVING** Calories: 166; Total Fat: 9.6g; Saturated Fat: 1.3g; Cholesterol: 0mg; Sodium: 300mg; Total Carbohydrates: 16.1g; Dietary Fiber: 4.4g; Sugars: 2.2g; Protein: 5.1g

# Eggplant, Spinach, & Goat Cheese Salad

*This salad is inspired by the Lisa Salad at Calabria Restaurant in Livingston, New Jersey. The restaurant goes out of their way to make sure that families on a gluten-free diet are well taken care of, and I sincerely appreciate it. And, I love their salads! Here's my homemade version of their classic salad.*

**YIELD: 6 SERVINGS**
Prep Time: 30 minutes
Total Time: 40 minutes

---

1 large eggplant, ends removed and cut into 1-inch pieces

2 tablespoons olive oil

½ teaspoon salt

½ teaspoon garlic powder

2 tablespoons white wine vinegar

1 garlic clove, peeled and finely minced

2 teaspoon lemon juice

1 teaspoon Dijon mustard

1 teaspoon sugar

¼ cup olive oil

1 (16-ounce) package fresh baby spinach leaves, rinsed and patted dry

1 pound button mushrooms, rinsed, patted dry, and thinly sliced

½ cup chopped fresh parsley, rinsed and patted dry

½ cup crumbled goat cheese

**1.** Preheat oven to 450°F. Line a baking sheet with foil and spray with nonstick spray. Spread the chopped eggplant evenly across the baking sheet and drizzle with olive oil, salt, and garlic powder. Rub the oil and seasonings in thoroughly. Roast for 20 to 25 minutes until golden. Cool completely.

**2.** In a small mixing bowl, whisk together the white wine vinegar, minced garlic, lemon juice, Dijon mustard, and sugar. Whisk in the olive oil until an emulsified dressing forms. Cover and refrigerate until ready to serve.

**3.** In a large bowl, toss together the cooled eggplant, spinach, mushrooms, parsley, and goat cheese. Toss the salad with the dressing before serving.

 **Dr. Bear Fun Fact!** Goat cheese has about half of the calories, fat, and cholesterol as cow's milk cheese. It usually has a stronger taste, too, so you don't need much to add loads of flavor!

*Nutritional data reflects one serving, based on a 6-serving yield.*

**PER SERVING**  Calories: 214; Total Fat: 16.4g; Saturated Fat: 3.6g; Cholesterol: 5.4mg; Sodium: 338.7mg; Total Carbohydrates: 9.9g; Dietary Fiber: 5.4g; Sugars: 3.7g; Protein: 7.4g

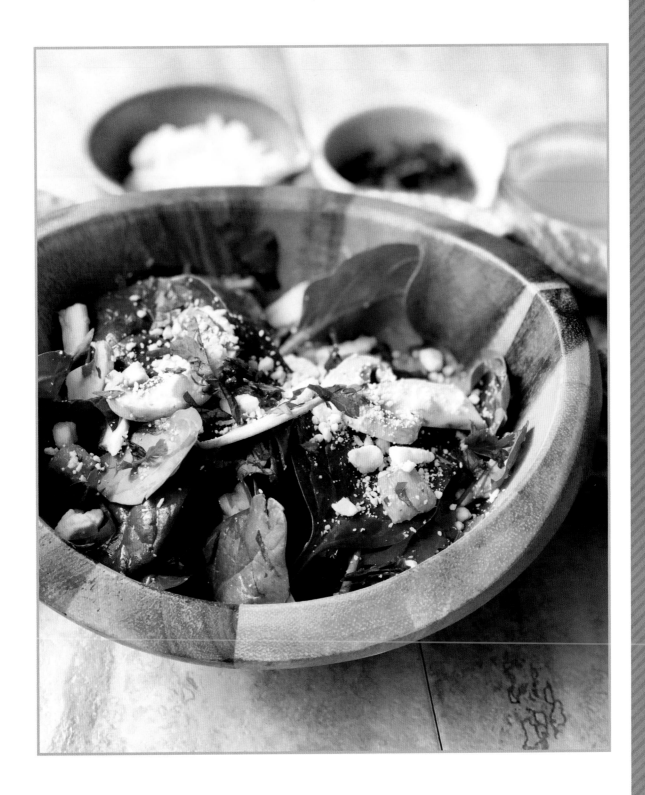

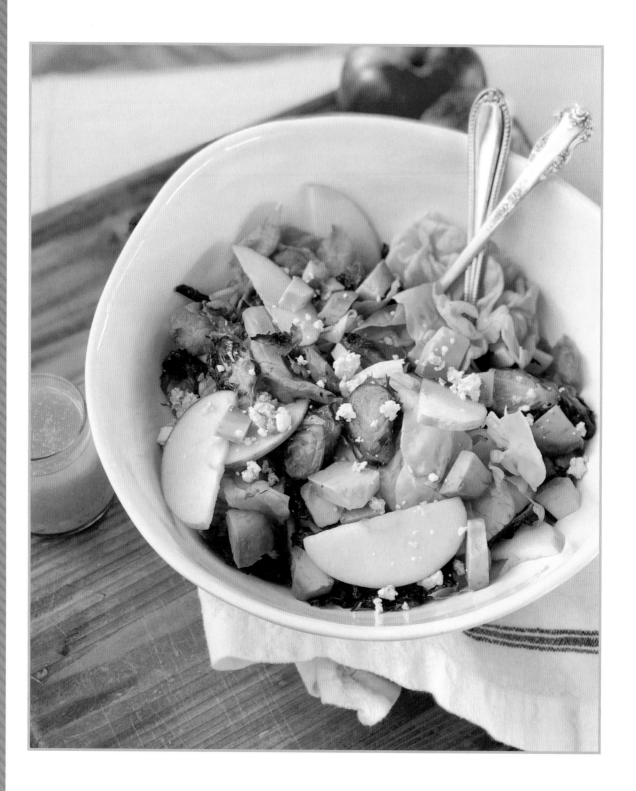

# Butter Lettuce with Blue Cheese Vinaigrette

*I love blue cheese dressing on butter lettuce. It just goes so well together. If you can't easily find butter lettuce, swap in a combination of chopped romaine and baby spinach.*

**YIELD: 6 SERVINGS**
Prep Time: 20 minutes
Total Time: 30 minutes

### For the Dressing

½ cup olive oil

½ cup crumbled blue cheese

¼ cup red wine vinegar

1 shallot, skin removed and finely minced

½ teaspoon salt

### For the Salad

1 pound shredded Brussels sprouts

2 tablespoons olive oil

1 teaspoon salt

1 teaspoon garlic powder

2 large heads butter lettuce, rinsed, patted dry, and chopped into bite-sized pieces

1 Honeycrisp apple, core removed, cut in half and thinly sliced

1 slightly firm avocado, skin and pit removed, chopped into cubes

**1.** Preheat oven to 425°F. Line a baking sheet with foil and set aside.

**2.** To make the dressing, combine the olive oil, blue cheese, red wine vinegar, shallot, and salt in small food processor. Pulse until a smooth mixture forms. If you like a chunkier blue cheese dressing, you can skip the food processor and whisk the ingredients together in a mixing bowl. Cover and refrigerate until ready to serve.

**3.** Place the shredded Brussels sprouts on the prepared baking sheet and toss with olive oil, salt, and garlic powder. Roast for 15 to 20 minutes until golden brown, tossing at least once during roasting. Remove from oven and cool completely.

**4.** To assemble the salad, toss together the chopped butter lettuce, cooled Brussels sprouts, sliced apple, and avocado in a large salad bowl. Drizzle the blue cheese dressing over the salad and toss to combine. Serve immediately.

 **Dr. Bear Fun Fact!** We call it "butter lettuce" because it's so tender it melts in your mouth—like butter!

*Nutritional data reflects one serving, based on a 6-serving yield.*

**PER SERVING** Calories: 339; Total Fat: 29.6g; Saturated Fat: 5.8g; Cholesterol: 8.4mg; Sodium: 744.3mg; Total Carbohydrates: 15.6g; Dietary Fiber: 5.9g; Sugars: 5.9g; Protein: 6.4g

# Taco Salad with Creamy Cilantro Lime Dressing

*As written, this taco salad is a vegetarian dish, but it also goes great topped with ground beef, shredded chicken, or grilled steaks.*

**YIELD: 6 SERVINGS**
Prep Time: 15 minutes
Total Time: 25 minutes

---

**For the Creamy Cilantro Lime Dressing**

¾ cup sour cream

½ cup fresh cilantro leaves, rinsed and patted dry

2 tablespoons olive oil

2 tablespoons lime juice

Zest of 1 lime

1 teaspoon ground cumin

1 teaspoon sugar

½ teaspoon salt

**For the Salad**

1 head romaine lettuce, rinsed, patted dry, and chopped

1 (15-ounce) can black beans, drained and rinsed

1 cup crumbled queso fresco cheese

1 cup chopped jicama

1 cup sweet yellow corn

1 red onion, skin removed and thinly sliced

Corn chips, for garnish

Chopped fresh cilantro leaves, rinsed and patted dry, for garnish

**1.** To make the dressing, combine the sour cream, cilantro, olive oil, lime juice, lime zest, cumin, sugar, and salt in a food processor. Purée until smooth. Cover and refrigerate until ready to serve.

**2.** In a large bowl, toss together the chopped lettuce, black beans, crumbled cheese, jicama, corn, and onion. Drizzle the dressing over the salad and toss to combine.

**3.** Place heaping portions of the salad into serving bowls. Garnish with corn chips and additional chopped cilantro, if desired.

 **Dr. Bear Fun Fact!** Despite resembling potatoes and other root vegetables, jicama is actually a member of the bean family!

*Nutritional data reflects one serving without garnishes, based on a 6-serving yield.*

**PER SERVING** Calories: 315; Total Fat: 16.6g; Saturated Fat: 6.4g; Cholesterol: 32.5mg; Sodium: 714mg; Total Carbohydrates: 31.4g; Dietary Fiber: 10.8g; Sugars: 5.9g; Protein: 12.9g

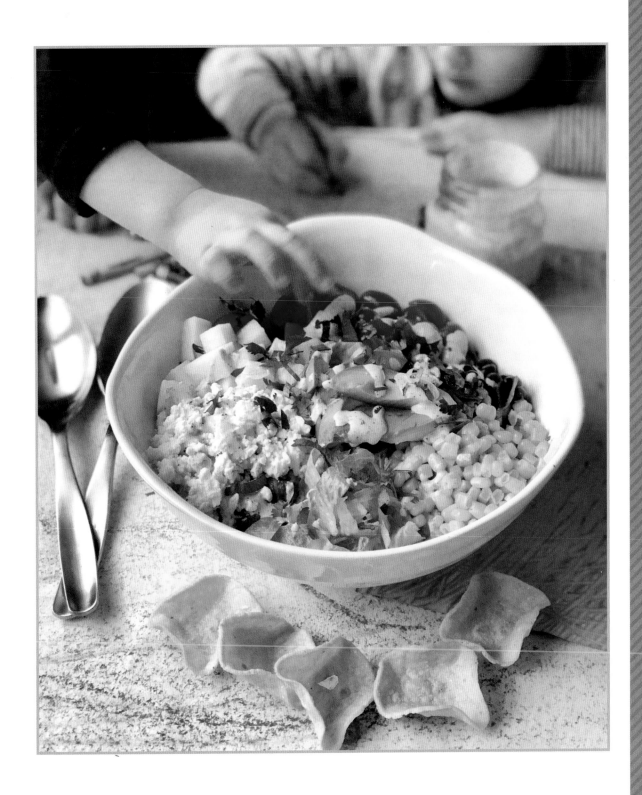

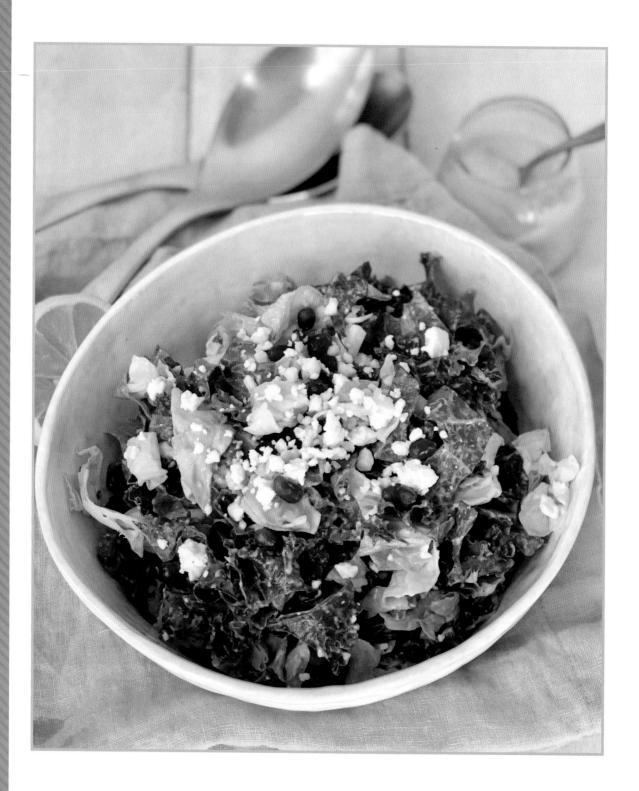

# Kale & Avocado No-Chovy Caesar Salad

*This Caesar salad is inspired by the Diplomat Resort beach-side restaurant in Hollywood, Florida. My taste buds were blown away by the combination of the slightly tart pomegranate arils with the mild Cotija cheese tossed in with the Caesar dressing. I just had to try it out at home. My kids won't go near a Caesar dressing with anchovies so this version has the same great flavors, sans fish.*

**YIELD: 6 SERVINGS**
Prep Time: 15 minutes
Total Time: 20 minutes

---

**For the No-Chovy Caesar Dressing**
1 avocado, skin and pit removed
½ cup olive oil
1 garlic clove, peeled
2 tablespoons mayonnaise
2 tablespoons lemon juice
1 tablespoon Dijon mustard
1 tablespoon red wine vinegar
1 tablespoon Worcestershire sauce
½ teaspoon salt

**For the Salad**
1 (5-ounce) package baby kale, rinsed, patted dry, and chopped
2 cups chopped romaine lettuce, rinsed and patted dry
½ cup pomegranate arils
1 cup crumbled Cotija cheese
1 avocado, skin and pit removed, chopped into small pieces

**1.** To make the dressing, combine all of the ingredients in a food processor. Purée until smooth. Cover and refrigerate until ready to serve.

**2.** To make the salad, toss together the chopped kale, chopped romaine lettuce, pomegranate arils, and crumbled cotija cheese. Drizzle the dressing over the top of the salad and toss to coat all of the ingredients.

**3.** Distribute the salad into serving bowls, and top each serving with a spoonful of chopped avocado.

**Dr. Bear Fun Fact!** The Caesar salad isn't an ancient Roman invention—it was actually created by an Italian immigrant named Caesar Cardini who owned restaurants in Mexico and the United States!

*Nutritional data reflects one serving, based on a 6-serving yield.*

**PER SERVING** Calories: 436; Total Fat: 40.4g; Saturated Fat: 10.6g; Cholesterol: 39.7mg; Sodium: 877.1mg; Total Carbohydrates: 11.4g; Dietary Fiber: 4.8g; Sugars: 2.9g; Protein: 9.8g

# Charred Halloumi & Citrus Salad with Honey Poppyseed Vinaigrette

*Halloumi cheese is made from a blend of sheep and goat's milk. It's very salty and tastes great when paired with citrus. Unlike other cheeses that melt, halloumi can be grilled or pan-seared. This salad is best when the fruit is chilled and the cheese is hot, but it holds up overnight and is still good for lunch the next day.*

**YIELD: 6 SERVINGS**
Prep Time: 15 minutes
Total Time: 20 minutes

---

### For the Honey Poppyseed Vinaigrette

½ cup olive oil

¼ cup honey

2 tablespoons white vinegar

1 tablespoon Dijon mustard

1 small shallot, skin removed and finely minced

2 teaspoons poppy seeds

½ teaspoon salt

### For the Halloumi and Salad

1 (8-ounce) package halloumi cheese, cut into ½-inch thick triangles

1 grapefruit, skin removed and sliced into thin wedges

2 navel oranges, skin removed and sliced into thin wedges

1 small red onion, skin removed and thinly sliced into half moons

5 fresh mint leaves, rinsed, patted dry, rolled, and thinly sliced

**1.** To make the dressing, whisk together the olive oil, honey, white vinegar, Dijon mustard, chopped shallot, poppy seeds, and salt in a glass bowl. Cover and refrigerate until ready to serve.

**2.** To cook the halloumi, heat a large skillet over medium-high heat. Lay the pieces of halloumi down in the skillet and cook, untouched, for about 3 to 4 minutes until it begins to brown. Flip the cheese over and cook an additional 3 to 4 minutes. Remove from heat and set aside.

**3.** To assemble the salad, arrange the grapefruit and orange slices on a serving plate. Top with slices of red onion and the cooked halloumi cheese.

**4.** Drizzle the dressing over the salad and sprinkle the mint leaves on top before serving.

 **Dr. Bear Fun Fact!** Poppy seeds are rich sources of Vitamin $B_1$, calcium, manganese, magnesium, and phosphorus!

*Nutritional data reflects one serving, based on a 6-serving yield.*

**PER SERVING**  Calories: 382; Total Fat: 29g; Saturated Fat: 9.4g; Cholesterol: 28.6mg; Sodium: 659.2mg; Total Carbohydrates: 23.1g; Dietary Fiber: 2.2g; Sugars: 19.3g; Protein: 9.3g

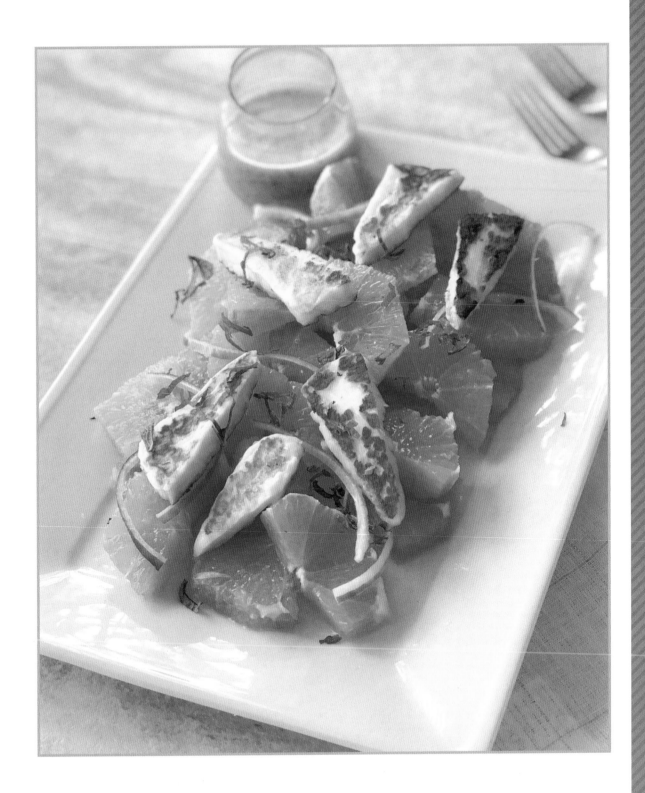

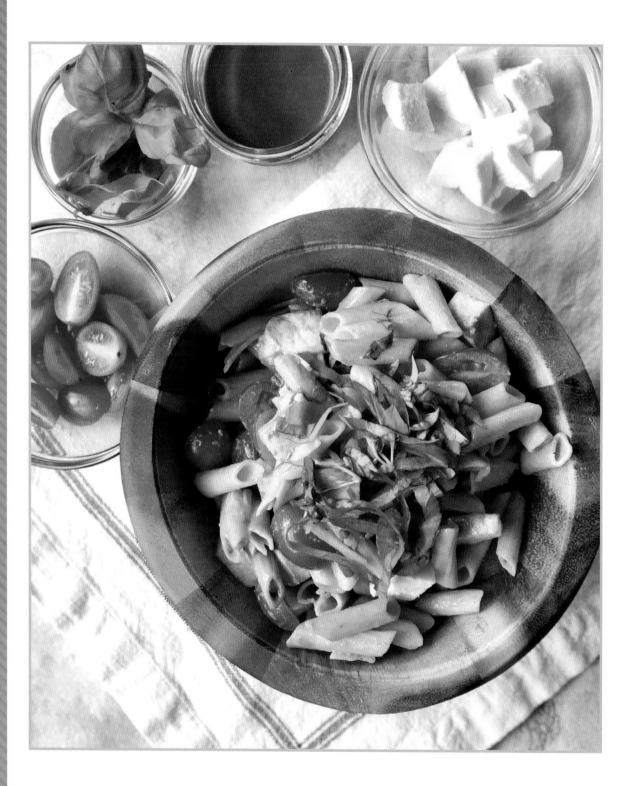

# Caprese Pasta Salad

*Use quinoa-based pasta to keep the texture of this pasta salad soft for longer. Save a little dressing for leftovers. You'll want to add a little more dressing on day two.*

**YIELD: 6–8 SERVINGS**
Prep Time: 20 minutes
Total Time: 30 minutes

—————————

### For the Dressing

¾ cup olive oil

½ cup balsamic vinegar

3 basil leaves, rinsed, patted dry, and roughly chopped

1 teaspoon fresh oregano leaves, rinsed and patted dry

3 tablespoons mayonnaise

2 tablespoons lemon juice

1 tablespoon Dijon mustard

1 tablespoon sugar

1 teaspoon salt

### For the Salad

1 (12-ounce) box gluten-free pasta

1 pint grape tomatoes, sliced in half

1 cup basil leaves, rinsed, patted dry, then rolled and thinly sliced

1 cup chopped fresh mozzarella

**1.** To make the dressing, combine the olive oil, balsamic vinegar, basil, oregano, mayonnaise, lemon juice, Dijon mustard, sugar, and salt in a small blender or food processor. Pulse until a smooth mixture forms. Cover and refrigerate until ready to serve with the salad.

**2.** To make the salad, cook the gluten-free pasta according to package instructions. Rinse with cold water and drain. Cool completely.

**3.** To assemble the salad, toss together the cooled pasta, tomatoes, basil, and mozzarella. Drizzle the dressing over the salad and toss to combine.

 **Dr. Bear Fun Fact!** The Caprese salad was created in Capri, Italy. It's also known as the "tricolore"— a nod to the three colors of the dish that complement the three colors of the Italian flag: red, green, and white.

*Nutritional data reflects one serving, based on an 8-serving yield.*

**PER SERVING** Calories: 463; Total Fat: 29.4g; Saturated Fat: 6.3g; Cholesterol: 16.9mg; Sodium: 497.1mg; Total Carbohydrates: 40.4g; Dietary Fiber: 2.4g; Sugars: 5.7g; Protein: 7.5g

# Mimi's Chicken Noodle Soup

*All of the credit for this soup goes to my mom, Connie, or, as my kid's call her, Mimi. As I was growing up, my mom made chicken rice soup all the time. It was the most comforting thing she ever made. She always used rice in the soup instead of noodles, but my kids really like noodles, so I swapped out the rice for thin rice noodles. Thanks, Mom, for sharing this family favorite.*

**YIELD: 4–6 SERVINGS**
Prep Time: 15 minutes
Total Time: 50 minutes

1 (8-ounce) package thin rice noodles

3 tablespoons olive oil, divided

2 boneless, skinless chicken breasts, rinsed and patted dry, cut in half

½ teaspoon salt, plus more for seasoning

1 cup chopped white onion, skin removed

1 cup chopped carrots, peeled and ends trimmed

½ cup chopped celery, rinsed, patted dry, and ends removed

4 cloves garlic, peeled and finely minced

1 tablespoon finely minced fresh ginger, peeled

1 cup chopped tomatoes

2 cups cubed butternut squash, ends removed and peeled

1 teaspoon Italian seasoning

8 cups chicken stock

*Nutritional data reflects one serving, based on a 6-serving yield.*

**PER SERVING** Calories: 351; Total Fat: 13g; Saturated Fat: 3g; Cholesterol: 44mg; Sodium: 723mg; Total Carbohydrates: 36g; Dietary Fiber: 5g; Sugars: 10.5g; Protein: 23g

**1.** Cook the rice noodles according to package instructions. Set aside.

**2.** In a large pot, heat 2 tablespoons olive oil over medium-high heat. Season the chicken breasts with salt and add to the hot oil. Cook for about 3 minutes per side until golden. Remove from the pot.

**3.** Add remaining 1 tablespoon of olive oil to the pot and heat over medium heat. Add the chopped onion, carrots, and celery and cook, stirring frequently, until the onions are soft and translucent, about 5 to 7 minutes.

**4.** Add the garlic and ginger and cook, stirring frequently, for about 1 minute. Add the chopped tomatoes, butternut squash, and Italian seasoning. Cook for 1 additional minute.

**5.** Add the chicken breasts back into the pot and add the chicken stock. Bring the soup to a boil over medium-high heat. Cover the soup, reduce heat to medium-low, and simmer for 20 to 30 minutes.

**6.** Carefully remove the chicken breasts from the pot and place on a cutting board. Using two forks, shred the chicken. Put the shredded chicken back into the pot.

**7.** Place a heaping portion of rice noodles in a serving bowl and ladle hot soup on top. Serve immediately.

 **Dr. Bear Fun Fact!** Research hasn't shown that chicken noodle soup has any medicinal properties, but it definitely seems to be just what the doctor ordered when we are sick!

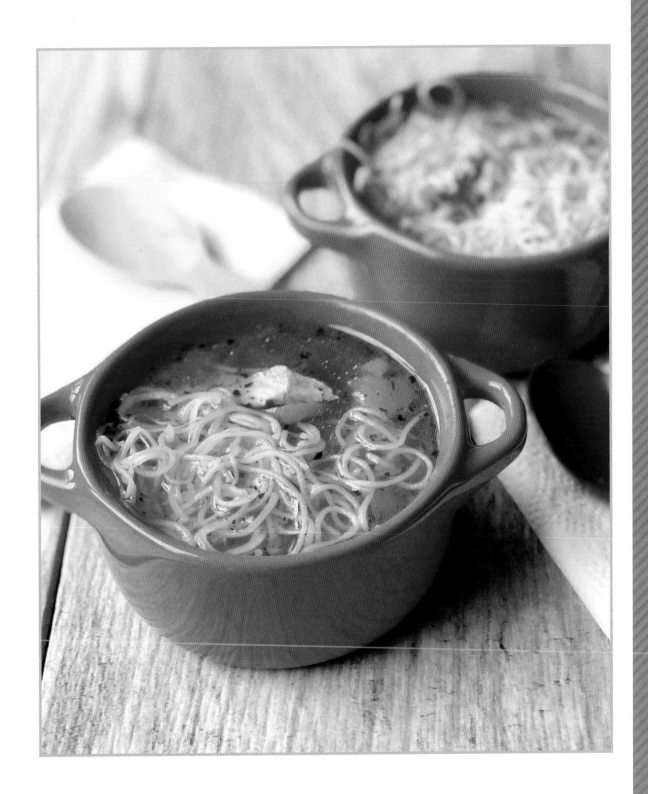

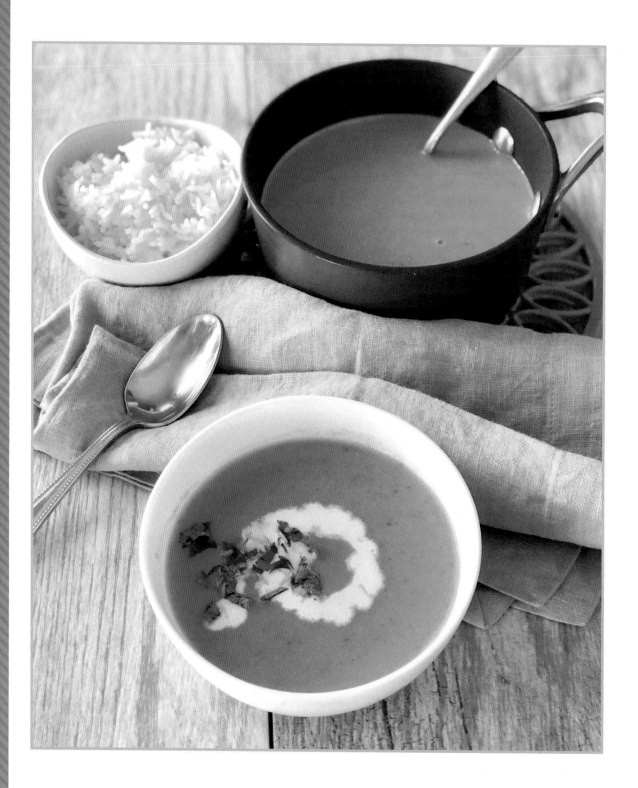

# Thai Pumpkin & Apple Soup

*This soup is plenty on its own, but if you're in the mood for a heartier soup, serve with sautéed shrimp. I like to dunk the steamed rice into the soup before taking a bite. It's delicious.*

**YIELD: 4 SERVINGS**
Prep Time: 10 minutes
Total Time: 25 minutes

---

1½ cups jasmine rice

2 tablespoons olive oil

2 cups finely chopped sweet yellow onion, skin removed

3 cloves garlic, peeled and very finely minced

1 tablespoon minced fresh ginger, peeled

1 cup pumpkin purée

1 cup Granny Smith apple, chopped and core removed

1 tablespoon brown sugar

1½ tablespoons red curry paste

3 cups coconut milk

2 cups vegetable broth

1 tablespoon fish sauce

1 tablespoon lime juice

½ teaspoon sea salt

Fresh cilantro leaves, rinsed, patted dry, and chopped, for garnish

**1.** Cook jasmine rice according to package instructions. Cover and keep warm until ready to serve.

**2.** In a large pot, heat olive oil over medium heat. Add the chopped onion and cook, stirring occasionally, until the onions are soft and translucent, about 5 to 7 minutes. Add the garlic and ginger and cook, stirring frequently until the garlic is very fragrant, for about 1 minute.

**3.** Add the pumpkin purée, chopped apples, brown sugar, and red curry paste and cook, stirring constantly, for about 1 additional minute.

**4.** Pour in the coconut milk, vegetable broth, and fish sauce, and bring to a boil over medium-high heat. Reduce heat to low, cover, and simmer for 10 minutes.

**5.** Remove the soup from heat and stir in the lime juice and sea salt.

**6.** Using an immersion blender, purée the soup until smooth. Taste and add more salt, if desired. If you don't have an immersion blender, carefully transfer to a food processor and purée until smooth.

**7.** Ladle the soup into serving bowl and serve with the steamed rice. Garnish with chopped cilantro.

**Dr. Bear Fun Fact!** Thai cuisine typically uses very little dairy—great news for those who are allergic to milk or lactose intolerant! Coconut milk provides an excellent creamy substitute.

*Nutritional data reflects one serving, based on a 4-serving yield.*

**PER SERVING** Calories: 426; Total Fat: 11.1g; Saturated Fat: 4.2g; Cholesterol: 0mg; Sodium: 1201mg; Total Carbohydrates: 74.7g; Dietary Fiber: 5.1g; Sugars: 12.9g; Protein: 8g

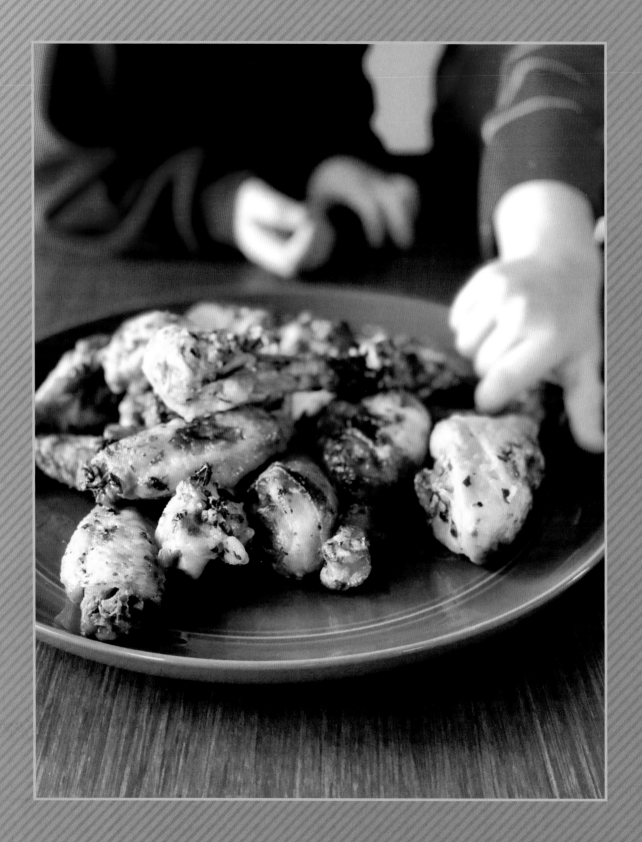

# 8

# Family Suppers

Kid-friendly participation steps are printed in **ORANGE**

# Basil Corn Risotto

*Risotto is one of my favorite foods, and this risotto is no exception. The base is the normal oil and butter combination with shallots, garlic, Arborio rice, and white wine. But what makes it really special is the addition of the cheesy lemon basil mixture and the boost in texture from the corn.*

**YIELD: 4 SERVINGS**

Prep Time: 20 minutes

Total Time: 50 minutes

---

2 tablespoons olive oil

2 tablespoons butter

2 shallots, skin removed and finely chopped

3 cloves garlic, peeled and finely minced

1½ cups Arborio rice

1½ cups white wine

3½ cups chicken stock or vegetable stock

½ cup packed fresh basil leaves, rinsed and patted dry

⅓ cup mascarpone cheese

¼ cup grated Parmesan cheese

Zest of 1 lemon

½ teaspoon salt

1 cup sweet corn kernels (fresh or frozen)

For garnish: additional basil leaves, thinly sliced

**1.** In a large, high-sided sauté pan, heat the olive oil and butter over medium heat.

**2.** When the butter is melted, add the shallots and cook, stirring frequently, for 2 to 3 minutes until soft. Add the garlic and cook 1 additional minute until fragrant.

**3.** Add the rice and stir to coat with the oil mixture. Cook, stirring frequently, until the rice is fragrant and somewhat translucent, about 3 to 5 minutes.

**4.** Pour in the white wine and cook for about 3 to 5 minutes until the liquid is almost absorbed.

**5.** Add the chicken stock and cook, stirring occasionally, until the liquid is almost absorbed, about 15 to 20 minutes.

**6.** While the risotto is cooking, combine the basil leaves, mascarpone, Parmesan, lemon zest, and salt in a small food processor and purée until smooth. Set aside.

**7.** When most of the liquid from the rice is absorbed, stir in the corn kernels, and cook for about 5 minutes until the corn is soft and bright in color.

**8.** Remove the risotto from heat, and gently stir the mascarpone mixture into the hot rice.

**9.** Top with additional chopped basil, if desired, and serve immediately.

 **Dr. Bear Fun Fact!** Basil is a very important ingredient in Italian cuisine. It's packed with nutrients like Vitamins A, B$_6$, C, and K!

*Nutritional data reflects one serving, based on a 4-serving yield.*

**PER SERVING** Calories: 671.7; Total Fat: 25.5g; Saturated Fat: 11.2g; Cholesterol: 45.6mg; Sodium: 983.2mg; Total Carbohydrates: 84.4g; Dietary Fiber: 4.1g; Sugars: 7.5g; Protein: 17.6g

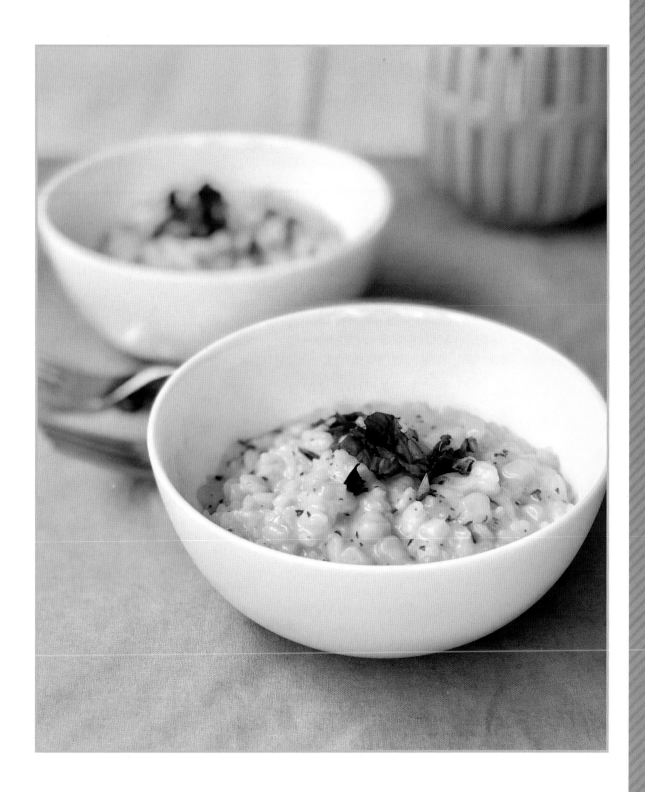

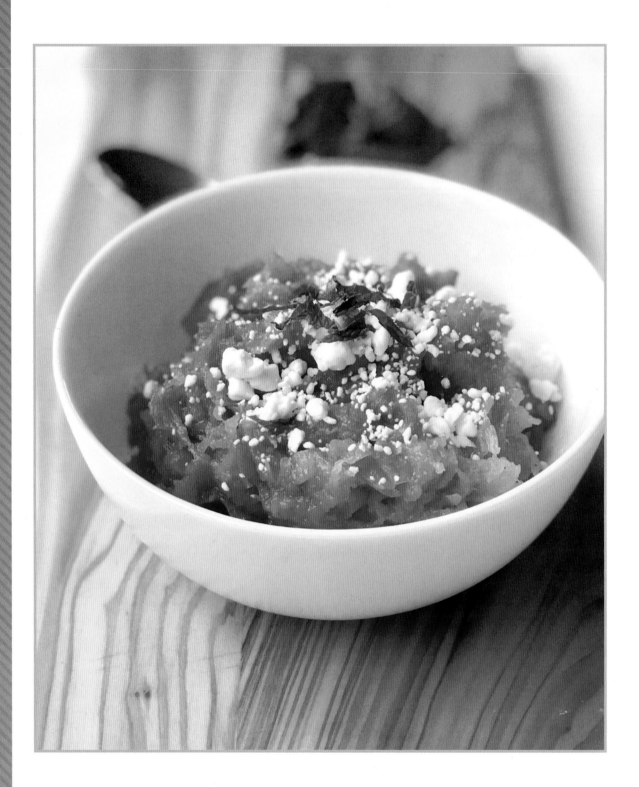

# Butternut Squash & Caramelized Onion Risotto

*This recipe is one of my favorites that utilize a "recipe base." Make the Butternut Squash & Caramelized Onion Mash ahead of time so when you go to make dinner, all you need to do is stir it into the simple risotto. This risotto is excellent paired with seared scallops.*

**YIELD: 4 SERVINGS**
Prep Time: 20 minutes
Total Time: 50 minutes

---

2 tablespoons olive oil

2 tablespoons butter, divided

3 cloves garlic, peeled and finely minced

1½ cups Arborio rice

1½ cups white wine

3½ cups chicken stock or vegetable stock

1 cup Butternut Squash & Caramelized Onion Mash (page 226)

½ cup shaved Parmesan, divided

1. In a large, high-sided sauté pan, heat the olive oil and 1 tablespoon butter over medium heat.

2. When the butter is melted, add the garlic and cook, stirring frequently, for 1 minute until fragrant.

3. Add the rice and stir to coat with the oil mixture. Cook, stirring frequently, until the rice is fragrant and somewhat translucent, about 3 to 5 minutes.

4. Pour in the white wine and cook for about 3 to 5 minutes until the liquid is almost absorbed.

5. Add the chicken stock and cook, stirring occasionally, until the liquid is almost absorbed, about 15 to 20 minutes.

6. Add remaining 1 tablespoon of butter into the risotto and stir until melted and creamy.

7. Stir the Butternut Squash & Caramelized Onion Mash into the risotto and mix until well combined.

8. Sprinkle about ¼ cup of the Parmesan cheese over the risotto and stir gently until fully combined.

9. Top with remaining shaved Parmesan cheese before serving.

 **Dr. Bear Fun Fact!** For a cheesier flavor, try adding some pecorino or asiago cheese. They have a stronger flavor and can deepen the flavor profile!

*Nutritional data reflects one serving, based on a 4-serving yield.*

**PER SERVING** Calories: 606; Total Fat: 23.2g; Saturated Fat: 7.2g; Cholesterol: 26mg; Sodium: 977.3mg; Total Carbohydrates: 73.3g; Dietary Fiber: 4.2g; Sugars: 9.1g; Protein: 15.7g

# Creamy Roasted Tomato Risotto

*My go-to Pink Pasta Sauce makes a splash in this creamily delicious risotto! Grilled chicken or shrimp are great protein additions to this tasty dish.*

**YIELD: 4 SERVINGS**
Prep Time: 20 minutes
Total Time: 50 minutes

---

2 tablespoons olive oil

2 tablespoons butter, divided

3 cloves garlic, peeled and minced

1½ cups Arborio rice

1½ cups white wine

3½ cups chicken stock
   or vegetable stock

1 cup Creamy Pink Pasta Sauce
   (page 329)

½ cup shaved Parmesan, divided

**1.** In a large, high-sided sauté pan, heat the olive oil and 1 tablespoon butter over medium heat.

**2.** When the butter is melted, add the garlic and cook, stirring frequently, for 1 minute until fragrant.

**3.** Add the rice and stir to coat with the oil mixture. Cook, stirring frequently, until the rice is fragrant and somewhat translucent, about 3 to 5 minutes.

**4.** Pour in the white wine, and cook for about 3 to 5 minutes until the liquid is almost absorbed.

**5.** Add the chicken stock and cook, stirring occasionally, until the liquid is almost absorbed, about 15 to 20 minutes.

**6.** Add remaining 1 tablespoon of butter into the risotto and stir until melted and creamy.

**7.** Stir the Creamy Pink Pasta Sauce into the risotto and mix until well combined.

**8.** Sprinkle about ¼ cup of Parmesan cheese over the risotto and stir gently until fully combined. Top with remaining shaved Parmesan cheese before serving.

 **Dr. Bear Fun Fact!** Arborio rice is the most common form of rice used in risotto. It's starchier than most rice, which makes it a great choice for hearty meals like risotto.

*Nutritional data reflects one serving, based on a 4-serving yield.*

**PER SERVING** Calories: 622; Total Fat: 27.7g; Saturated Fat: 9.5g; Cholesterol: 35.4mg; Sodium: 881.6mg; Total Carbohydrates: 64.4g; Dietary Fiber: 2.7g; Sugars: 5.7g; Protein: 16.1g

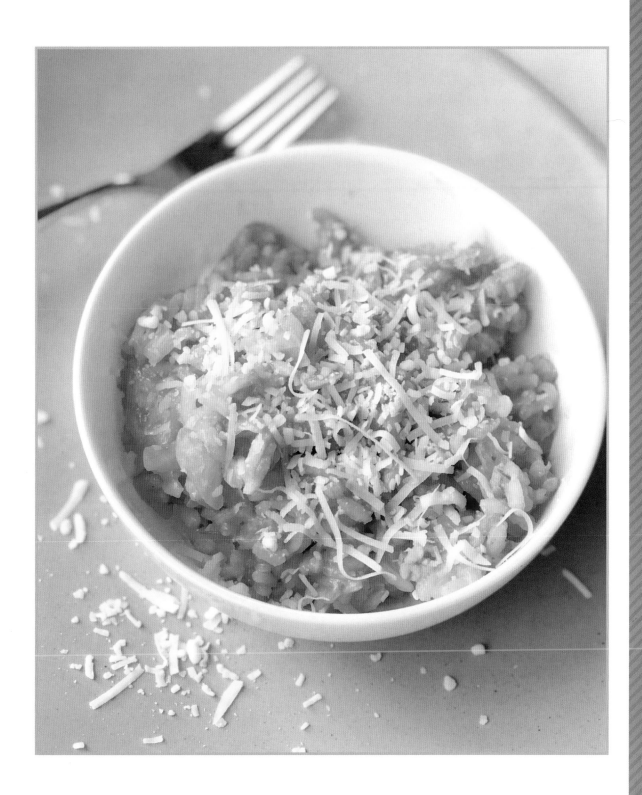

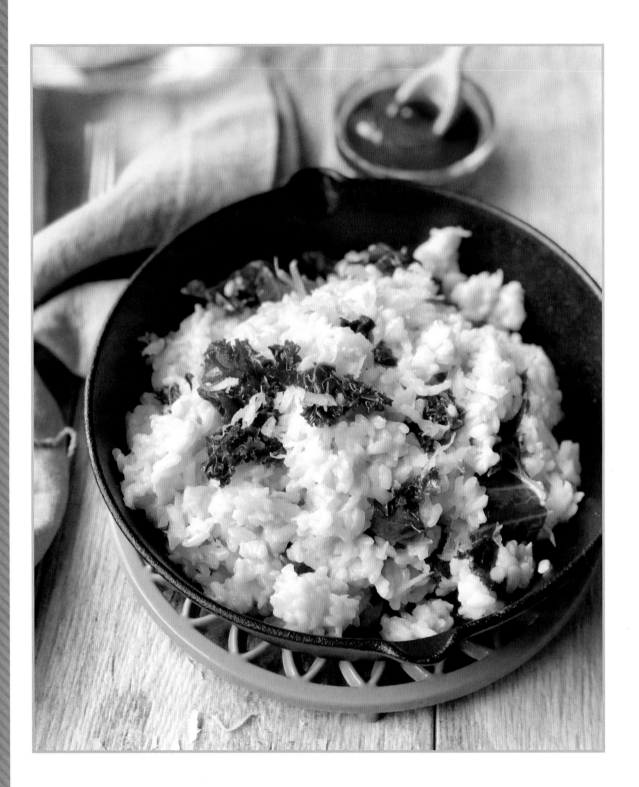

# Coconut Ginger Kale Risotto

*This risotto offers a nice change from the typical Italian-flavored risottos. It pairs well with grilled chicken or seafood with a drizzle of the Sweet Tamari Glaze.*

**YIELD: 4 SERVINGS**
Prep Time: 15 minutes
Total Time: 45 minutes

2 tablespoons butter

2 tablespoons olive oil

3 shallots, skin removed and finely chopped

3 cloves garlic, peeled and finely minced

1 tablespoon finely minced fresh ginger, peeled

1½ cups Arborio rice

1 cup white wine

2 (15-ounce) cans coconut milk

½ cup water

5 cups chopped kale, rinsed and patted dry

½ cup shredded coconut

1 teaspoon salt

**1.** In a large, high-sided sauté pan, heat the butter and olive oil over medium heat.

**2.** When the butter is melted, add in the shallots and cook, stirring frequently, for 2 to 3 minutes until soft. Add the garlic and ginger and cook 1 additional minute until fragrant.

**3.** Add the Arborio rice and stir to coat with the oil mixture. Cook, stirring frequently, until the rice is fragrant and somewhat translucent, about 3 to 5 minutes.

**4.** Pour in the white wine and cook for about 3 to 5 minutes until the liquid is almost absorbed.

**5.** Add the coconut milk and water and bring to a boil over medium-high heat, stirring frequently. Reduce heat to medium-low and cook, stirring occasionally, until the liquid is almost absorbed, about 15 to 20 minutes.

**6.** To finish the risotto, stir in the kale, shredded coconut, and salt.

**7.** Spoon the risotto into serving bowls and serve hot.

**Dr. Bear Fun Fact!** Kale is one of the best superfoods you can find! It's loaded with Vitamins A, C, and K, calcium, antioxidants, iron, and magnesium. Our bodies easily absorb these nutrients from kale unlike many other leafy greens.

*Nutritional data reflects one serving, based on a 4-serving yield.*

**PER SERVING** Calories: 608.3; Total Fat: 25.1g; Saturated Fat: 13.9g; Cholesterol 15.3mg; Sodium: 656.5mg; Total Carbohydrates: 80.3g; Dietary Fiber: 5.9g; Sugars: 5.4g; Protein: 12.7g

# Basic Roasted Chicken

*Simple and delicious. Make a double version of this recipe on Sunday evening, and you'll have chicken to use in recipes for the week.*

**YIELD: 4–6 SERVINGS**
Prep Time: 5 minutes
Total Time: 50 minutes

---

4 boneless, skinless chicken breasts, rinsed and patted dry

3 tablespoons olive oil

1 teaspoon salt

1½ teaspoons garlic powder

**1.** Preheat oven to 375°F. Line a baking sheet with foil and place the chicken breasts on top of the foil.

**2.** Brush the olive oil over all sides of the chicken and season evenly with salt and garlic powder.

**3.** Roast for 30 to 35 minutes until the juices run clear. Let the chicken cool for about 10 minutes, then use a fork to shred the chicken.

 **Dr. Bear Fun Fact!** There are more chickens in the world than any other bird species!

*Nutritional data reflects one serving, based on a 5-serving yield.*

**PER SERVING** Calories: 241; Total Fat: 12.4g; Saturated Fat: 2.3g; Cholesterol: 81.6mg; Sodium: 546.2mg; Total Carbohydrates: 0.7g; Dietary Fiber: 0.1g; Sugars: 0g; Protein: 29.8g

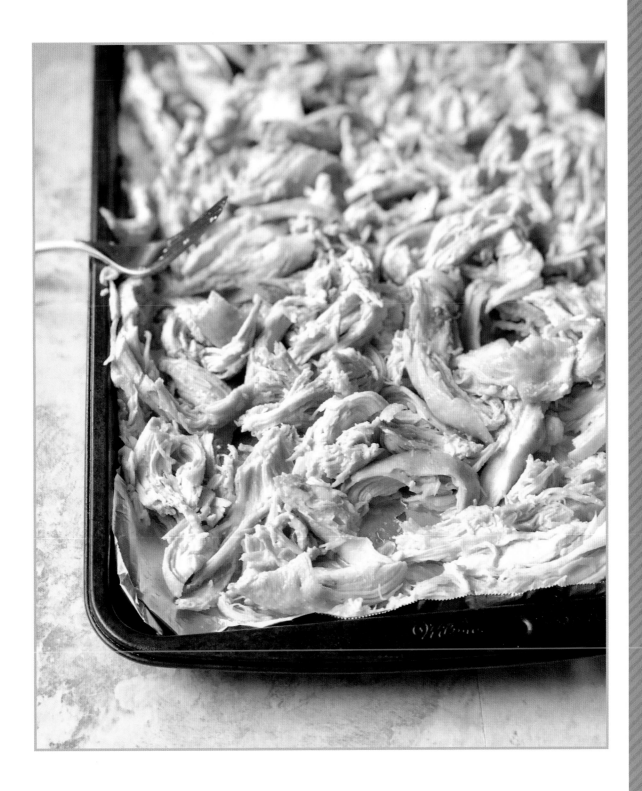

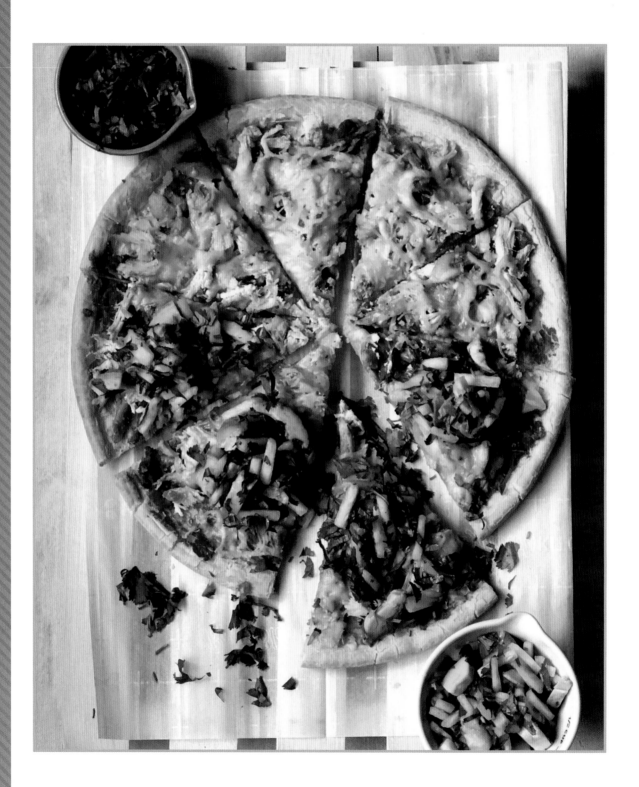

# Mexican Pizza with Rotisserie Chicken & Pineapple Avocado Salsa

*When I was pregnant with my first son, Brandon, all I wanted to eat was pizza and tacos... sometimes at the same time. So, I started making Mexican Pizzas. Be sure to pick an enchilada sauce that is thickened with a gluten-free ingredient. Several varieties contain wheat flour.*

**YIELD: 1 (12-INCH) PIZZA (8 SERVINGS)**

Prep Time: 15 minutes
Total Time: 35 minutes

---

1 (12-inch) gluten-free pizza crust

1 cup refried beans

2 cups shredded rotisserie or roasted chicken

1½ cups shredded cheddar jack cheese

⅔ cup finely chopped pineapple, skin and top removed

⅓ cup chopped fresh cilantro leaves, rinsed and patted dry

Juice of 1 lime

1 avocado, skin and pit removed, cut into bite-sized pieces

½ cup mild red enchilada sauce for garnish

1. Preheat oven to 375°F. Line a baking sheet with parchment paper and set gluten-free pizza crust on top.

2. Spread the refried beans evenly over the pizza crust, leaving the ends uncovered. Evenly sprinkle the chicken on top of the beans and then top with the shredded jack cheese.

3. Bake the pizza for 15 to 20 minutes until the cheese is melted and golden.

4. While the pizza bakes, make the pineapple topping. In a glass mixing bowl, toss together the chopped pineapple, cilantro, lime juice, and avocado. Cover and refrigerate until ready to serve.

5. Remove the pizza from the oven and slice into 8 slices.

6. Drizzle enchilada sauce over the top.

7. Ask your kiddos if they want their slices topped with the pineapple avocado salsa. If yes, top all pieces of pizza with the salsa. If not, try putting some on the side and letting the little ones try it! You might be surprised at how much they enjoy this sweet and tangy addition.

 **Dr. Bear Fun Fact!** One avocado has 4 grams of protein, making it the fruit with the highest protein content!

*Nutritional data reflects one slice, based on an 8-serving yield using the Basic Roasted Chicken Recipe.*

**PER SERVING** Calories: 360; Total Fat: 21.6g; Saturated Fat: 9g; Cholesterol: 61.6mg; Sodium: 691.2mg; Total Carbohydrates: 22.1g; Dietary Fiber: 3.5g; Sugars: 3g; Protein: 21.7g

# Thai Chili Chicken Pizzas with Rotisserie Chicken & Tangy Cucumber Slaw

*This recipe is inspired by my friend Margot from the Potomac MOMS Club. When my youngest son, Leo, was born, the group organized a meal train for our family. It was an amazing gesture, since everyone made sure to only deliver gluten-free food to us. One of my favorite meals was pizzas piled high with an amazing Thai chili slaw. This recipe is my recreation of that dish. Thanks, Margot!*

**YIELD: 4 (8-INCH) PIZZAS (8 SERVINGS)**
Prep Time: 15 minutes
Total Time: 35 minutes

———————

3 tablespoons honey

3 tablespoons apple cider vinegar

2 cups matchstick-cut cucumbers, rinsed, patted dry, and ends removed

2 cups matchstick-cut carrots

½ cup chopped scallions, ends removed

½ cup chopped peanuts,

½ teaspoon crushed red pepper flakes

4 Udi's Gluten-Free 8" Pizza Crusts

1 cup duck sauce

2 cups shredded part-skim milk mozzarella cheese

2 cups shredded cooked rotisserie or roasted chicken

**1.** Preheat oven to 375°F. Line two baking sheets with foil or parchment paper and set aside.

**2.** In a glass mixing bowl, whisk together the honey and apple cider vinegar until smooth. Toss in the cucumbers and carrots and mix well. Cover and refrigerate until ready to serve.

**3.** In a second glass mixing bowl, toss together the scallions, peanuts, and red pepper flakes. Cover and refrigerate until ready to serve.

**4.** Place the gluten-free pizza crusts on prepared baking sheets and spread the duck sauce evenly across the surfaces of the crusts.

**5.** Top with shredded mozzarella cheese and rotisserie chicken and bake for 12 to 15 minutes until cheese is melted and golden.

**6.** Remove the pizza from the oven and slice each pizza into 4 slices.

**7.** Ask your kids if they want their slices topped with the cucumber slaw. If yes, top all pieces of pizza with the slaw. If not, try putting some on the side and letting the little ones try it! They might just enjoy this crunchy addition!

*Nutritional data reflects one serving (2 slices), based on an 8-serving yield.*

**PER SERVING** Calories: 482; Total Fat: 19g; Saturated Fat: 5g; Cholesterol: 42mg; Sodium: 843mg; Total Carbohydrates: 59g; Dietary Fiber: 4g; Sugars: 29g; Protein: 22g

 **Dr. Bear Fun Fact!** Don't worry, there's no duck in your duck sauce! It's really just a mix of fruit, vinegar, and chili. It's called "duck sauce" because it used to be served only with a fried duck dish at Chinese restaurants.

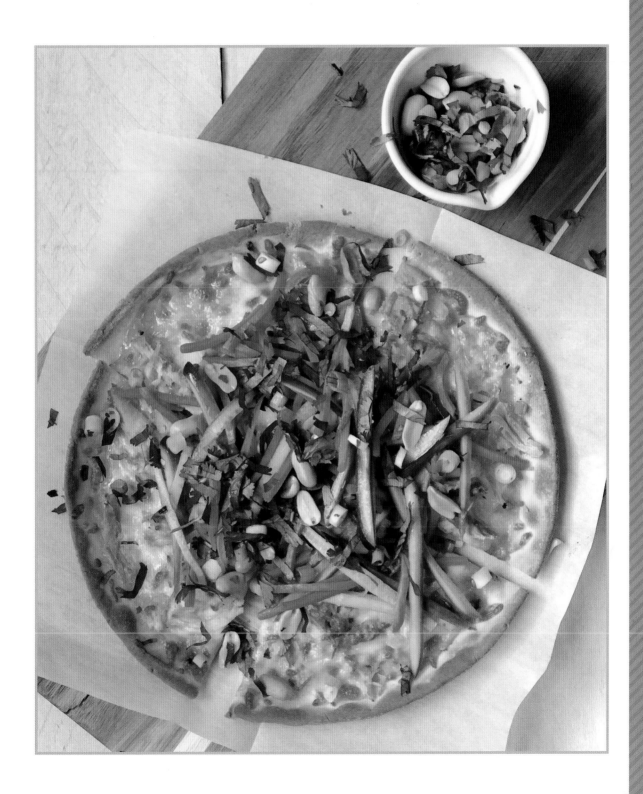

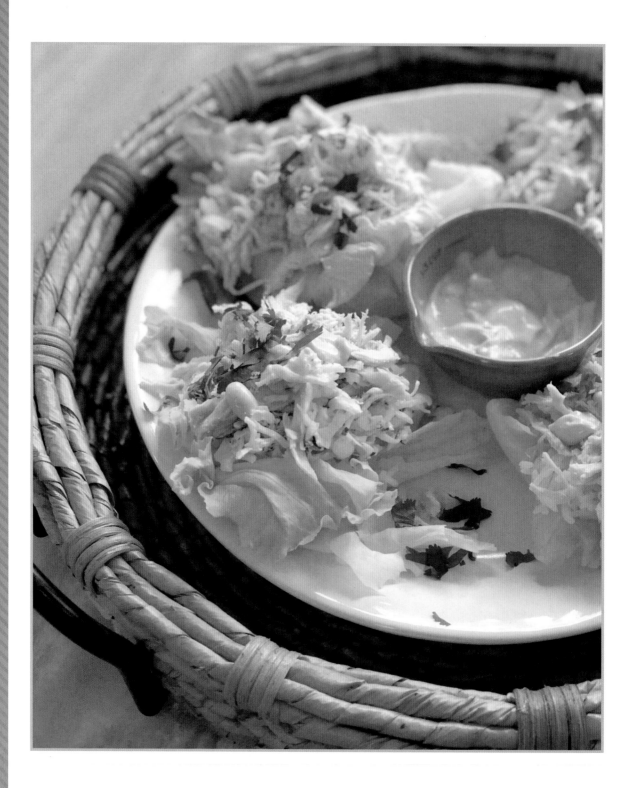

# Lettuce Wraps with Rotisserie Chicken, Creamy Slaw, & Sriracha Mayo

*Lettuce cups are like a tortilla, but made of lettuce. Rinse the lettuce and carefully pull the leaves off in whole pieces, then pile them high with the toppings. I recommend using Boston Bibb Lettuce, but you can also use romaine as a substitute.*

**YIELD: 12 LETTUCE CUPS
(4 SERVINGS)**
Prep Time: 20 minutes
Total Time: 30 minutes

---

1½ cups jasmine rice

2¼ cups water

½ teaspoon salt

1 cup mayonnaise

½ tablespoon sriracha (more or less depending on desired spice level)

2 teaspoons lime juice

1 (14-ounce) package shredded cabbage coleslaw mix

½ cup finely chopped fresh cilantro leaves, rinsed and patted dry

12 Boston Bibb lettuce cups, rinsed and patted dry

4 cups shredded rotisserie or roasted chicken

2 limes, cut into quarters, for serving

*Nutritional data reflects one serving of 3 lettuce cups, based on a 4-serving yield.*

**PER SERVING** Calories: 925; Total Fat: 57g; Saturated Fat: 9g; Cholesterol: 118mg; Sodium: 1346mg; Total Carbohydrates: 61g; Dietary Fiber: 4g; Sugars: 4g; Protein: 42g

**1.** In the bowl of a rice cooker, combine the rice, water, and salt. Cook the rice according to package instructions. If you don't have a rice cooker, combine the rice, water, and salt in a medium-sized pot. Bring to a boil over high heat, then reduce heat to medium-low, cover, and simmer for about 12 to 15 minutes until water is fully absorbed. Remove from heat, fluff with a fork, and leave covered until ready to serve.

**2.** While the rice cooks, start making the mayo and slaw. In a large mixing bowl, whisk together the mayonnaise, sriracha, and lime juice. Set aside.

**3.** In another large mixing bowl, toss together the slaw mix and cilantro. Drizzle approximately ½ cup of the sriracha mayo mixture over the slaw and toss together well. Reserve remaining sriracha mayo for garnish.

**4.** To assemble the lettuce wraps, fill each lettuce leaf cup with a small scoop of rice. Top with a heaping portion of the slaw and then the rotisserie chicken. Garnish with a drizzle of the sriracha mayo and serve with lime quarters.

 **Dr. Bear Fun Fact!** Every sriracha is slightly different! Usually, chile pepper, vinegar, garlic, sugar, and salt are among the main ingredients. The exact origin of the sauce is debated, but generally agreed that it was created about 100 years ago in a small town in Thailand called Si Racha.

# Rotisserie Chicken & Butternut Squash Enchiladas

*These enchiladas are the most requested dinner in my house. They are sweet and spicy and everything in between.*

**YIELD: 12 ENCHILADAS
(6 SERVINGS)**
Prep Time: 15 minutes
Total Time: 60 minutes

**For the Enchilada Sauce**

1 (16-ounce) jar green tomatillo salsa

1¼ cups sour cream

1 cup cilantro leaves, rinsed and patted dry

1 teaspoon ground cumin

½ teaspoon paprika

**For the Enchiladas**

12 soft white corn tortillas

1½ cups Butternut Squash & Caramelized Onion Mash (page 226)

2 cups shredded rotisserie or roasted chicken

2 cups shredded Monterey Jack cheese, divided

Optional garnishes: guacamole, sour cream, pico de gallo, corn chips

**1.** Preheat oven to 350°F. Spray a 9-by-13-inch glass baking dish with nonstick spray and set aside.

**2.** In a blender or food processor, purée together the tomatillo salsa, sour cream, cilantro, cumin, and paprika.

**3.** Pour the sauce into a mixing bowl that is wide enough to dip a tortilla into and set aside.

**4.** To assemble the enchiladas, set up an assembly line with ingredients in bowls in the following order: corn tortillas, enchilada sauce, Butternut Squash and Caramelized Onion Mash, rotisserie chicken, shredded cheese. Use tongs or spoons for each ingredient to make it easier to assemble. Also, set up a cutting board to lay tortillas on for assembly.

**5.** Take one corn tortilla and dip it into the tomatillo enchilada sauce, and let the excess sauce drip off. Spoon 1 teaspoon of the Butternut Squash & Caramelized Onion Mash into the tortilla and spread out evenly. Add about 1 tablespoon of shredded chicken and a pinch of shredded cheese. Roll up the enchilada and place in the prepared baking dish. Repeat with remaining 11 tortillas.

**6.** Pour the remaining enchilada sauce over the top of the enchiladas and sprinkle with remaining shredded cheese. Bake for 30 to 35 minutes until the sauce is bubbly and the cheese on top is golden.

**7.** Serve with your favorite enchilada accompaniments such as guacamole, pico de gallo, and corn chips, if so desired.

**Dr. Bear Fun Fact!** What in the world is a "tomatillo?" They're actually part of the same family as tomatoes, but they're grown primarily in Mexico! They are green and have a slightly less sweet taste than their red cousins. They're great in salsas!

*Nutritional data reflects one serving without garnishes, based on a 6-serving yield using the Basic Roasted Chicken Recipe.*

**PER SERVING** Calories: 614.1; Total Fat: 33g; Saturated Fat: 14g; Cholesterol: 94mg; Sodium: 1143mg; Total Carbohydrates: 51g; Dietary Fiber: 8g; Sugars: 18g; Protein: 29g

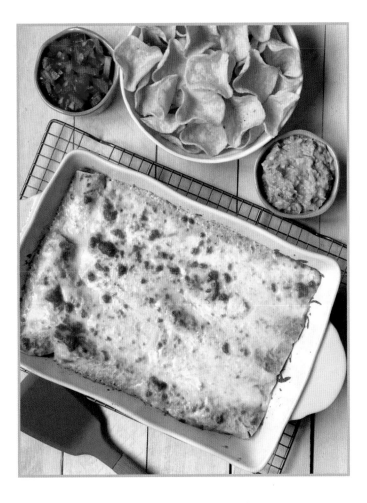

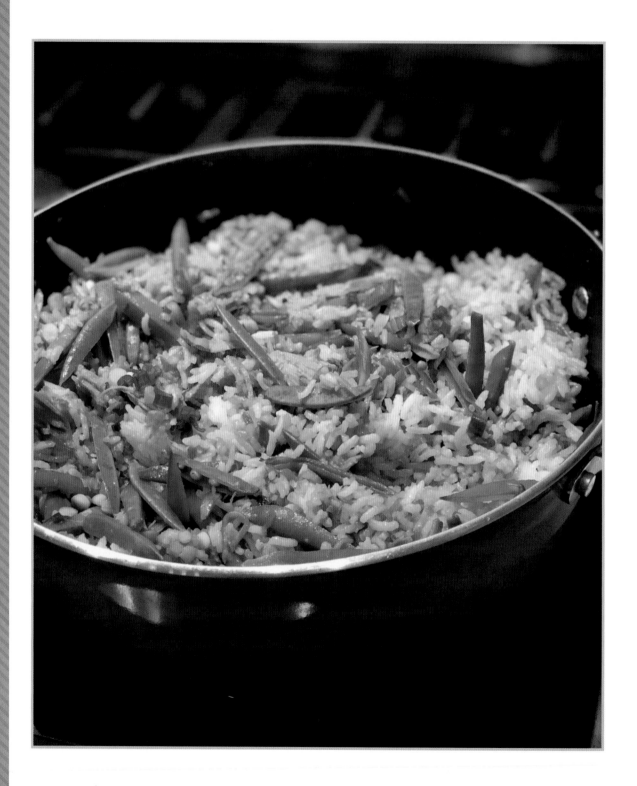

# Ginger Soy Fried Rice with Rotisserie Chicken & Sugar Snap Peas

*This fried rice is excellent with chicken but also goes great with beef or shrimp too. Also, let's be honest, fried rice is for cleaning out the refrigerator. Toss in any veggies you have on hand.*

**YIELD: 4 SERVINGS**
Prep Time: 15 minutes
Total Time: 45 minutes

---

1½ cups jasmine rice

3 cups water

½ cup gluten-free soy sauce

2 tablespoons rice wine vinegar

2 tablespoons brown sugar

4 tablespoons vegetable oil, divided

3 cups shredded rotisserie
  or roasted chicken

5 cloves garlic, peeled and finely
  minced

1 tablespoon finely minced fresh
  ginger, peeled

1 cup shredded cabbage, rinsed and
  patted dry

1 cup shredded carrots, ends removed
  and peeled

4 scallions, ends removed and finely
  chopped

1 (8-ounce) package sugar snap peas,
  sliced in half lengthwise

*Nutritional data reflects one serving,
based on a 4-serving yield.*

**PER SERVING** Calories: 654; Total Fat: 25g;
Saturated Fat: 4g; Cholesterol: 71mg; Sodium:
1499mg; Total Carbohydrates: 68g; Dietary
Fiber: 4g; Sugars: 10g; Protein: 35g

**1.** In the bowl of a rice cooker, add the rice and water. If you don't have a rice cooker, combine the rice and water in a medium-sized pot. Bring to a boil over high heat, then reduce heat to medium-low, cover, and simmer for about 15 to 18 minutes until water is fully absorbed. Remove from heat, fluff with a fork, then leave covered until ready to use in the fried rice.

**2.** In a glass measuring cup, whisk together the soy sauce, rice wine vinegar, and brown sugar. Set aside.

**3.** While the rice is cooking, in a large, high-sided sauté pan or wok, heat 2 tablespoons vegetable oil over medium-high heat. Add the shredded chicken and cook, stirring frequently, for about 3 minutes. Add the remaining vegetable oil, garlic, and ginger and cook, stirring frequently, for about 1 minute until fragrant.

**4.** Add the gluten-free soy sauce mixture and mix to combine. Cook, stirring frequently, until the liquid is bubbling, about 2 minutes.

**5.** Add the cabbage, carrots, and scallions and cook, stirring frequently, until the vegetables begin to soften, about 3 to 5 minutes. Add the sugar snap peas and cook for about 1 minute.

**6.** Slowly add the cooked rice into the chicken and vegetables mixture, about ¼ cup at a time, stirring well after each addition. Repeat until all of the rice is added.

**7.** Taste and season with salt, if desired.

 **Dr. Bear Fun Fact!** Can't find rice wine vinegar? No worries—rice vinegar is the same thing!

# Citrus and Cilantro Pulled Chicken with Rice & Beans

*This citrus and cilantro sauce transforms Basic Roasted Chicken into a dinner with Cuban flare.*

**YIELD: 4 SERVINGS**

Prep Time: 10 minutes

Total Time: 20 minutes (not including making condiments for serving)

---

4 cloves garlic, peeled

1 cup cilantro leaves, rinsed and patted dry

Zest of 1 orange

¾ cup orange juice

¼ cup gluten-free soy sauce

3 tablespoons olive oil

1 teaspoon cornstarch

1 teaspoon ground cumin

½ teaspoon finely chopped fresh oregano leaves, rinsed and patted dry

¼ teaspoon salt

4 cups shredded rotisserie or roasted chicken

1 recipe Garlic Rice & Black Beans (page 229)

Optional garnishes: guacamole, salsa, sour cream, corn chips

**1.** In a small food processor, combine the garlic, cilantro, orange zest, orange juice, gluten-free soy sauce, olive oil, cornstarch, ground cumin, oregano, and salt. Purée until a smooth mixture forms. Set aside.

**2.** Set a large skillet over medium-high heat. Pour in the puréed sauce mixture and bring to a slow simmer. Add the shredded rotisserie chicken and toss with the sauce. Cook, stirring frequently, for about 5 to 7 minutes until the sauce thickens and clings to the chicken.

**3.** Serve the chicken with the Garlic Rice & Black Beans, guacamole, salsa, sour cream, and/or corn chips.

 **Dr. Bear Fun Fact!** Cornstarch is a popular ingredient in gluten-free foods. Although it's used in small quantities, it helps to thicken sauces and soups.

*Nutritional data reflects one serving, based on a 4-serving yield using the Basic Roasted Chicken Recipe. (Nutritional data does not include garnishes.)*

**PER SERVING** Calories: 754; Total Fat: 33.1g; Saturated Fat: 12.3g; Cholesterol: 94mg; Sodium: 2114.1mg; Total Carbohydrates: 72g; Dietary Fiber: 10.2g; Sugars: 4.5g; Protein: 41.1g

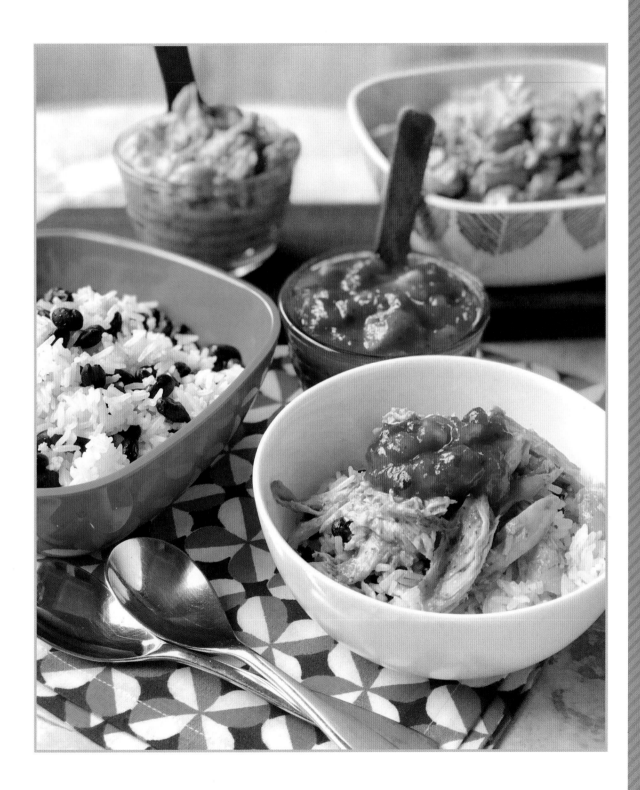

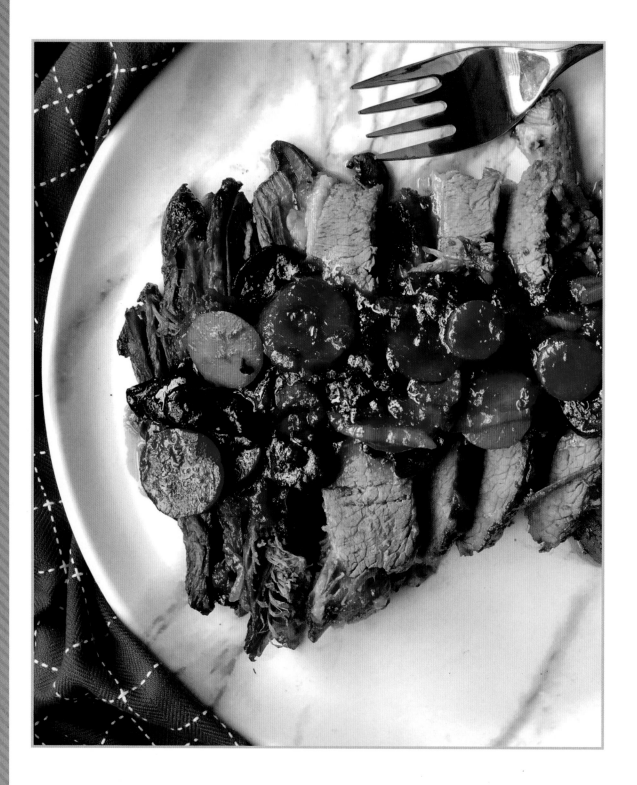

# Cider Braised Beef Brisket

*I'm famous in my family for this recipe. My cousins on my dad's side have decided I'm required to make it every year for Passover. I happily oblige, but I also make it other times of the year too! Don't worry, the alcohol in the hard cider cooks out.*

**YIELD: 8 SERVINGS**
Prep Time: 15 minutes
Total Time: 4 hours, 30 minutes

---

4 pounds beef brisket

1 teaspoon salt

1 teaspoon garlic powder

2 cups thinly sliced yellow onions, skin removed

1 cup thinly sliced button mushrooms, rinsed and patted dry

1 cup chopped carrots, ends removed and peeled

1 cup chopped celery, rinsed, patted dry, and ends removed

1½ cups tomato sauce

1½ cups gluten-free hard cider

1 cup brown sugar

½ cup gluten-free soy sauce

¼ cup apple cider vinegar

¼ cup Worcestershire sauce

1. Preheat oven to 350°F. Spray the bottom and sides of a roasting pan with nonstick spray.

2. Place the brisket in the bottom of the roasting pan and sprinkle with salt and garlic powder. Arrange the onions, mushrooms, carrots, and celery on top and around the sides of the brisket.

3. In a mixing bowl, whisk together the tomato sauce, gluten-free hard cider, brown sugar, gluten-free soy sauce, apple cider vinegar, and Worcestershire sauce. Pour the sauce evenly over the brisket.

4. Cover the brisket with foil and cook for 3 hours, 30 minutes. Remove the foil from the brisket and cook an additional 30 minutes until the brisket is fork tender.

5. Let the brisket rest for about 15 minutes in the pan before carving. Slice the brisket against the grain and serve garnished with the remaining sauce and vegetables.

 **Dr. Bear Fun Fact!** The moment you put your fork into this brisket, you'll notice that it falls apart easily. That's a result of the slow cooking process, which tenderizes meat and makes it fall right off the bone!

*Nutritional data reflects one serving, based on an 8-serving yield.*

**PER SERVING** Calories: 617; Total Fat: 20.7g; Saturated Fat: 7.8g; Cholesterol: 204.1mg; Sodium: 1212.1mg; Total Carbohydrates: 32.4g; Dietary Fiber: 2.3g; Sugars: 25.7g; Protein: 72.3g

# Slow Cooker Brisket Burrito Bowls with Jalapeño Lime Slaw

*This recipe is similar to my traditional brisket with some subtle changes in seasoning and, of course, a different cooking method. Start the brisket cooking in the morning, and you will come home from work with your house smelling AMAZING. To cut down on carbs, try replacing the rice with steamed "riced" cauliflower.*

**YIELD: 6 SERVINGS**
Prep Time: 15 minutes
Total Time: 4–6 hours (depending on
   slow cooker settings)

3 pounds beef brisket, cut into 6 pieces

2 cups thinly sliced yellow onions,
   skin removed

2 cups thinly sliced button mushrooms,
   rinsed and patted dry

1½ cups tomato sauce

1½ cups gluten-free lager beer

1 cup brown sugar

½ cup gluten-free low sodium soy sauce

¼ cup apple cider vinegar

¼ cup Worcestershire sauce

1 teaspoon ground cumin

½ teaspoon chili powder

1½ cups jasmine rice

3 cups water

1 recipe Jalapeño Lime Coleslaw
   (page 233)

1 cup crumbled queso fresco cheese

Chopped fresh cilantro leaves, rinsed
   and patted dry, for garnish

**1.** Spray the bottom and sides of the slow cooker with nonstick spray. Place the brisket in the bottom of the slow cooker and arrange onions and mushrooms on top and around the sides of the brisket.

**2.** In a mixing bowl, whisk together tomato sauce, gluten-free beer, brown sugar, gluten-free soy sauce, apple cider vinegar, Worcestershire sauce, cumin, and chili powder. Pour the sauce over the brisket.

**3.** Cover the brisket and cook on high for 4 to 6 hours until the brisket is fork tender. It should pull apart very easily with a fork.

**4.** While the brisket cooks, combine the rice and water in the bowl of a rice cooker. Cook the rice according to package instructions. If you don't have a rice cooker, combine the rice and water in a medium-sized pot. Bring to a boil over high heat, then reduce heat to medium-low, cover, and simmer for about 15 to 18 minutes until water is fully absorbed. Remove from heat, fluff with a fork, and leave covered until ready to use.

**5.** While the rice cooks, transfer the brisket to a cutting board and, using two forks, shred the meat. Once shredded, place the meat back into the roasting pan with the gravy so it can absorb more of the sauce. (It's so good!)

**6.** To assemble the bowls, place a scoop of rice into each bowl. Top with a generous portion of shredded brisket and then a scoop of the Jalapeño Lime Coleslaw. Sprinkle queso fresco on top and garnish with chopped cilantro. If your kids aren't into all of the ingredients being combined together, place each ingredient in separate spots on the same plate. My kids won't eat everything combined, but they devour this meal when the portions are separated!

 **Dr. Bear Fun Fact!** Worcestershire sauce is actually made from fish! It gives a savory flavor to any meat it marinates. Always make sure to double-check that the brand you buy is gluten-free!

*Nutritional data reflects one serving, based on a 6-serving yield.*

**PER SERVING** Calories: 890; Total Fat: 28g; Saturated Fat: 11g; Cholesterol: 171mg; Sodium: 1834mg; Total Carbohydrates: 94g; Dietary Fiber: 6g; Sugars: 46g; Protein: 60g

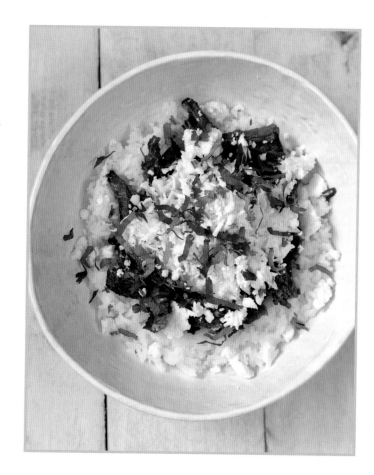

# Pumpkin Mascarpone Manicotti

*When I was diagnosed with celiac disease fifteen years ago, I was lucky to find one type of gluten-free pasta at the grocery store. Today, there are dozens of gluten-free pastas made from a variety of grains that come in every shape and size. I was particularly excited when Jovial introduced a gluten-free manicotti. Now I can make gluten-free stuffed pasta! I use a piping bag to fill the pasta, and it's a little bit neater this way, but the easiest method is shoving it in with your finger. Plus, the kids love helping with this messy step!*

**YIELD: 4 SERVINGS**
Prep Time: 20 minutes
Total Time: 60 minutes

---

1 (7-ounce) package gluten-free manicotti

2 tablespoons olive oil

3 shallots, skin removed and roughly chopped

1 apple, core removed and chopped into bite-sized pieces

2 cups chicken broth

1 (15-ounce) can pumpkin purée

1 (8-ounce) container mascarpone

Zest of 2 lemons, divided

3 tablespoons maple syrup

1 teaspoon salt, divided

1 (15-ounce) container ricotta cheese

4 cups packed fresh baby spinach leaves, rinsed and patted dry, roughly chopped

½ cup shredded Parmesan cheese, divided

1 cup shredded mozzarella cheese, divided

**1.** Preheat oven to 375°F. Spray a 9-by-13-inch glass baking dish with nonstick spray and set aside.

**2.** Cook gluten-free manicotti according to package instructions. Drain and set aside.

**3.** To make the pumpkin mascarpone sauce, in a high-sided sauté pan or pot, heat olive oil over medium heat. Add the shallots and cook, stirring frequently until softened, about 5 minutes. Add the apples and cook for 2 to 3 minutes, just until soft. Add the chicken broth and cook until the mixture comes to a simmer.

**4.** Stir in the pumpkin purée, mascarpone, maple syrup, zest of 1 lemon, and ½ teaspoon salt and mix until well combined.

**5.** Remove the pot from the heat and, using an immersion blender, purée the mixture until smooth. If you don't have an immersion blender, transfer the mixture to a blender or food processor and pulse until smooth. Set aside.

**6.** In a medium-sized mixing bowl, mix together the ricotta cheese, chopped spinach, remaining lemon zest, ¼ cup Parmesan cheese, ¼ cup mozzarella cheese, and remaining ½ teaspoon salt. Set aside.

**7.** To assemble the manicotti, start by spreading a thin layer of the pumpkin mascarpone sauce (about 3 table-spoons) into the bottom of the prepared baking dish.

**8.** Fill each manicotti shell with about 3 teaspoons of the ricotta filling. You can put the filling into a piping bag or just use a spoon and your fingers to push the filling inside. Place the filled shells into the prepared baking dish. Repeat until all manicotti are filled.

**9.** Pour the pumpkin mascarpone sauce over the top of the stuffed manicotti and then sprinkle remaining mozzarella across the top of the sauce.

**10.** Bake for 25 to 30 minutes until the sauce is bubbling and the cheese is golden.

 **Dr. Bear Fun Fact!** "Manicotti" means "little sleeve" in Italian! It's perfect for stuffed pasta dishes like this one with mascarpone, which is Italian cream cheese!

*Nutritional data reflects one serving, based on a 4-serving yield.*

**PER SERVING** Calories: 967; Total Fat: 60g; Saturated Fat: 32g; Cholesterol: 166mg; Sodium: 1625mg; Total Carbohydrates: 80g; Dietary Fiber: 7g; Sugars: 24g; Protein: 32g

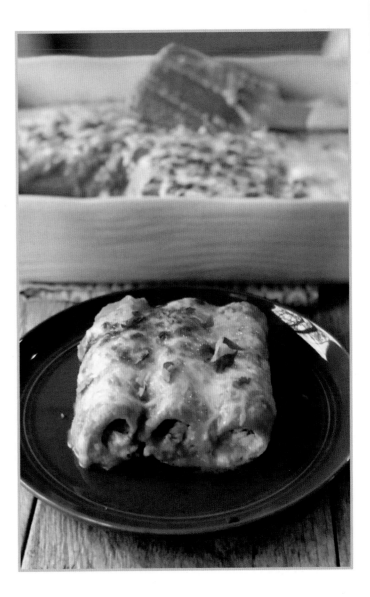

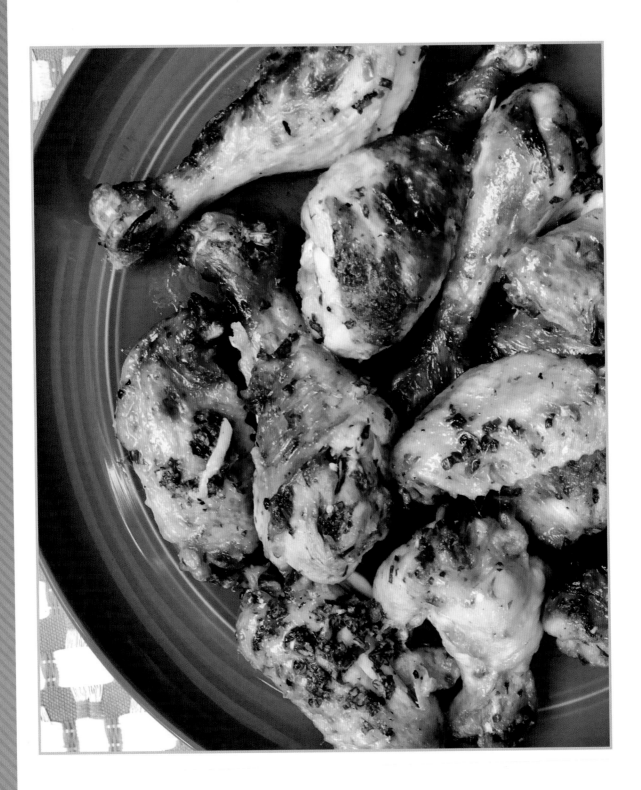

# Lemony Garlicky Buttery Chicken Wings

*These wings can be baked or fried. My personal choice is to use the air fryer. Simply follow the same instructions, but cook in the air fryer at 400°F for 20 minutes.*

**ERVINGS**
1 hour 15 minutes
Total Time: 1 hour 45 minutes

---

½ cup olive oil

6 cloves garlic, peeled

2 lemons

¼ cup roughly chopped basil leaves, rinsed and patted dry, divided

¼ cup roughly chopped fresh oregano leaves, rinsed and patted dry, divided

½ teaspoon red pepper flakes

¾ teaspoon salt, divided

1 pound chicken wings

1 pound chicken drumsticks

¼ cup butter

**1.** In a small skillet, heat olive oil over medium heat. Add garlic cloves and cook, stirring frequently until garlic is soft and lightly browning, about 1 to 2 minutes. Remove from heat and cool for about 5 minutes.

**2.** While the garlic oil cools, zest and juice the 2 lemons, keeping the zest and juice in separate bowls. Set aside.

**3.** In a blender or food processor, pulse the cooled oil and garlic, lemon juice, half of the chopped basil, half of the chopped oregano, red pepper flakes, and ½ teaspoon salt.

**4.** Place the chicken wings and drumsticks in a large bowl or zip-top bag, and pour the marinade over the meat. Refrigerate for at least one hour before cooking.

**5.** While the chicken is absorbing the lemony, garlicky flavors, make the compound butter. In a food processor, pulse together the butter and the remaining lemon zest, basil, oregano, and salt. Set aside.

**6.** To cook the chicken, preheat oven to 425°F. Line a baking sheet with foil. Remove the chicken from the marinade and place on prepared baking sheet. Bake for 25 to 30 minutes until the wings and drumsticks reach an internal temperature of 165°F.

**7.** Remove from the oven and transfer the wings and drumsticks to a large mixing bowl. Add the lemon butter and toss to coat the chicken pieces. Serve immediately.

*Nutritional data reflects one serving, based on a 4-serving yield.*

**PER SERVING** Calories: 752; Total Fat: 67g; Saturated Fat: 19g; Cholesterol: 211mg; Sodium: 926mg; Total Carbohydrates: 6g; Dietary Fiber: 2g; Sugars: 1g; Protein: 36g

**Dr. Bear Fun Fact!** Garlic doesn't just pack a punch in flavor—it also packs a punch in nutrition! Studies have shown that higher garlic consumption can help lower cholesterol and prevent dementia and high blood pressure.

# Herbed Fontina & Asparagus Tart

*This tart is perfect for taking to parties. It looks so pretty and elegant and is bursting with flavor.*

**YIELD: 4 SERVINGS**
Prep Time: 15 minutes
Total Time: 35 minutes

---

1 sheet gluten-free puff pastry (pictured is GeeFree Gluten-Free Puff Pastry sheets)

¼ cup olive oil

6 cloves garlic, peeled

2 teaspoons chopped fresh rosemary, rinsed and patted dry

2 teaspoons chopped fresh thyme, rinsed and patted dry

¼ teaspoon salt

1 pound asparagus, ends trimmed

2 cups shredded fontina cheese, divided

1 egg

1 teaspoon water

1. Preheat oven to 375°F. Line a plate with paper towels and set aside. Set out a baking sheet and cut a piece of parchment paper to fit properly on the baking sheet.

2. Dust the parchment paper with gluten-free all-purpose flour and set the puff pastry sheet on top of the floured parchment paper. Carefully roll the pastry dough into a 9-by-14-inch rectangle, approximately. Carefully transfer the parchment and puff pastry to the baking sheet. Partially bake for about 8 minutes until starting to turn golden. Remove from oven and set aside.

3. While the puff pastry is in the oven, purée the olive oil, garlic, rosemary, thyme, and salt in a small food processor until a smooth mixture forms. Set aside.

4. Fill a large skillet about halfway with water and heat over medium-high heat. Once boiling, add the asparagus and cook for about 2 to 3 minutes until the asparagus is softened and bright green. Remove from water and dry on paper towel lined plate.

5. Remove puff pastry from the oven and, using a brush, spread about ¾ of the olive oil mixture across the surface of the dough. Sprinkle half of the fontina cheese across the surface of the puff pastry.

6. Arrange the asparagus on top of the cheese. If your kids will eat asparagus, cover the entire puff pastry. If they are a little skeptical, leave part of the tart with just the plain cheese (but remember to encourage them to taste the asparagus!)

7. Brush remaining olive oil mixture over the top of the asparagus and sprinkle remaining cheese on top.

**8.** In a small bowl, whisk together the egg and water to make an egg wash. Brush the egg wash across the exposed parts of the puff pastry crust.

**9.** Bake for 10 to 15 minutes until the cheese is melted and golden. Serve immediately.

 **Dr. Bear Fun Fact!** Italians say that true fontina cheese gets its taste and quality from the high altitude of the Alps, where the cows graze.

*Nutritional data reflects one serving, /based on a 4-serving yield.*

**PER SERVING** Calories: 613; Total Fat: 44g; Saturated Fat: 21g; Cholesterol: 104mg; Sodium: 905mg; Total Carbohydrates: 39g; Dietary Fiber: 4g; Sugars: 6g; Protein: 19g

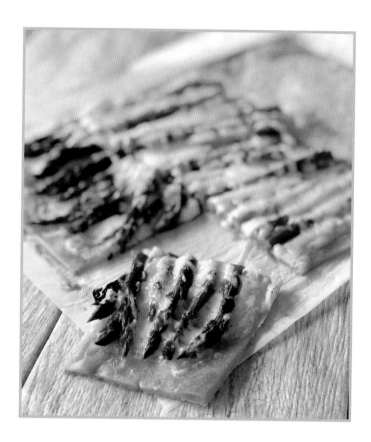

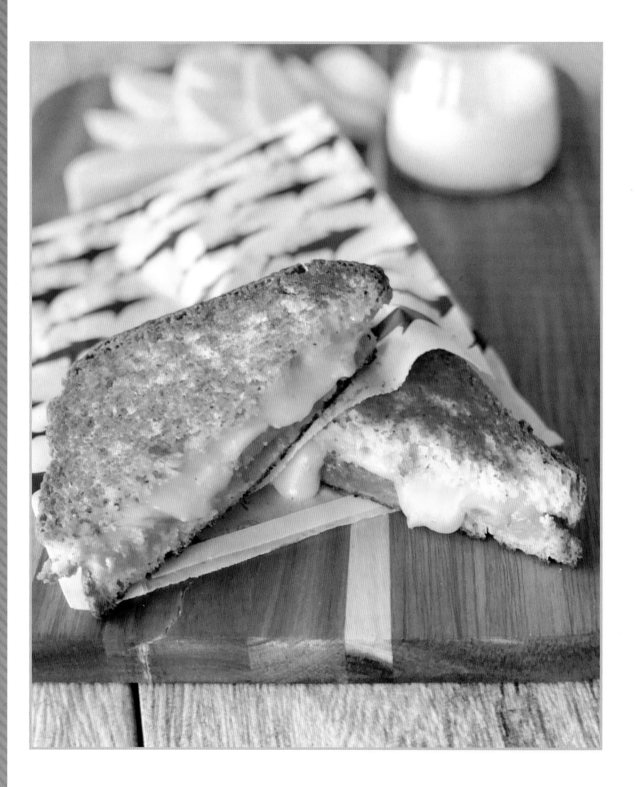

# Grilled Cheese with Butternut Squash & Gruyère

*This recipe came to life on a day that I was starving and needed a quick lunch. In just moments, I had what I consider a grown-up grilled cheese that my kids also really liked!*

**YIELD: 4 SERVINGS**
Prep Time: 5 minutes
Total Time: 15 minutes

———————

8 teaspoons butter

8 slices gluten-free sandwich bread

½ cup Butternut Squash & Caramelized Onion Mash (page 226)

4 slices Gruyère cheese

2 Granny Smith apples, core removed and thinly sliced

**1.** Spread about 1 teaspoon butter onto one side of each slice of bread. Place 4 pieces of bread with the buttered side down into a large skillet.

**2.** On the non-buttered side of each piece of bread in the pan, spread 2 tablespoons of the Butternut Squash & Caramelized Onion Mash. Top with one slice of Gruyère cheese.

**3.** Close the sandwiches with the remaining 4 pieces of bread, keeping the buttered side of the bread facing outward (non-buttered side is touching the cheese).

**4.** Cover and cook the sandwiches over low heat for about 4 to 6 minutes until you can see the cheese beginning to melt. Using a spatula, flip the sandwiches to cook the opposite side for about 4 additional minutes.

**5.** Serve with sliced Granny Smith apples.

 **Dr. Bear Fun Fact!** This recipe is a great way to add vegetables to a kid favorite! Try adding a gluten-free tomato soup on the side if you want to increase the meal's size.

*Nutritional data reflects one serving, based on a 4-serving yield.*

**PER SERVING** Calories: 650; Total Fat: 39.8g; Saturated Fat: 20.5g; Cholesterol: 90.6mg; Sodium: 683.7mg; Total Carbohydrates: 57.8g; Dietary Fiber: 4.5g; Sugars: 13.8g; Protein: 13.6g

# Skirt Steak Tacos with Goat Cheese Avocado Cream

*This is one of those recipes to keep in your back pocket for a super busy night when you're craving a home cooked meal but have little energy to make it. My kids love helping with the assembly, especially spreading the "yummy green sauce" on the tortillas.*

**YIELD: 12 TACOS (4 SERVINGS)**
Prep Time: 15 minutes
Total Time: 30 minutes

---

2 avocados, skin and pit removed

⅓ cup goat cheese crumbles

Juice of 2 limes

½ cup cilantro leaves, plus more for garnish, rinsed and patted dry

2 tablespoons olive oil

4 boneless petite sirloin steaks (about 6 ounces each)

1 teaspoon salt

1 teaspoon garlic powder

2 cups thinly sliced button mushrooms, rinsed and patted dry

1 cup finely chopped sweet yellow onion, skin removed

2 cloves garlic, peeled and finely minced

1 teaspoon cumin

12 corn tortillas

**1.** In the bowl of a small food processor, combine the avocado, goat cheese, lime juice, and cilantro leaves. Pulse together until a smooth mixture forms. Cover and refrigerate until ready to serve.

**2.** In a large skillet, heat olive oil over high heat. Season the steaks on both sides with salt and garlic powder and place in the hot pan. Cook for about 2 to 3 minutes per side, just to get a good sear on the steaks. Remove the steaks from the pan and transfer to a cutting board. Let them rest.

**3.** To the same pan the steaks were cooked in, add the chopped mushrooms and yellow onions. Cook, stirring occasionally, until the onions are soft and beginning to brown, about 5 to 7 minutes.

**4.** While the mushrooms and onions are cooking, chop the steaks into bite-sized pieces.

**5.** Add the garlic and cumin to the mushroom and onion mixture and cook, stirring frequently for 1 minute.

**6.** Add the steak pieces back into the pan with the mushrooms and onions and toss to combine. Remove from heat and set aside.

**7.** Heat a separate large skillet over medium-high heat. Add the tortillas to the pan and heat for about 2 minutes per side until the tortillas begin to brown. Work in batches so as not to overcrowd the pan.

**8.** To assemble the tacos, spread a thin layer of the avocado goat cheese sauce on a tortilla. Top with a heaping portion of the steak mixture and garnish with cilantro, if desired.

**Dr. Bear Fun Fact!** Skirt steak and flank steak are different cuts of meat from two different parts of the cow, but are often confused with each other. Don't worry—you can still use flank steak for this recipe if you can't find skirt steak!

*Nutritional data reflects one serving of 3 tacos, based on a 4-serving yield.*

**PER SERVING** Calories: 684; Total Fat: 30g; Saturated Fat: 7g; Cholesterol: 136mg; Sodium: 884mg; Total Carbohydrates: 49g; Dietary Fiber: 10g; Sugars: 4g; Protein: 61g

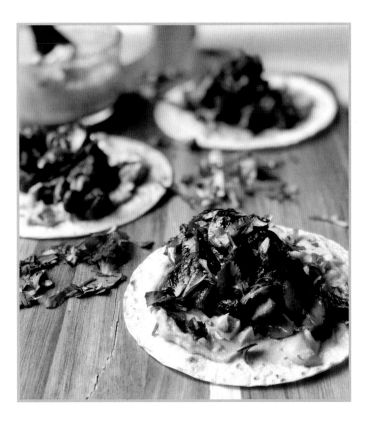

# Shrimp Tacos with Roasted Red Pepper Sauce

*Despite the sauce coming from a roasted red pepper, these tacos are actually not spicy at all! They're the perfect spice level for grown-ups and kids.*

**YIELD: 12 TACOS (4 SERVINGS)**
Prep Time: 25 minutes
Total Time: 50 minutes

---

**For the Roasted Red Pepper Sauce**

1 red pepper

1 tablespoon olive oil

¼ teaspoon salt

1 shallot, skin removed and roughly chopped

12 basil leaves, rinsed and patted dry

Zest of 1 lemon

Juice of 1 lemon

**For the Shrimp and Tacos**

2 tablespoons olive oil

1½ pounds shrimp, peeled and deveined

½ cup finely chopped red onion, skin removed

½ cup finely chopped fresh cilantro leaves, plus more for garnish, rinsed and patted dry

12 corn tortillas

Guacamole or avocado slices for garnish

1 cup Cotija cheese, for garnish

**1.** To make the sauce, preheat oven to 400°F. Line a baking sheet with foil and place the red pepper on the baking sheet.

**2.** Drizzle the red pepper with olive oil and salt and rub with your fingers to fully coat the pepper. Roast for 20 to 25 minutes until the pepper is soft and beginning to brown. Remove from oven and cool completely.

**3.** Once the red pepper is cooled, discard the stem and seeds. Place the remaining red pepper flesh in a food processor or blender. Add the shallots, basil leaves, lemon zest, and lemon juice and purée until a smooth sauce forms. Set aside.

**4.** To make the shrimp, heat the olive oil over medium-high heat. Add the shrimp and red onion and cook for about 4 to 6 minutes until the shrimp are pink and beginning to brown.

**5.** Pour the red pepper sauce over the shrimp and toss to combine. Bring the sauce to a boil and let the sauce reduce slightly. Remove from heat and toss in the cilantro.

**6.** Heat a separate large skillet over medium-high heat. Add the tortillas to the pan and heat for about 2 minutes per side until the tortillas begin to brown. Work in batches so as not to overcrowd the pan.

**7.** To assemble the tacos, place the heated tortillas on a plate. Put a heaping scoop of shrimp in the center of each taco and then top with guacamole, Cotija cheese, and chopped cilantro.

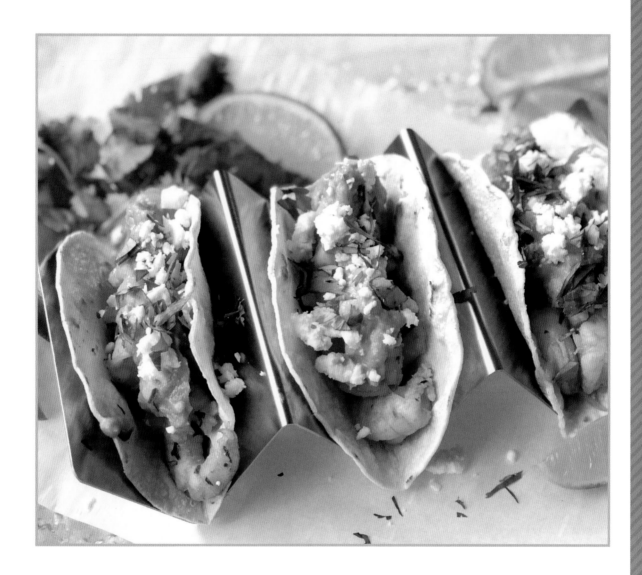

 **Dr. Bear Fun Fact!** Bell peppers are the only members of the pepper family that do not contain capsaicin, the natural chemical that makes peppers spicy!

*Nutritional data reflects one serving of 3 tacos, based on a 4-serving yield. (Nutritional data does not include garnishes.)*

**PER SERVING** Calories: 579.4; Total Fat: 23.8g; Saturated Fat: 8.1g; Cholesterol: 354.2mg; Sodium: 885.6mg; Total Carbohydrates: 40.4g; Dietary Fiber: 5.5g; Sugars: 4.5g; Protein: 53.4g

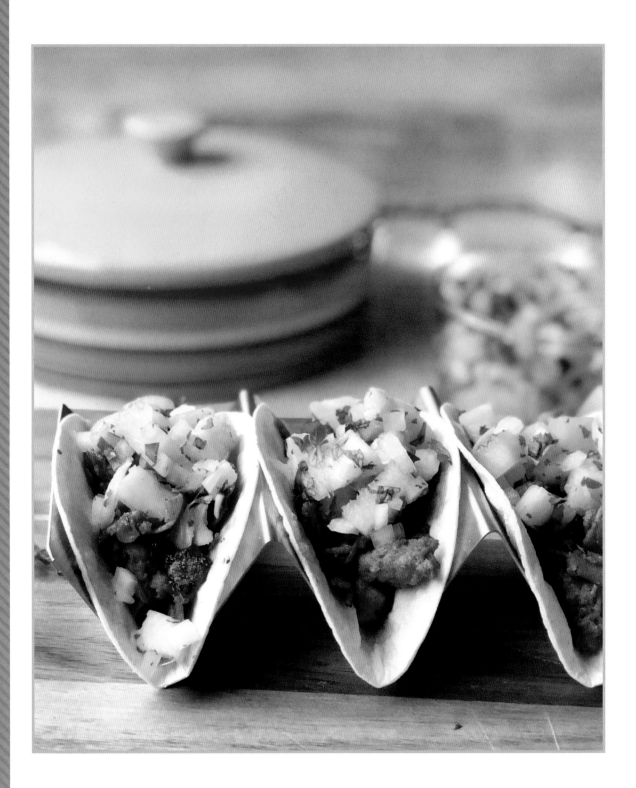

# Sausage & Bacon Tacos with Pineapple Pico

*I'm a big fan of emptying the refrigerator so nothing goes to waste. I developed these tacos because I had an open package of bacon and a few pieces of sweet Italian sausage in my refrigerator. They both have strong flavors on their own so pair nicely with a mild pineapple pico.*

**YIELD: 12 TACOS (6 SERVINGS)**
Prep Time: 15 minutes
Total Time: 45 minutes

### For the Pineapple Pico

2 cups finely chopped pineapple, skin and top removed

½ cup finely chopped white onion, skin removed

½ cup finely chopped cilantro leaves, rinsed and patted dry

Juice of 1 lime

### For the Taco Filling

2 tablespoons olive oil

1 pound sweet Italian sausage

1 (8-ounce) package bacon, roughly chopped

1 cup finely chopped white onion, skin removed

2 cups chopped tomatoes

2 teaspoons paprika

2 teaspoons ground cumin

1 teaspoon chili powder

½ teaspoon salt

12 corn tortillas

**1.** To make the pineapple pico, toss together the chopped pineapple, white onion, cilantro, and lime juice in a glass mixing bowl. Cover and refrigerate until ready to serve.

**2.** To make the taco filling, heat olive oil over medium-high heat in a large skillet. Add the sweet Italian sausage and cook, stirring to break up the meat into small pieces, for about 5 minutes or until the sausage is no longer pink.

**3.** Add the chopped bacon and onion and cook, stirring occasionally, until the bacon and sausage are browned and the onions are soft, about 5 to 7 minutes.

**4.** Add the chopped tomatoes, paprika, cumin, chili powder, and salt and cook, stirring occasionally, until the tomatoes are soft, about 5 minutes.

**5.** Heat a separate large skillet over medium-high heat. Add the tortillas to the pan and heat for about 2 minutes per side until the tortillas begin to brown. Work in batches so as not to overcrowd the pan.

**6.** To assemble the tacos, place a heaping portion of the sausage and bacon mixture on each corn tortilla and top with pineapple pico.

 **Dr. Bear Fun Fact!** Leftover pineapple slices? Try grilling them for a sweet dessert! Grilling fruit caramelizes its sugars, creating sweet, healthy treats.

*Nutritional data reflects one serving of 2 tacos, based on a 6-serving yield.*

**PER SERVING** Calories: 500; Total Fat: 26.1g; Saturated Fat: 7.9g; Cholesterol: 60.1mg; Sodium: 1306.3mg; Total Carbohydrates: 39.3g; Dietary Fiber: 5.4g; Sugars: 10.1g; Protein: 29.5g

# Ground Beef Tacos with Cheddar Cheese

*My son Brandon loves beef tacos, but I still can't get him to eat the tacos fully assembled. So, I plate with purpose and put the plain taco shell on his plate with a scoop of beef and a pile of cheese and tomatoes.*

**YIELD: 12 TACOS (4 SERVINGS)**

Prep Time: 5 minutes

Total Time: 25 minutes

---

2 tablespoons olive oil

1½ pounds ground beef

1 cup chopped white onion, skin removed

3 cloves garlic, peeled and finely minced

2 teaspoons ground cumin

1 teaspoon salt

12 hard corn tortilla shells

1 cup shredded cheddar cheese

For garnish: shredded lettuce, chopped tomatoes, and sour cream

**1.** In a large skillet, heat olive oil over medium-high heat. Add the ground beef and cook, stirring to break the beef up into small pieces, for about 5 to 7 minutes until the beef is no longer pink.

**2.** Add the chopped onion and cook, stirring occasionally, until the onions are soft and translucent and the beef is beginning to brown. Add the minced garlic, ground cumin, and salt and cook, stirring frequently, for 1 to 2 more minutes.

**3.** To assemble the tacos, spoon a heaping portion of the ground beef into the hard corn tortilla shells. Top with shredded cheddar cheese and garnish with lettuce, tomatoes, and sour cream, if desired.

 **Dr. Bear Fun Fact!** The biggest taco ever made was 1,654 pounds in Mexicali, Mexico!

*Nutritional data reflects one serving of 3 tacos, based on a 4-serving yield. (Nutritional data does not include garnishes.)*

**PER SERVING** Calories: 775; Total Fat: 44.6g; Saturated Fat: 17.8g; Cholesterol: 179.7mg; Sodium: 909.9mg; Total Carbohydrates: 38.9g; Dietary Fiber: 4.8g; Sugars: 2.7g; Protein: 53.9g

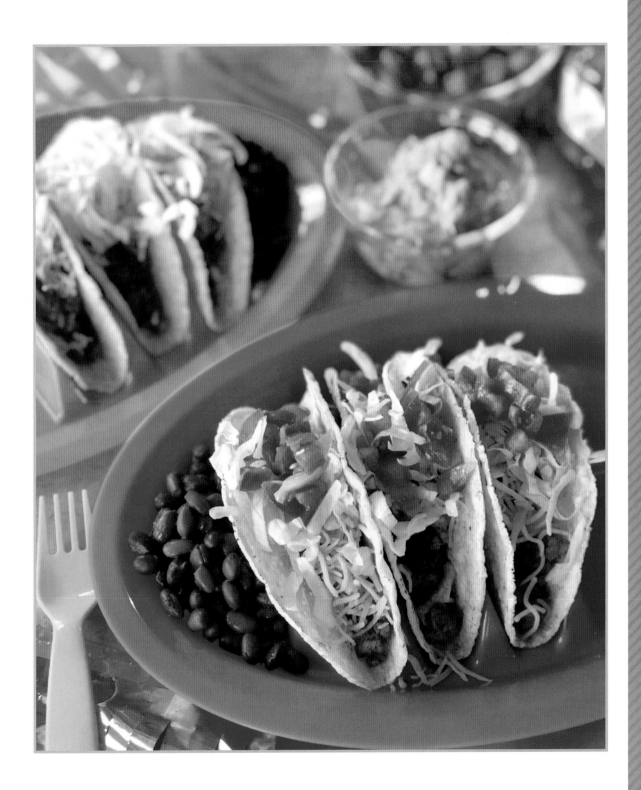

# Pink Pasta (aka Salmon Spaghetti)

*I lucked out and am thankful every day that I can always get my kids to eat salmon. This pink fish is a great source of protein and omega-3 fatty acids as well as vitamin B$_{12}$ and vitamin D.*

**YIELD: 4 SERVINGS**
Prep Time: 25 minutes
Total Time: 40 minutes

---

**For the Pink Sauce**

1 pint grape tomatoes

2 cloves garlic, peeled

3 tablespoons olive oil, divided

½ teaspoon salt

2 shallots, skin removed and roughly chopped

12 basil leaves, rinsed and patted dry

Zest of 1 lemon

Juice of 1 lemon

1 teaspoon sugar

3 tablespoons mascarpone cheese

**For the Pasta**

1 (12-ounce) package gluten-free spaghetti pasta

2 tablespoons butter

1 teaspoon olive oil

½ teaspoon salt

3 (6-ounce) salmon fillets

Grated parmesan cheese, for garnish

*Nutritional data reflects one serving, based on a 4-serving yield.*

**PER SERVING** Calories: 783; Total Fat: 34g; Saturated Fat: 10g; Cholesterol: 120mg; Sodium: 571mg; Total Carbohydrates: 75g; Dietary Fiber: 5g; Sugars: 7g; Protein: 39g

1. To make the sauce, preheat oven to 400°F. Line a baking sheet with foil. Drizzle the tomatoes with 2½ tablespoons olive oil and salt and toss to evenly coat all of the tomatoes. Spread the tomatoes evenly across the foil.

2. Place the garlic cloves on a piece of foil and drizzle with remaining olive oil and a pinch of salt. Wrap up the garlic and place on baking tray with tomatoes. Roast for 15 to 20 minutes until the tomatoes are soft and beginning to brown. Remove from oven and cool completely.

3. Once the tomatoes are cooled, combine the tomatoes and garlic and all remaining liquids from the cooking juices in a food processor or blender. Add the shallots, basil leaves, lemon zest, lemon juice, sugar, and mascarpone and purée until a smooth sauce forms.

4. While the tomatoes are cooking and cooling, cook the gluten-free spaghetti according to package instructions. Drain and set aside.

5. To make the salmon, heat butter and olive oil together in a large skillet over medium-high heat. Season the salmon fillets on both sides with salt and add to the pan. Cook for 4 to 6 minutes per side until the salmon is opaque and easily flakes.

6. Reduce heat to medium-low and, using two forks, shred the salmon in the pan into bite-sized pieces. Pour the pink tomato sauce over the salmon and gently stir to combine. Bring the sauce and salmon to a simmer and gently toss in the cooked gluten-free spaghetti.

7. Serve garnished with grated parmesan cheese.

 **Dr. Bear Fun Fact!** Salmon are pink due to their diet! The more krill and shrimp they eat, they get pinker!

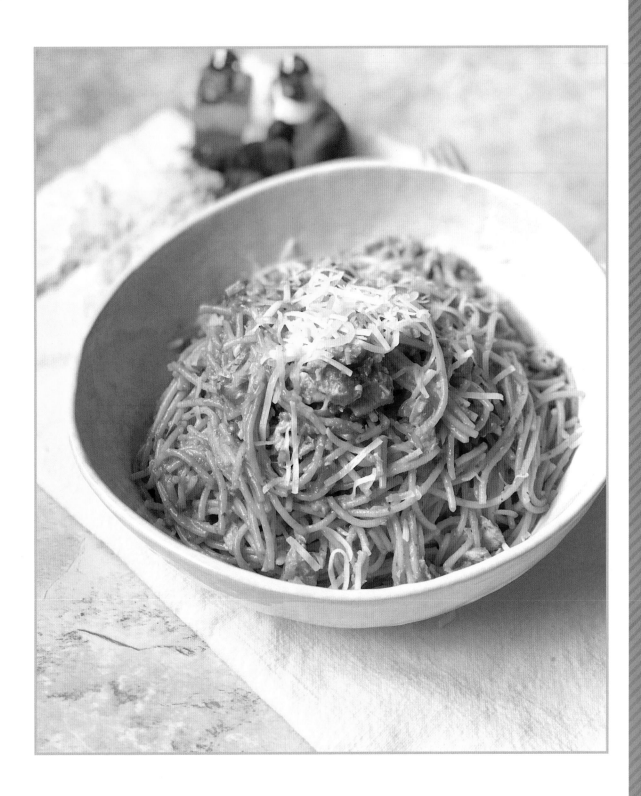

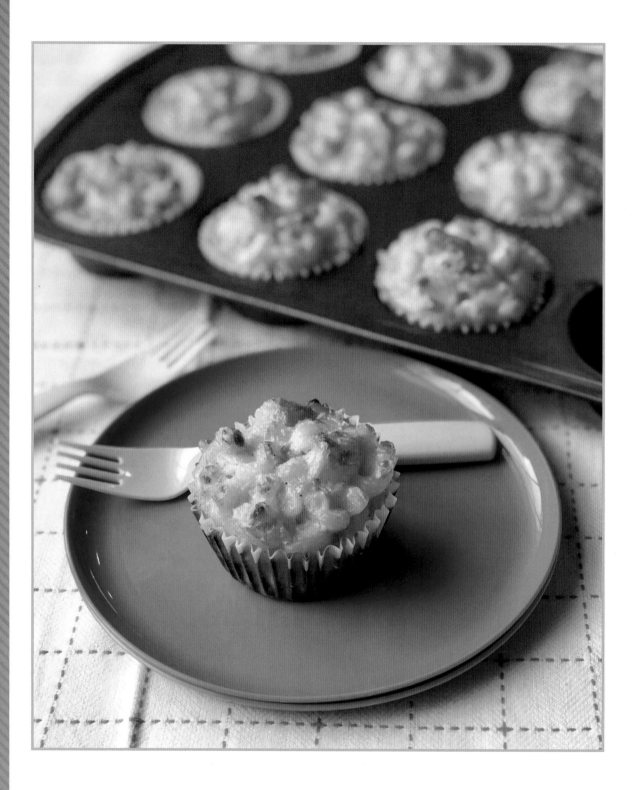

# Baked Squash Macaroni & Cheese Cups

*If you don't have the Butternut Squash & Caramelized Onion Mash on hand, you can replace it with 1 cup of pumpkin purée and 2 tablespoons maple syrup.*

**YIELD: 15 MUFFINS**
Prep Time: 15 minutes
Total Time: 40 minutes

---

1 (8-ounce) box gluten-free elbow pasta

1 tablespoon butter

1 tablespoon cornstarch

1 cup milk (1 or 2 percent works best)

1 cup grated Gruyère cheese

½ cup grated sharp cheddar cheese

½ cup mascarpone

2 cups Butternut Squash & Caramelized Onion Mash (page 226)

1½ teaspoons Dijon mustard

½ teaspoon nutmeg

½ teaspoon salt

2 eggs, lightly beaten

¼ cup grated Parmesan cheese

**1.** Preheat oven to 375°F. Line a 12-cup muffin pan with liners or lightly spray the muffin cups with a nonstick spray and set aside.

**2.** Cook gluten-free pasta according to package instructions. Drain and set aside in a large mixing bowl.

**3.** While the pasta is cooking, in a medium-size pot, heat butter over medium-high heat. Whisk in the cornstarch and cook, whisking constantly, for 1 minute.

**4.** Slowly whisk in the milk and cook, whisking constantly, until the mixture thickens, about 3 to 5 minutes. The mixture should coat the back of a spoon.

**5.** Once the milk mixture is thick, stir in the grated Gruyère, sharp cheddar cheese, and mascarpone. Stir constantly until the cheese has melted. Stir in the Butternut Squash & Caramelized Onion Mash, Dijon mustard, nutmeg, and salt. Mix until well combined.

**6.** Remove the pan from the heat and stir in the eggs. Pour this mixture over the top of the cooked gluten-free elbow pasta and stir together until well combined.

**7.** Divide the mixture evenly among the prepared muffin cups and sprinkle each top with grated Parmesan cheese. Bake for 24 to 28 minutes or until lightly browned.

 **Dr. Bear Fun Fact!** Pasta and cheese recipes have been recorded as early as the fourteenth century!

*Nutritional data reflects one muffin, based on a 15-muffin yield.*
**PER SERVING** Calories: 254; Total Fat: 15g; Saturated Fat: 7.2g; Cholesterol: 56.2mg; Sodium: 426.7mg; Total Carbohydrates: 22.3g; Dietary Fiber: 1.7g; Sugars: 5.2g; Protein: 8.5g

# Almond Crusted Chicken Tenders with Homemade Honey Mustard & BBQ Sauces

*Like most kids, both of my boys love chicken tenders, especially this homemade version. They're dipped in a thin coating of almond flour that's gently seasoned with garlic and paprika. I included both dipping sauces because my kids are split on which one they like best!*

**YIELD: 4 SERVINGS**
Prep Time: 5 minutes
Total Time: 20 minutes

---

**For the Sweet & Tangy BBQ Sauce**

⅓ cup ketchup

2 tablespoons Worcestershire sauce

1 tablespoon apple cider vinegar

1 tablespoon honey

½ tablespoon brown sugar

½ teaspoon lemon juice

½ teaspoon garlic powder

½ teaspoon paprika

¼ teaspoon salt

**For the Honey Mustard Sauce**

2 tablespoons Dijon mustard

2 tablespoons mayonnaise

2 tablespoons honey

½ teaspoon red wine vinegar

**For the Chicken**

½ cup almond flour

1 teaspoon salt

1 teaspoon garlic powder

½ teaspoon paprika

1½ pounds boneless, skinless chicken tenders, rinsed and patted dry

4 tablespoons vegetable oil

**1.** To make the BBQ sauce, in a small sauce pot set over medium heat, whisk together ketchup, Worcestershire sauce, apple cider vinegar, honey, brown sugar, lemon juice, garlic powder, paprika, and salt. Bring to a simmer and then reduce heat to low. Let simmer for 5 minutes. Cool completely or serve warm.

**2.** To make the honey mustard sauce, whisk together the Dijon mustard, mayonnaise, honey, and red wine vinegar in a small glass bowl. Cover and refrigerate until ready to serve.

**3.** To make the chicken tenders, whisk together the almond flour, salt, garlic powder, and paprika. Dip each chicken tender into the mixture and coat well.

**4.** In a large sauté pan, heat vegetable oil over medium-high heat. Cook the chicken in the oil for 2 to 4 minutes per side until golden brown and the internal temperature reaches 165°F. Remove from pan and drain excess oil before serving with dipping sauces.

**Dr. Bear Fun Fact!** Similar sauces were created throughout history, but the Worcestershire sauce we're familiar with was created by the Lea & Perrins company in 1838! It's named after the English county in which it was invented—Worcestershire!

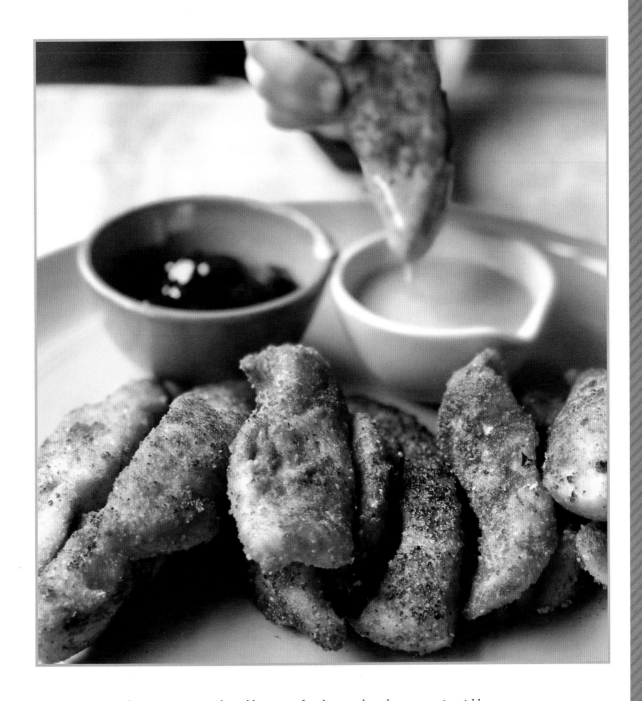

*Nutritional data reflects one serving with 2 tablespoons of each sauce, based on a 4-serving yield.*

**PER SERVING** Calories: 640; Total Fat: 34g; Saturated Fat: 5.7g; Cholesterol: 147.6mg; Sodium: 1309.4mg; Total Carbohydrates: 26.3g; Dietary Fiber: 2.1g; Sugars: 20.6; Protein: 56.4g

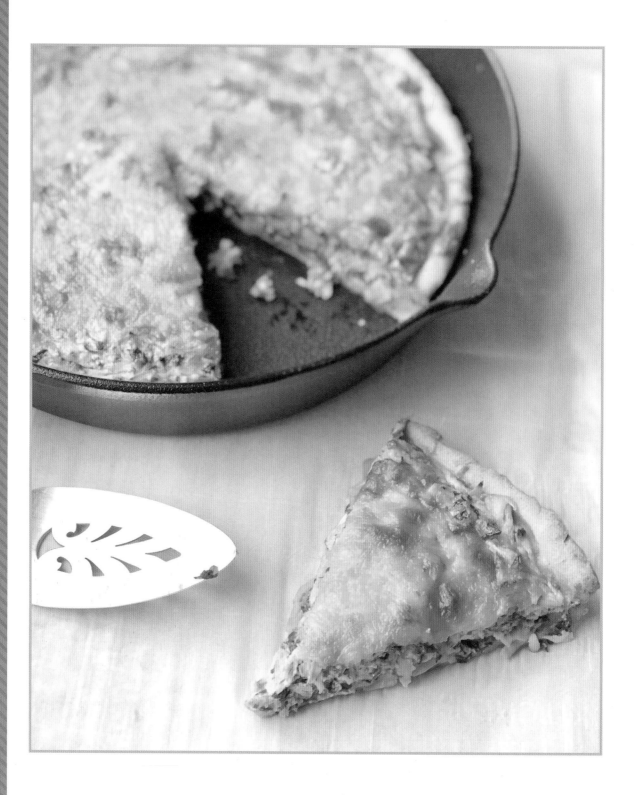

# Zucchini, Spinach, & Artichoke Deep Dish Pizza

*This recipe turns spinach artichoke dips into pizza! There are several brands of premade gluten-free pizza dough. Pictured here I used the Wholly Wholesome Gluten-Free Dough Ball.*

**YIELD: 1 (12-INCH) PIZZA (10 SERVINGS)**
Prep Time: 15 minutes
Total Time: 50 minutes

---

1 (14-ounce) package gluten-free pizza dough

2 eggs

½ cup mayonnaise

½ cup sour cream

½ cup grated Parmesan cheese

1 cup shredded Monterey Jack cheese, divided

2 cups frozen spinach, thawed and drained

1 (14-ounce) can artichoke hearts, drained and roughly chopped

1 cup shredded zucchini, ends removed

**1.** Preheat oven to 375°F. Spray a 12-inch cast iron skillet with nonstick spray. If you don't have a cast iron skillet, you can use a spring form pan or a round cake pan.

**2.** Grease your hands and place the pizza dough into the skillet. Gently stretch the dough until it covers the entire bottom of the pan and up the sides about 2 inches. Partially bake the dough for 5 minutes.

**3.** While the dough is par-baking, whisk together the eggs, mayonnaise, sour cream, Parmesan cheese, and ½ cup Monterey Jack cheese in a large mixing bowl.

**4.** Using a spoon or spatula, stir in the spinach, artichoke hearts, and shredded zucchini. Mix until well combined.

**5.** Remove the partially baked crust from the oven and pour the spinach mixture into the crust.

**6.** Bake for 30 to 35 minutes until the center of the pizza is set and the cheese is golden.

 **Dr. Bear Fun Fact!** Artichokes are a great source of folate, a type of B vitamin your body requires!

*Nutritional data reflects one slice, based on a 10-slice yield.*

**PER SERVING** Calories: 298; Total Fat: 18.7g; Saturated Fat: 6.6g; Cholesterol: 58.6mg; Sodium: 551.4mg; Total Carbohydrates: 25.9g; Dietary Fiber: 7g; Sugars: 2.4g; Protein: 10.1g

# Sheet Pan Steak & Veggies with Paprika Herb Butter

*Sheet pan meals are an easy way to have a home-cooked meal in very little time. Using just one or two pans, you can quickly toss together ingredients that cook at roughly the same speed for a tasty meal. The best part is that sheet pan meals typically use naturally gluten-free ingredients like beef, poultry, seafood, vegetables, and potatoes, so they're perfect for a gluten-free diet!*

**YIELD: 4 SERVINGS**
Prep Time: 15 minutes
Total Time: 30 minutes

---

**For the Paprika Butter**

½ cup butter

2 cloves garlic, peeled and finely minced

1 teaspoon paprika

¼ cup fresh cilantro leaves, rinsed and patted dry

¼ cup fresh parsley, rinsed and patted dry

½ teaspoon salt

**For the Steak & Vegetables**

4 (6-ounce) steaks (pictured are boneless petite sirloin steaks)

2 teaspoons sea salt, divided

2 teaspoons garlic powder, divided

2 large sweet potatoes, peeled and chopped into bite-sized pieces

2 zucchini, ends removed and chopped into bite-sized pieces

1 pound green beans, stems removed

1 red onion, skin removed, cut in half and thinly sliced

4 tablespoons olive oil

1 lemon

**1.** Preheat oven to 350°F. Line two baking sheets with parchment paper or foil and set aside.

**2.** To make the paprika butter, combine the butter, garlic cloves, paprika, cilantro, parsley, and salt in a small food processor. Pulse until a smooth butter forms. If you like a slightly chunkier butter, combine the ingredients in a glass bowl, and use a fork to mash together. Cover and refrigerate until ready to serve.

**3.** Arrange the 4 pieces of steak on one half of one sheet pan. In a small bowl, mix together 1 teaspoon sea salt and 1 teaspoon garlic powder. Sprinkle this mixture on both sides of each steak.

**4.** In a large mixing bowl, toss together the chopped sweet potatoes, zucchini, green beans, and red onion. Drizzle the olive oil and remaining sea salt and garlic powder over the vegetables and toss to evenly coat. Arrange the vegetables on the remaining sheet pan and additional half sheet pan with the steaks.

**5.** Bake for 20 minutes, then increase oven temperature to broil setting and broil for about 5 to 8 minutes until steaks are browning.

**6.** Remove from oven and squeeze the juice of one lemon over the vegetables. Toss to combine.

**7.** To serve, place a heaping portion of vegetables on each plate. Top with a piece of steak and garnish with a scoop of the paprika butter. You want the butter to melt over the steak and the vegetables.

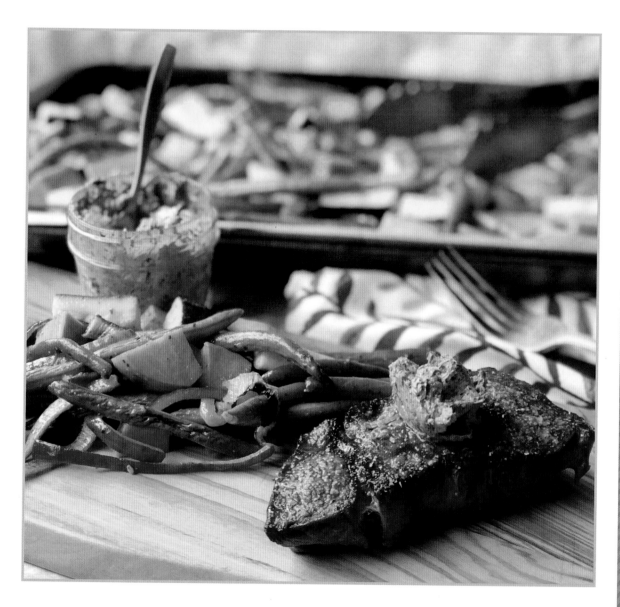

 **Dr. Bear Fun Fact!** Green beans are picked before they're fully ripe. If you let them ripen, you would get dry beans. You could put those in a chili!

*Nutritional data reflects one serving, based on a 4-serving yield.*

**PER SERVING** Calories: 831; Total Fat: 52.9g; Saturated Fat: 22.5g; Cholesterol: 214.1mg; Sodium: 1778mg; Total Carbohydrates: 36g; Dietary Fiber: 8.9g; Sugars: 13.3g; Protein: 58.8g

# Chinese Ginger Chicken Lettuce Wraps

*Boston Bibb lettuce is my favorite lettuce to use for lettuce wraps. It's a tad bit sweet and crispy, but it also bends well to wrap up around the fillings. If kids aren't into the assembled version of the lettuce wrap, try starting out by serving them the individual components on a plate…then work up to it all together.*

**YIELD: 4 SERVINGS**
Prep Time: 15 minutes
Total Time: 40 minutes

---

1 cup jasmine rice

½ cup finely chopped fresh cilantro leaves, rinsed and patted dry

½ cup finely chopped fresh mint leaves, rinsed and patted dry

½ cup chopped roasted, unsalted peanuts

¼ cup gluten-free reduced sodium soy sauce

¼ cup gluten-free hoisin sauce

1 tablespoon mirin

1 tablespoon brown sugar

2 tablespoons vegetable oil

1½ pounds ground chicken

2 cups thinly sliced button mushrooms, rinsed and patted dry

4 cloves garlic, peeled and finely minced

2 tablespoons finely minced fresh ginger, peeled

1½ cups shredded cabbage, rinsed and patted dry

12 lettuce cups, rinsed and patted dry (Boston Bibb lettuce works best)

1. Steam jasmine rice according to package instructions. Set aside and keep warm.

2. In a glass mixing bowl, stir together the chopped cilantro, mint, and peanuts. Cover and refrigerate until ready to serve.

3. In a glass mixing cup, whisk together the gluten-free soy sauce, gluten-free hoisin sauce, mirin, and brown sugar. Set aside until ready to use.

4. In a large skillet, heat vegetable oil over medium-high heat. Add the ground chicken and mushrooms and cook, stirring to break up the chicken into small pieces, for about 5 to 7 minutes or until the chicken is no longer pink.

5. Add the minced garlic and ginger and cook, stirring occasionally, for about 1 to 2 minutes until the garlic and ginger are very fragrant. Add the salt and stir to combine.

6. Pour the sauce over the meat mixture and stir to combine. Cook, stirring occasionally, until the sauce reduces by approximately half, about 5 minutes. Stir in the shredded cabbage and remove from heat.

7. To assemble the lettuce wraps, spread a small amount of rice into the bottom of each lettuce cup. Then place a heaping portion of the meat mixture on top and garnish with a spoonful of the cilantro, mint, and peanut mixture.

 **Dr. Bear Fun Fact!** Mirin is a type of Japanese rice wine. If you have trouble finding it, try "aji-mirin" by brands like Kikkoman or use a mixture of one tablespoon of rice vinegar to ½ teaspoon sugar.

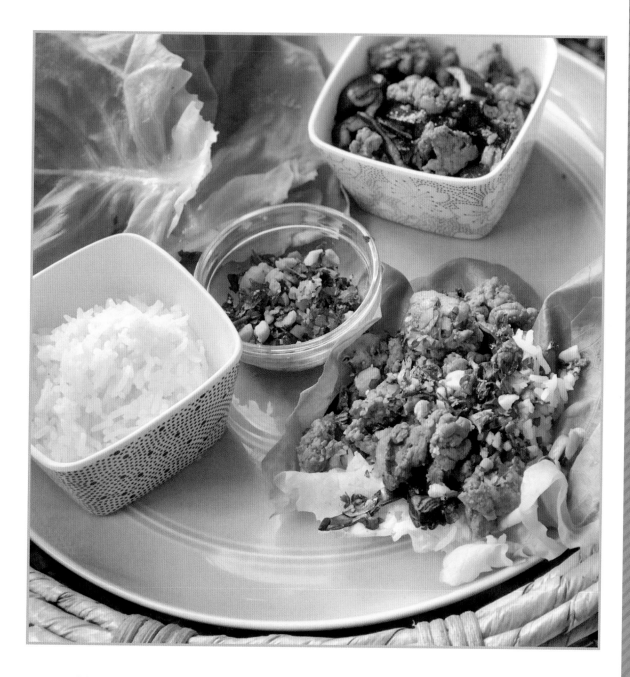

*Nutritional data reflects one serving, based on a 4-serving yield.*

**PER SERVING**  Calories: 757; Total Fat: 35.5g; Saturated Fat: 8g; Cholesterol: 182.5mg; Sodium: 1213.1mg; Total Carbohydrates: 57.6g; Dietary Fiber: 5.8g; Sugars: 11.1g; Protein: 53.1g

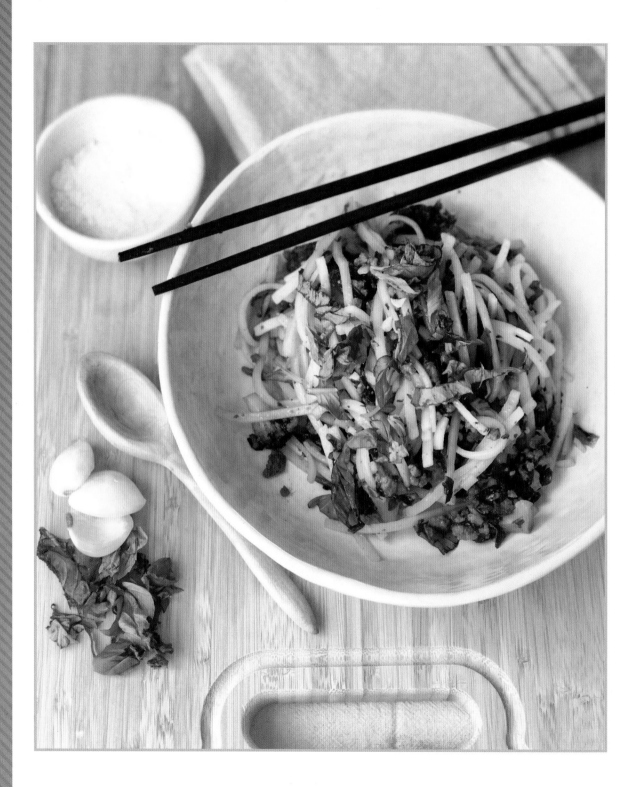

# Stir Fried Rice Noodles with Ground Beef & Basil

*Before I was diagnosed with celiac disease, I was a huge fan of the classic Thai dish pad see ew. Unfortunately, most restaurants use gluten-containing soy sauce and oyster sauce in the dish, making it off-limits for my gluten-free diet. Thankfully, there are now several manufacturers producing both soy sauce and oyster sauce using gluten-free ingredients, so I can enjoy a homemade version of this Thai delicacy.*

**YIELD: 4 SERVINGS**
Prep Time: 10 minutes
Total Time: 30 minutes

---

1 (14-ounce) package Pad Thai style rice noodles

½ cup gluten-free soy sauce

⅓ cup gluten-free oyster sauce

¼ cup water

3 tablespoons brown sugar

2½ tablespoons rice vinegar

2 tablespoons vegetable oil

1½ pounds ground beef

4 cloves garlic, peeled and finely minced

1 cup roughly chopped basil leaves, rinsed, patted dry, and divided

4 cups packed chopped Chinese broccoli, rinsed and patted dry

1. Prepare the rice noodles according to package instructions. Drain and set aside.

2. In a glass measuring cup, whisk together the gluten-free soy sauce, gluten-free oyster sauce, water, brown sugar, and rice vinegar. Set aside.

3. In a large, high-sided skillet or wok, heat vegetable oil over high heat. Add the ground beef and cook, stirring frequently to break the beef into small pieces, until the beef is no longer pink and starting to brown.

4. Reduce heat to medium and add the minced garlic and half of the basil. Cook, stirring occasionally, until the garlic is fragrant, about 2 minutes.

5. Add the Chinese broccoli and pour half of the sauce over the top. Cook, gently tossing all of the ingredients together, until the broccoli is soft, about 2 minutes. Add the noodles and remaining sauce and toss to combine until the sauce is clinging to the noodles, about 2 minutes.

6. Toss in the remaining basil and serve immediately.

*Nutritional data reflects one serving, based on a 4-serving yield.*

**PER SERVING** Calories: 932; Total Fat: 36g; Saturated Fat: 12g; Cholesterol: 150mg; Sodium: 1890mg; Total Carbohydrates: 94g; Dietary Fiber: 3g; Sugars: 10g; Protein: 55g

 **Dr. Bear Fun Fact!** Oyster sauce was invented by accident! In 1888, a Chinese man named Lee Kum Sheung, left oysters cooking on the stove for too long. When he tasted the dark brown sauce that had formed as a result, he started serving it at his teahouse! When shopping for oyster sauce, make sure to buy one using gluten-free tamari.

# Sweet Tamari Glazed Salmon

*This is the easiest dinner to make, and your family will think you spent hours slaving away in the kitchen. Just look at the gorgeous photo!*

**YIELD: 4 SERVINGS**
Prep Time: 10 minutes
Total Time: 25 minutes

---

6 tablespoons butter, divided
4 (6-ounce) salmon fillets
1 teaspoon salt
1 teaspoon garlic powder
¾ cup apricot preserves
⅓ cup gluten-free tamari soy sauce

**1.** In a large skillet, heat 2 tablespoons butter over high heat. Season each salmon fillet with ¼ teaspoon salt and ¼ teaspoon garlic powder.

**2.** Add the salmon to the pan and sear for about 3 minutes per side until starting to brown and the salmon is cooked through. Transfer salmon to a plate and cover with foil.

**3.** To the same pan used for the salmon, add remaining butter, apricot preserves, and soy sauce to the pan and whisk vigorously to combine.

**4.** Add the salmon back to the skillet with the sauce and baste the sauce over the salmon. Reduce heat to low and let the salmon sit in the sauce for about 3 minutes. Serve immediately.

 **Dr. Bear Fun Fact!** What's the difference between tamari and soy sauce? Both sauces are made from fermented soy beans, but tamari is more often found in Japan. Tamari tends to be darker, richer, thicker, and less salty than its Chinese cousin, soy sauce.

*Nutritional data reflects one serving, based on a 4-serving yield.*

**PER SERVING** Calories: 623; Total Fat: 31.2g; Saturated Fat: 12.9g; Cholesterol: 166.5mg; Sodium: 1360.8mg; Total Carbohydrates: 39.9g; Dietary Fiber: 0.3g; Sugars: 26.1g; Protein: 45.3g

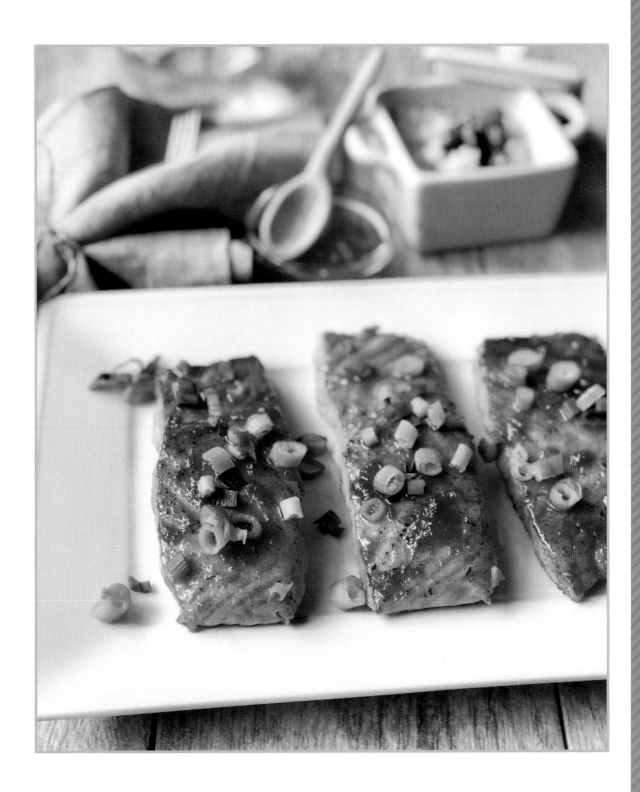

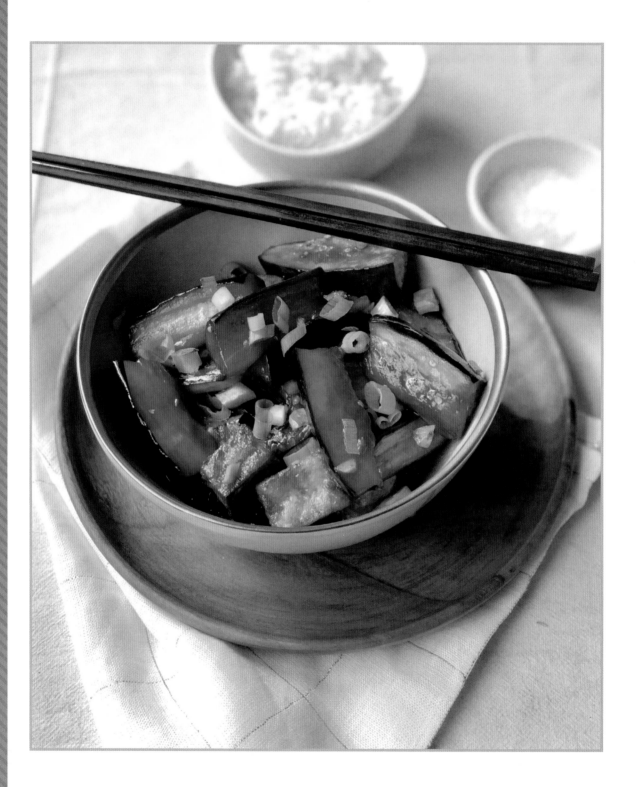

# Garlic Eggplant & Tofu Stir Fry

*I'm pretty sure my family will eat anything that's fried, including tofu. If your kids are a little wary about the brown sauce, keep the fried tofu separate and offer them the sauce on the side as a dip.*

**YIELD: 4 SERVINGS**
Prep Time: 15 minutes
Total Time: 30 minutes

---

1½ cups jasmine rice

¾ cup cornstarch

1 (14-ounce) package extra firm tofu, pressed dry with paper towels and chopped into bite-sized pieces

1 large eggplant, ends removed and chopped into bite-sized pieces

⅓ cup gluten-free soy sauce

4 tablespoons brown sugar

2 tablespoons gluten-free oyster sauce

1 tablespoon minced fresh ginger, peeled

1 tablespoon minced garlic, peeled

½ teaspoon red pepper flakes

4 tablespoons vegetable oil

½ cup chopped fresh basil leaves, rinsed and patted dry

**1.** Cook the jasmine rice according to package instructions. Cover and set aside until ready to serve.

**2.** Spread the cornstarch out on a dinner plate and roll the pieces of tofu and eggplant in the cornstarch to coat all sides.

**3.** In a glass measuring cup, whisk together the gluten-free soy sauce, brown sugar, oyster sauce, ginger, garlic, and red pepper flakes. Set aside.

**4.** In a large, high-sided skillet, heat the oil over medium-high heat. Add the tofu and eggplant and cook, tossing frequently, until the tofu and eggplant are crispy and golden. Use a slotted spoon to transfer the tofu and eggplant to a paper-towel-lined plate. Set aside.

**5.** To the same pan set over medium heat, pour the soy sauce and spices mixture and stir with a whisk constantly for about 2 minutes until the mixture thickens.

**6.** Reduce heat to low and add the tofu, eggplant, and basil into the pan. Toss to coat with the sauce.

**7.** Place a scoop of jasmine rice into a bowl. Top with a heaping portion of the eggplant and tofu mixture.

 **Dr. Bear Fun Fact!** Tofu is made from condensed soy milk. It provides lots of protein and contains all nine essential amino acids.

*Nutritional data reflects one serving, based on a 4-serving yield.*

**PER SERVING** Calories: 625.2; Total Fat: 19.7g; Saturated Fat: 3.3g; Cholesterol: 0mg; Sodium: 882.5mg; Total Carbohydrates: 94.8g; Dietary Fiber: 6.6g; Sugars: 16.5g; Protein: 18.1g

# Cod with Bok Choy & Ginger Cilantro Butter

*A simple compound butter brings big flavors to mildly flavored cod. I love serving this cod on top of steamed rice because it absorbs the wonderful flavors, but you could also use a gluten-free baguette to sop up the luscious butter.*

**YIELD: 4 SERVINGS**

Prep Time: 15 minutes

Total Time: 40 minutes

---

1½ cups jasmine rice

½ cup butter

½ cup fresh cilantro leaves, rinsed and patted dry

Zest of 1 lemon

2 scallions, ends removed and roughly chopped

1 tablespoon minced fresh ginger, peeled

1 clove garlic, peeled

4 teaspoons sesame oil, divided

1 teaspoon salt

3 cups thinly sliced shitake mushrooms, rinsed and patted dry

3 cups chopped bok choy, rinsed, patted dry

4 (6-ounce) boneless, skinless cod fillets

1 lemon, sliced into 8 thin round slices

**1.** Cook jasmine rice according to package instructions. Keep covered and warm until ready to serve.

**2.** Preheat oven to 450°F. Line a baking sheet with parchment paper and set out 4 large pieces of parchment to make packets for cooking the fish. Set aside.

**3.** In a food processor, combine the butter, cilantro, lemon zest, scallions, ginger, garlic, 2 teaspoons sesame oil, and salt and purée until smooth. Cover and refrigerate until ready to serve.

**4.** To assemble the cooking packets, place ¾ cup of mushrooms and ¾ cup of bok choy in the center of each piece of parchment. Place a cod fillet on top of each mound of vegetables. Sprinkle a pinch of salt and set two lemon slices on top of each cod fillet. Drizzle about ½ teaspoon of sesame oil over each fillet.

**5.** Fold the sides of the parchment together with the fish mixture in the middle. To seal the packets, start at the top corner and folder the paper toward you to create a seal. Press each fold as you go to seal the packets well, otherwise steam will escape. Bake for 14 to 16 minutes until the fish is cooked through.

**6.** Carefully open the sealed pouches and top with a generous portion of the ginger cilantro butter. You want the butter to melt down and around the fish and veggies.

**7.** Serve the fish and vegetables along with the cooked jasmine rice.

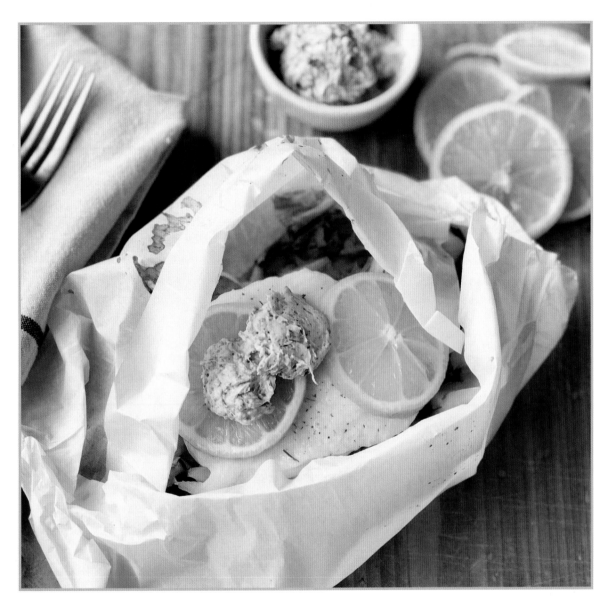

 **Dr. Bear Fun Fact!** Bok choy is a type of Chinese cabbage. It has been cultivated for 5,000 years! It contains high levels of Vitamins A and C.

*Nutritional data reflects one serving, based on a 4-serving yield.*

**PER SERVING** Calories: 680; Total Fat: 29.9g; Saturated Fat: 15.5g; Cholesterol: 154.6mg; Sodium: 767.3mg; Total Carbohydrates: 54.5g; Dietary Fiber: 2.1g; Sugars: 2.4g; Protein: 47g

# Thai Chicken Meatball Bowls

*These meatballs are a favorite in my house. I usually make a double batch and keep them in the freezer for a quick weeknight meal. They can be heated in the microwave in about a minute.*

**YIELD: 4 SERVINGS**
Prep Time: 15 minutes
Total Time: 45 minutes

### For the Chicken Meatballs

1½ cups jasmine rice
  (divided after cooking)
4 cloves garlic, peeled
3 shallots, skin removed and
  roughly chopped
½ cup fresh cilantro leaves,
  rinsed and patted dry
1 pound ground chicken
2 eggs
1½ tablespoons fish sauce
1 tablespoon sweet red chili sauce
Zest of 1 lime
1 teaspoon salt

### For the Cucumber Carrot Slaw

2 tablespoons lime juice
2 tablespoons gluten-free soy sauce
1 tablespoon rice vinegar
2 teaspoons sesame oil
2 cups matchstick-cut cucumbers,
  rinsed, patted dry, ends removed
2 cups matchstick-cut carrots
½ cup chopped unsalted peanuts
½ cup finely chopped fresh cilantro
  leaves, rinsed and patted dry
¼ cup finely chopped fresh mint
  leaves, rinsed and patted dry

**1.** In the bowl of a rice cooker, cook the rice according to package instructions. Once finished cooking, fluff with a fork. Scoop ¾ cup of rice out of the pot and set aside to cool. Then leave remaining rice covered until ready to serve. If you don't have a rice cooker, combine the rice and water in a medium-sized pot. Bring to a boil over high heat, then reduce heat to medium-low, cover, and simmer for about 15 to 18 minutes until water is fully absorbed.

**2.** Preheat oven to 450°F. Line two baking sheets with foil and set aside.

**3.** To make the meatballs, combine the garlic, shallots, and cilantro in a food processor. Pulse until finely chopped. Add the ground chicken, ¾ cup of the cooked and cooled rice, and eggs and pulse until well mixed.

**4.** Add the fish sauce, sweet red chili sauce, lime zest, and salt and pulse until the ingredients form a coarse paste.

**5.** Roll the chicken mixture into balls about 1-inch in diameter and place on prepared baking sheets. Bake for 10 to 12 minutes until cooked through.

**6.** While the meatballs are baking, make the slaw. In a glass mixing bowl, whisk together the lime juice, soy sauce, rice vinegar, and sesame oil. Add the cucumbers and carrots and toss to combine. Cover and refrigerate until ready to serve.

**7.** In a small bowl, mix together the chopped peanuts, cilantro, and mint. Cover and refrigerate until ready to serve.

**8.** To assemble the bowls, place a scoop of steamed rice in each bowl. Top with 5 meatballs and a scoop of the cucumber and carrot mixture. Be sure to get some of the sauce as well. Garnish with the peanut and herb mixture.

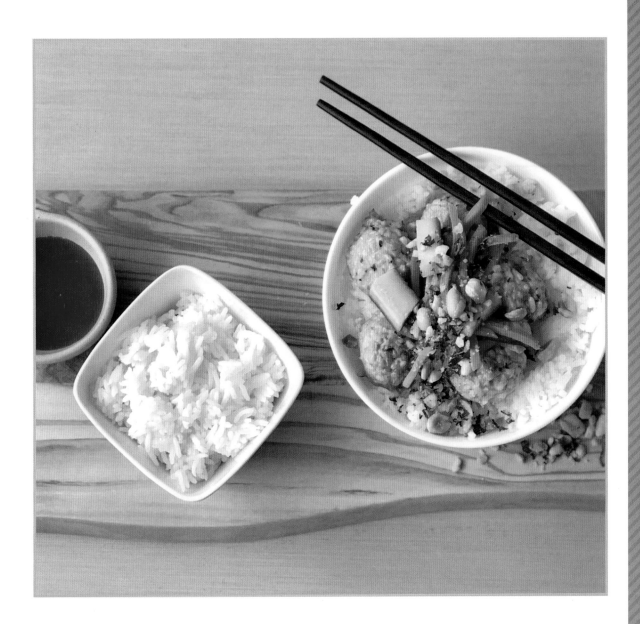

 **Dr. Bear Fun Fact!** Fish sauce is normally gluten-free, since it typically contains only fish and salt as the ingredients. Always check the label, though!

*Nutritional data reflects one serving, based on a 4-serving yield.*

**PER SERVING** Calories: 628; Total Fat: 23.7g; Saturated Fat: 5.3g; Cholesterol: 179.6mg; Sodium: 1631.7mg; Total Carbohydrates: 70g; Dietary Fiber: 5.9g; Sugars: 8.4g; Protein: 35g

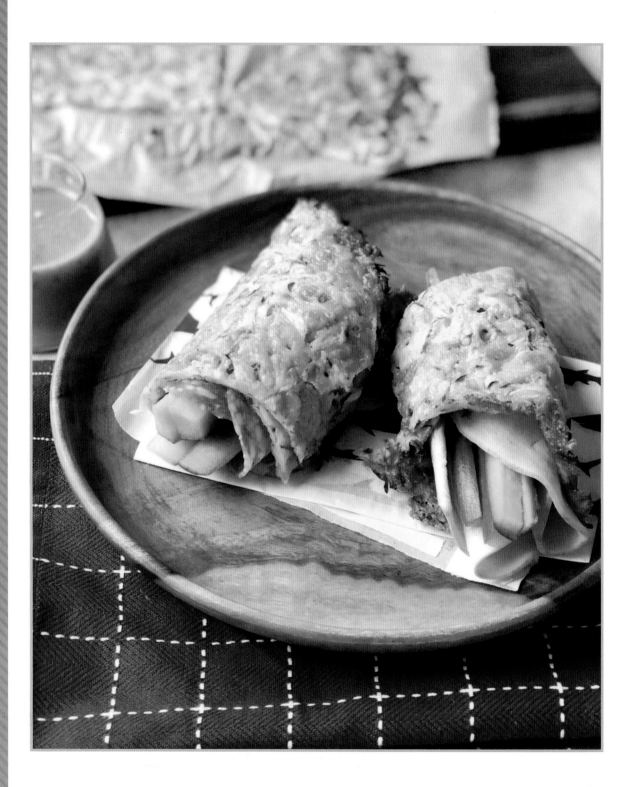

# Cheesy Zucchini Wraps

*My friend Jackie Kestler made these for me as a crispy cracker to use as a scooper for hummus. She gave them to me on a very busy day, so of course I waited far too long to eat them, and by the time I got around to it they weren't crispy anymore. Thank goodness, because now we have the Cheesy Zucchini Wrap! These wraps are a welcome change from the crumbly gluten-free tortilla options in grocery stores and taste excellent as a deli sandwich wrap with cucumbers, salami, turkey, and the Honey Mustard Dipping Sauce (page 319).*

**YIELD: 6 WRAPS**
Prep Time: 10 minutes
Total Time: 30 minutes

4 eggs
2 large zucchinis, ends removed and shredded
4 cups shredded cheddar cheese
½ teaspoon salt

**1.** Preheat oven to 450°F. Line three cookie sheets with parchment paper and, using a dark marker, draw 6 (6-inch) circles on the paper. Flip the parchment over. You should still be able to see the outline of the circles.

**2.** In a large mixing bowl, whisk the eggs together. Add the shredded zucchini, cheddar cheese, and salt and mix together well.

**3.** Evenly divide the mixture between the 6 circles on the parchment and press the mixture firmly down. Bake for 12 minutes. Rotate the pans in the oven and bake an additional 5 minutes.

**4.** Cool the wraps completely before removing from the tray. Assemble the wraps with your desired fillings.

 **Dr. Bear Fun Fact!** One zucchini has more potassium content than one banana!

*Nutritional data reflects one wrap without fillings, based on a 6-wrap yield.*

**PER SERVING** Calories: 368; Total Fat: 28.6g; Saturated Fat: 15.3g; Cholesterol: 184mg; Sodium: 733.4mg; Total Carbohydrates: 6g; Dietary Fiber: 1.1g; Sugars: 3.4g; Protein: 22.2g

# Creamy Tomato Pasta with Ground Beef

*This recipe is extremely versatile. I like using a store-bought marinara sauce that has basil in it, but any gluten-free marinara sauce will do.*

**YIELD: 4 TO 6 SERVINGS**
Prep Time: 5 minutes
Total Time: 25 minutes

---

1 tablespoon olive oil

1 pound ground beef

1 cup heavy cream

1 cup skim milk

2 cups tomato basil marinara sauce

1 teaspoon paprika

1 teaspoon salt

½ teaspoon pepper

1 (12-ounce) package gluten-free elbow pasta

1 cup shredded Parmesan cheese, divided

**1.** In a large, high-sided skillet, heat olive oil over medium-high heat. Add the ground beef and cook, stirring frequently to break the meat into small pieces, for about 5 to 7 minutes until the meat is no longer pink and starts to brown.

**2.** Pour out any excess liquid in the pan and then add heavy cream, milk, tomato sauce, paprika, salt, and pepper. Cook, stirring occasionally, until the mixture comes to a simmer.

**3.** Add the dry gluten-free pasta and stir until well combined. Cover the pan and cook over medium-low heat for 8 to 10 minutes until the pasta is tender. Stir about halfway through.

**4.** When the pasta is tender, remove the pan from heat and add ½ cup of the shredded Parmesan cheese and stir to combine well.

**5.** Scoop the pasta into serving dishes and garnish with remaining Parmesan cheese.

 **Dr. Bear Fun Fact!** Hungarians are famous for their paprika, but the peppers that are used to make it originate from the Americas!

*Nutritional data reflects one serving, based on a 6-serving yield.*

**PER SERVING** Calories: 689; Total Fat: 37.2g; Saturated Fat: 17g; Cholesterol: 126.5mg; Sodium: 1032.5mg; Total Carbohydrates: 53.4g; Dietary Fiber: 2.5g; Sugars: 6g; Protein: 32.7g

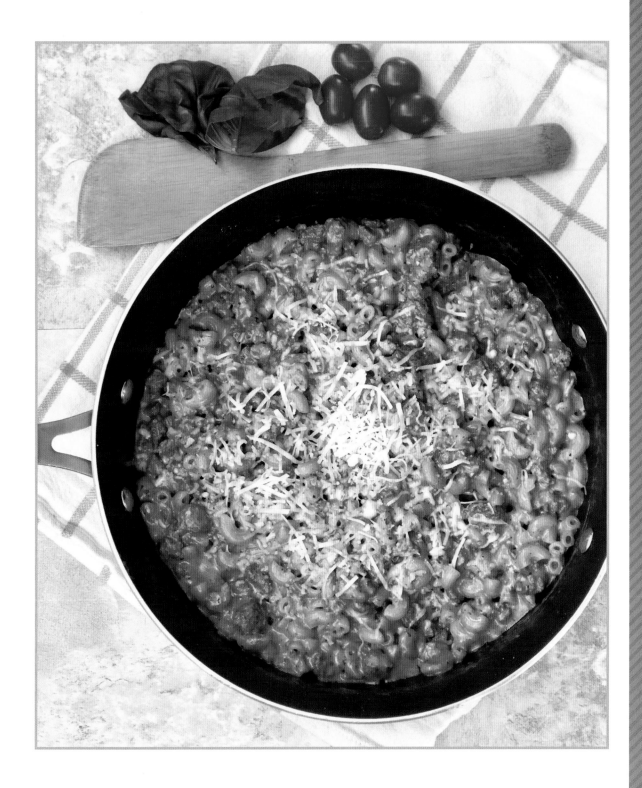

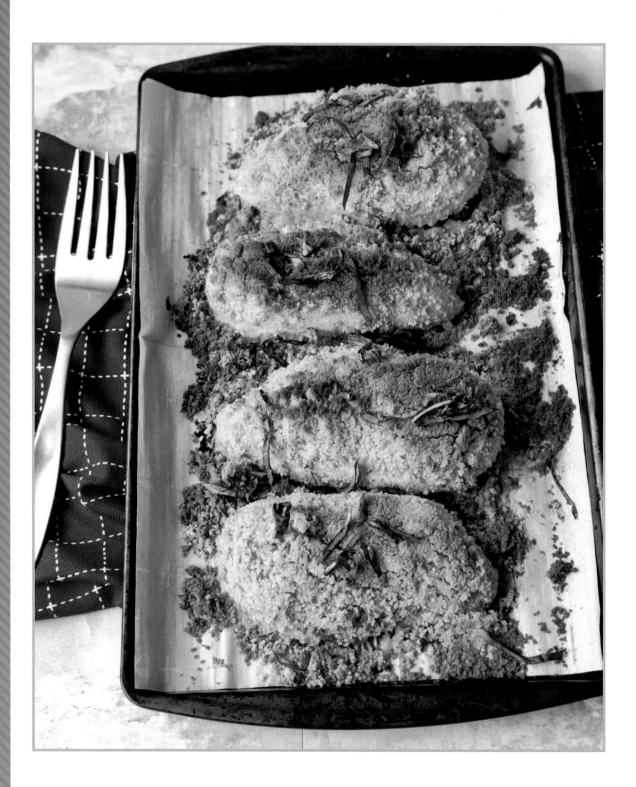

# Crispy Basil Dijon Crusted Chicken Breasts

*...ile chicken breasts are typically dipped in an egg wash before breading, if you have an egg ...ergy, that doesn't work! I came up with this idea when my egg-allergic friend Stefanie came over ...r dinner. And, I have to say, I like this version more. The creamy Dijon provides a flavorful base for adhering the breadcrumbs.*

**YIELD: 4 SERVINGS**
Prep Time: 15 minutes
Total Time: 40 minutes

---

4 boneless, skinless chicken breasts, rinsed and patted dry

⅓ cup crème fraîche

2 teaspoons Dijon mustard

2 teaspoons honey

1 teaspoon apple cider vinegar

1¾ cups gluten-free breadcrumbs

½ cup butter, room temperature

10 basil leaves, plus more for garnish, rinsed and patted dry

2 cloves garlic, peeled

Zest of 1 lemon

½ teaspoon salt

**1.** Preheat oven to 375°F. Line a baking sheet with parchment paper and place the chicken breasts on top. Set aside.

**2.** In a small glass bowl, whisk together the crème fraîche, Dijon mustard, honey, and apple cider vinegar. Spread this mixture evenly over the entire surface of each chicken breast.

**3.** In the bowl of a food processor, combine the gluten-free breadcrumbs, butter, basil leaves, garlic, lemon zest, and salt. Pulse until the mixture is combined and crumbly.

**4.** Use your hands to press the crumbly bread-crumb mixture over the top and sides of the chicken breasts.

**5.** Bake for 20 to 25 minutes until the chicken juices run clear and the chicken reaches an internal temperature of 165°F. Serve immediately.

 **Dr. Bear Fun Fact!** In addition to fantastic flavor, basil provides excellent sources of Vitamins A, $B_6$, C, and K!

*Nutritional data reflects one serving, based on a 4-serving yield.*

**PER SERVING** Calories: 662; Total Fat: 34.8g; Saturated Fat: 20g; Cholesterol: 171.7mg; Sodium: 1312.3mg; Total Carbohydrates: 46.2g; Dietary Fiber: 2.9g; Sugars: 3.5g; Protein: 36.3g

# Air Fried Old Bay Shrimp Bowls with Lemon Cilantro Aioli

*I'm absolutely obsessed with my air fryer. It cooks food so quickly and makes it wonderfully crispy without using oil. If you don't have an air fryer, don't worry. You can make this dinner in your oven. Just cook at 400°F for 10 to 15 minutes. Or, heat oil in a large skillet and fry until golden on all sides.*

**YIELD: 5 SERVINGS**
Prep Time: 20 minutes
Total Time: 45 minutes

---

**For the Lemon Cilantro Aioli**

½ cup mayonnaise

½ cup fresh cilantro leaves, plus more for garnish, rinsed and patted dry

¼ cup lemon juice

3 scallions, ends removed and roughly chopped

½ teaspoon salt

**For the Shrimp & Bowls**

1½ cups jasmine rice

1 cup corn starch

1 tablespoon Old Bay seasoning

Zest of 1 lemon

1¼ cups sparkling water.

1½ pounds (31 to 40 count) shrimp, peeled and deveined, patted dry

3 cups slaw mix

3 cups chopped butter lettuce, rinsed and patted dry

**1.** To make the lemon cilantro aioli, in a food processor, combine the mayonnaise, cilantro leaves, lemon juice, scallions, and salt. Purée until a smooth mixture forms. Cover and refrigerate until ready to serve.

**2.** Cook the rice according to package instructions. Cover and set aside until ready to assemble the bowls.

**3.** To make the shrimp, whisk together the cornstarch, Old Bay seasoning, lemon zest, and sparkling water in a large mixing bowl until a smooth batter forms. Place the shrimp in the batter and toss to combine.

**4.** Prepare the air fryer tray according to the appliance instructions for cooking shrimp. The instructions for my Cuisinart Air fryer suggest air frying the coated shrimp at 400°F for 8 to 10 minutes until golden and crispy.

**5.** While the shrimp are air frying, toss together the slaw mix and chopped butter lettuce in a large mixing bowl. Drizzle half of the lemon cilantro aioli over the top and toss to combine.

**6.** To assemble the bowls, place a scoop of rice in the bottom of each bowl. Top with a heaping portion of the slaw and lettuce mixture and then a scoop of air fried shrimp. Garnish with additional aioli and cilantro.

 **Dr. Bear Fun Fact!** Old Bay Seasoning is a staple in spice cabinets across the mid-Atlantic region of the United States. It's most popularly used to season crabs, shrimp, and French fries.

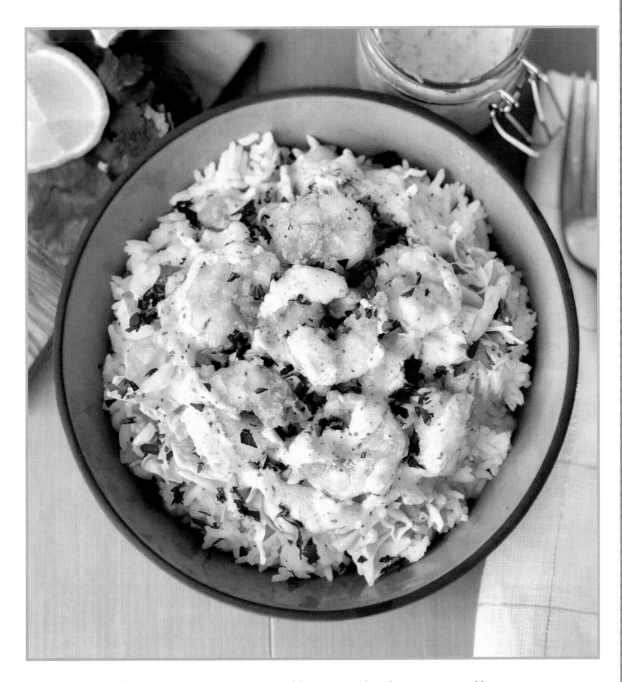

*Nutritional data reflects one serving with 2 tablespoons of dipping sauce, based on a 5-serving yield.*

**PER SERVING** Calories: 435; Total Fat: 5.9g; Saturated Fat: 1.1g; Cholesterol: 173.8mg; Sodium: 1046.3mg; Total Carbohydrates: 67.6g; Dietary Fiber: 1.9g; Sugars: 1.7g; Protein: 23.2g

# Penne with Veggie "Vodka Sauce" & Quinoa Chicken Meatballs

*Kids love meatballs. It doesn't matter if you use ground chicken, turkey, or beef, as long as they are rolled up in a cute little ball, most kids will eat them! Instead of using breadcrumbs, these meatballs are bound together using cooked quinoa, which adds protein, fiber, and essential amino acids. The sauce is a full serving of veggies puréed into a delicious sauce.*

**YIELD: 28–32 MEATBALLS (6 SERVINGS)**
Prep Time: 30 minutes
Total Time: 60 minutes

---

**For the Veggie Vodka Sauce**

1 pint grape tomatoes

1 eggplant, ends removed, sliced in half moons

12 baby carrots

1 sweet yellow onion, skin removed and thickly sliced

6 tablespoons olive oil, divided

1½ teaspoons salt plus a pinch

6 cloves garlic, peeled

1 teaspoon Italian seasoning

½ teaspoon paprika

½ cup chicken stock

**For the Meatballs & Pasta**

1 (12-ounce) package gluten-free penne pasta

1 pound ground chicken

1 egg, lightly beaten

1 cup cooked quinoa

½ cup part-skim ricotta cheese

¼ cup shredded Parmesan cheese, plus more for garnish

¼ cup chopped fresh parsley, rinsed and patted dry

Zest of 1 lemon

1 teaspoon salt

¼ cup olive oil

½ cup chicken or vegetable broth

**1.** Preheat oven to 450°F. Line a baking sheet with parchment paper and spread the tomatoes, eggplant, carrots, and onion slices out evenly across the pan. Drizzle 3 tablespoons of olive oil over the vegetables and rub to fully coat. Sprinkle 1½ teaspoons salt across the tops of the vegetables.

**2.** Place the garlic cloves in a small piece of foil. Drizzle 1 teaspoon olive oil and a pinch of salt over the garlic. Close the foil and place the wrapped garlic on the baking sheet next to the vegetables. Roast for 18 to 22 minutes until the vegetables are soft and golden.

**3.** Transfer the cooked vegetables and garlic to a food processor. Drizzle remaining olive oil, Italian seasoning, paprika, and chicken stock over the vegetables and purée until a smooth sauce forms. Set aside.

**4.** Bring a large pot of water to a boil over high heat. Cook gluten-free pasta according to package instructions. Drain and set aside.

**5.** To make the meatballs, mix together ground chicken, egg, cooked quinoa, ricotta cheese, shredded Parmesan cheese, chopped parsley, lemon zest, and salt in a large mixing bowl. Once combined, form into 1-inch meatballs.

**6.** To cook the meatballs, heat olive oil over medium heat. Add the meatballs and cook, turning frequently, until lightly browned, about 5 to 7 minutes. Remove the meatballs from the pan and put on a plate.

**7.** In the same pan used to make the meatballs, pour in the pasta sauce and whisk the chicken or vegetable broth in while heating over medium heat. Bring the mixture to a simmer, stirring frequently, and then add the meatballs back into the sauce. Spoon the sauce over the meatballs and cook for 3 to 4 more minutes to let the sauce soak into the meatballs.

**8.** Serve the meatballs and sauce over the cooked gluten-free pasta. Garnish with Parmesan cheese.

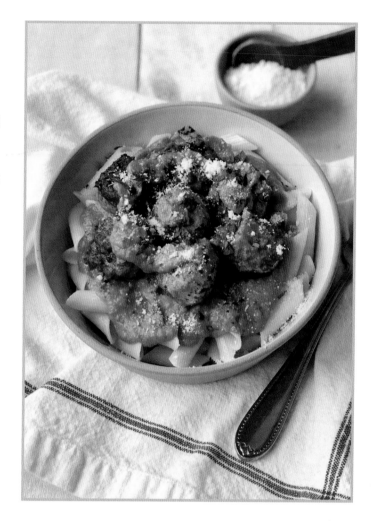

 **Dr. Bear Fun Fact!** Many think meatballs are an Italian dish, but meatballs are a food tradition all around the world! It's believed that they were first created in either Ancient Rome or Ancient Persia.

*Nutritional data reflects one serving of 5 meatballs, based on a 30-meatball yield.*

**PER SERVING** Calories: 678; Total Fat: 35g; Saturated Fat: 7g; Cholesterol: 102mg; Sodium: 1197mg; Total Carbohydrates: 67g; Dietary Fiber: 6g; Sugars: 8g; Protein: 26g

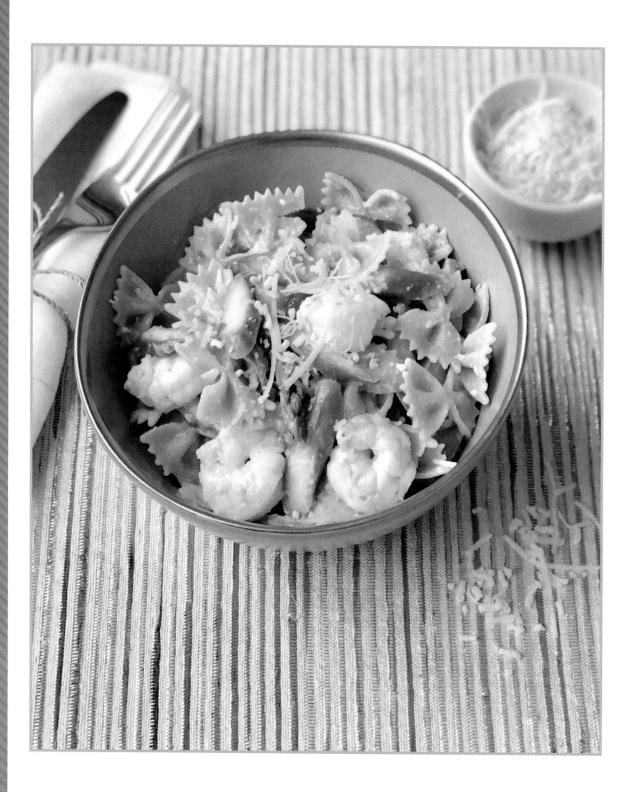

# Creamy Lemon Sautéed Shrimp & Asparagus with Bowtie Pasta

*My kids call this dish "Daddy Noodles" because it's my husband's go-to order in a restaurant even if it really isn't on the menu. And both of my boys happily eat it off of his plate. So, of course, I had to start making it at home. I hope your kids enjoy this recipe as much as mine do! While it's not the most glamorous job ever, my kids enjoy helping pull the shells off of the shrimp.*

**YIELD: 4 SERVINGS**
Prep Time: 10 minutes
Total Time: 30 minutes

---

1 (12-ounce) package gluten-free bowtie pasta

1 pound asparagus, trimmed and chopped into bite-sized pieces

1 tablespoon olive oil

1¼ pounds (21 to 25 count) shrimp, peeled and deveined

2 shallots, skin removed and finely minced

3 cloves garlic, peeled and finely minced

½ cup white wine

¾ cup chicken stock

½ cup lemon juice

1 (8-ounce) container mascarpone cheese

2 teaspoons lemon zest

1 teaspoon salt

Grated Parmesan cheese, for garnish

**1.** Fill a large pot with water and bring to a boil over high heat. Add the gluten-free bowtie pasta and cook according to package instructions, stirring occasionally. Add the asparagus pieces during the last 2 minutes of cooking. Drain pasta and asparagus under cold water and set aside.

**2.** In a large, high-sided skillet, heat olive oil over medium-high heat. Add the shrimp and cook, stirring occasionally, until the shrimp starts turning pink. Add the shallots and garlic and cook 2 to 3 minutes, stirring frequently.

**3.** Add the white wine to deglaze the pan and simmer until most of the liquid has evaporated. Add the chicken stock and lemon juice and bring to a rolling boil.

**4.** Reduce heat to medium and stir in the mascarpone cheese, lemon zest, and salt. Simmer, stirring constantly, for 3 to 4 minutes.

**5.** Toss the gluten-free bowtie pasta and asparagus into the shrimp mixture and stir to coat well. Divide the mixture into serving bowls and garnish with freshly grated Parmesan cheese.

 **Dr. Bear Fun Fact!** Mascarpone cheese is only made of two ingredients—heavy cream and lemon juice!

*Nutritional data reflects one serving, based on a 4-serving yield.*

**PER SERVING** Calories: 818; Total Fat: 34g; Saturated Fat: 17.5g; Cholesterol: 345.1mg; Sodium: 957.7mg; Total Carbohydrates: 78.4g; Dietary Fiber: 6g; Sugars: 6.9g; Protein: 48.6g

# Grilled Steak & Scallop Skewers with Herby Chimichurri

*Making skewers for dinner is a great way to let everyone have what they want for dinner without having to make four separate meals. Prepare all of the ingredients and let your kids pick what they want on their skewers. For example, Brandon will go surf and turf all the way by layering his skewer with steak and scallops. Leo won't touch the scallops but will stack his skewer with steak and zucchini. My husband and I like some of everything.*

**YIELD: 8 SKEWERS (4 SERVINGS)**
Prep Time: 10 minutes
Total Time: 30 minutes

---

**For the Herby Chimichurri**
½ cup olive oil
½ cup fresh cilantro leaves, rinsed and patted dry
½ cup fresh parsley leaves, rinsed and patted dry
⅓ cup red wine vinegar
1 tablespoon lemon juice
½ teaspoon salt

**For the Skewers**
8 wooden skewers, soaked in water
1 pound boneless top sirloin steak, cut into cubes
1 pound sea scallops, patted dry
4 zucchinis, ends removed and cut into 1-inch pieces
3 tablespoons olive oil
Juice of 1 lemon
1 teaspoon garlic powder
1 teaspoon salt

1. Combine all ingredients for the chimichurri in a food processor. Pulse until the ingredients are all well chopped and desired consistency is reached. This chimichurri can be as smooth or chunky as you'd like. Cover and refrigerate until ready to serve.

2. To make the skewers, thread the steak pieces, scallops, and zucchini, evenly dividing them amongst the 8 skewers.

3. In a small bowl, whisk together the olive oil, lemon juice, garlic powder, and salt. Brush this mixture thoroughly over the skewers.

4. Preheat the grill on high heat. Brush the grates with vegetable oil, then place the skewers onto the grates. Grill for about 3 to 5 minutes per side until the steak and scallops are cooked through and charred and the vegetables have softened.

5. Serve topped with the herby chimichurri.

**Dr. Bear Fun Fact!** Chimichurri originated in Argentina and Uruguay, likely from Basque settlers in the nineteenth century. The Basque word, "tximitxurri," can be loosely translated as "a mixture of several things in no particular order."

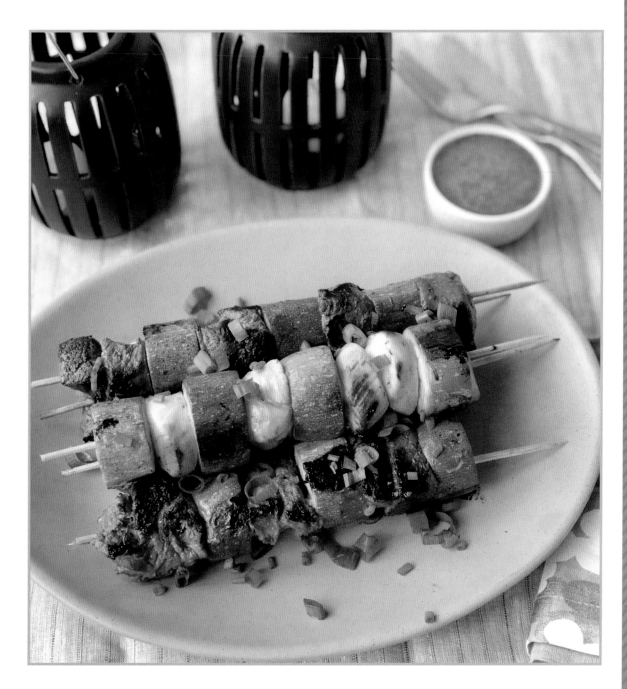

*Nutritional data reflects one serving with 2 tablespoons of Herby Chimichurri, based on a 4-serving yield.*

**PER SERVING**  Calories: 580; Total Fat: 30.8g; Saturated Fat: 5.7g; Cholesterol: 133.8mg; Sodium: 1599.4mg; Total Carbohydrates: 18g; Dietary Fiber: 3.5g; Sugars: 8.5g; Protein: 61.4g

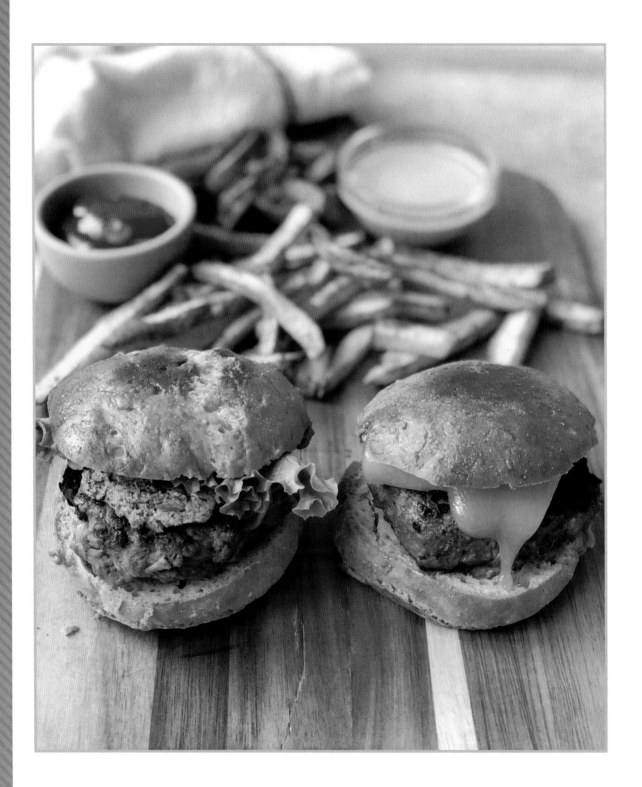

# Brandon's Blazin' Burgers

*My five-year-old son Brandon loves cheeseburgers. He would eat them every single day if I let him. Last year, I started trying some new techniques to squeeze more veggies into his diet and was pleasantly surprised that I got away with zucchini in the hamburgers. I piloted these burgers at a big family BBQ and found that every single kid ate the burgers, and no one mentioned the zucchini. So now, it's just the way I make burgers. The buns in the photo are from Rise Bakery in Washington, DC. I recommend finding hamburger buns at a bakery you like and stocking up on them.*

**YIELD: 6 SERVINGS**
Prep Time: 10 minutes
Total Time: 25 minutes

---

1⅓ pounds ground beef

1 cup shredded zucchini, ends removed

2 tablespoons Paprika & Herb Compound Butter (page 326)

½ teaspoon salt

6 gluten-free hamburger buns

Optional garnishes: sharp cheddar cheese, lettuce, tomatoes, sliced avocado, ketchup, Honey Mustard Dipping Sauce (page 319), etc.

1. Preheat grill to high heat.

2. In a large mixing bowl, mash together the ground beef, shredded zucchini, Paprika & Herb Compound Butter, and salt. Mix until very well combined.

3. Form the meat mixture into 6 evenly-sized hamburger patties.

4. Brush the grates on the grill with vegetable oil, place the hamburger patties on the grill, and cook for about 3 to 5 minutes. When you see the cook line reaching about halfway up, flip the burgers over and cook for an additional 3 to 5 minutes, depending on desired level of doneness. If you want melted cheese on the burger, place the sliced cheese on the burger during the last minute of cooking.

5. Serve on gluten-free buns with desired garnishes.

 **Dr. Bear Fun Fact!** While the history of the hamburger is unclear, the United States popularized the hamburger to specifically mean selling two slices of bread with meat in the middle.

*Nutritional data reflects one burger, based on a 6-burger yield.*

**PER SERVING** Calories: 455; Total Fat: 23.1g; Saturated Fat: 8.1g; Cholesterol: 89.3mg; Sodium: 683.3mg; Total Carbohydrates: 35.5g; Dietary Fiber: 4.1g; Sugars: 5.6g; Protein: 26.7g

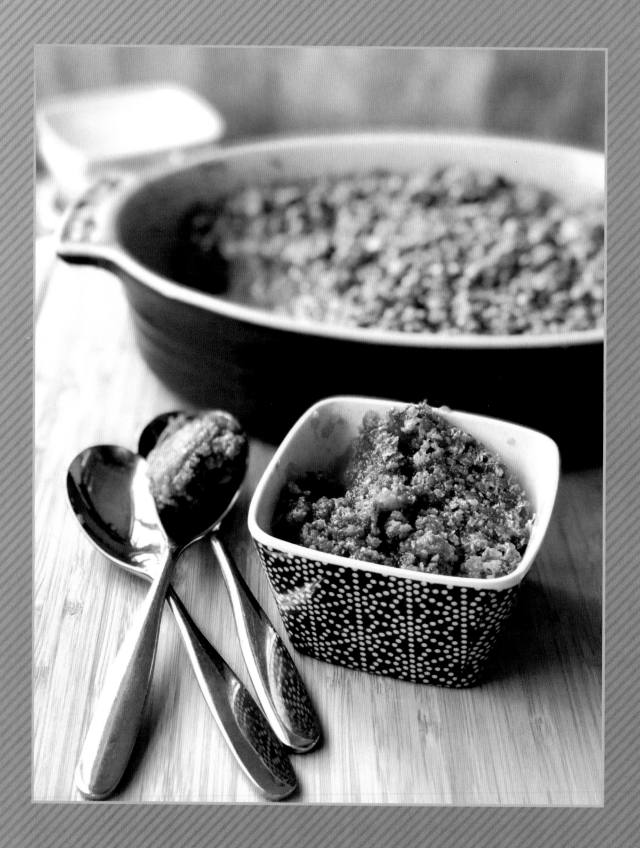

# 9

# Simple Side Dishes

Kid-friendly participation steps are printed in **ORANGE**

# Butternut Squash & Caramelized Onions Mash

*This is one of the most versatile dishes I make for my family. I serve it as a side, as part of a sandwich, a taco… the possibilities are endless! You'll see it in a number of recipes throughout the book. If you serve it as a side dish, top with crumbled goat cheese.*

**YIELD: 3 CUPS (6 SERVINGS)**
Prep Time: 10 minutes
Total Time: 45 minutes

---

2 pounds butternut squash, ends removed, peeled, and cut into 1-inch cubes

5 tablespoons olive oil, divided

1½ teaspoons salt, divided

¼ teaspoon paprika

1 large sweet yellow onion, skin removed, cut in half and thinly sliced

2 cloves garlic, peeled and thinly sliced

⅓ cup apple cider vinegar

⅓ cup maple syrup

Optional garnish: crumbled goat cheese

1. Preheat oven to 450°F. Line a baking sheet with foil and set aside.

2. In a large bowl, toss the cubed butternut squash with 3 tablespoons olive oil, 1 teaspoon salt, and paprika.

3. Arrange coated squash on the prepared baking sheet and roast for 25 minutes, stirring about halfway through cooking. The squash is done when it starts to brown and is soft.

4. While the squash cooks, add the remaining 2 tablespoons olive oil to a medium-sized skillet and heat over medium heat. Add the sliced onions and remaining ½ teaspoon salt and cook, stirring frequently, until the onions are very soft and beginning to brown, about 10 to 12 minutes.

5. Add the garlic and cook, stirring frequently until fragrant, for about 1 minute. Add the apple cider vinegar and maple syrup and cook, stirring frequently, until most of the liquid is absorbed, about 10 more minutes.

6. Combine the roasted squash and caramelized onions in a large mixing bowl. Mash the squash and onions together using a potato masher or fork. Leave as chunky or smooth as you like.

7. Serve the mash as a side dish garnished with crumbled goat cheese or use in the Butternut Squash & Caramelized Onion Risotto (page 147) or the Rotisserie Chicken & Butternut Squash Enchiladas (page 160).

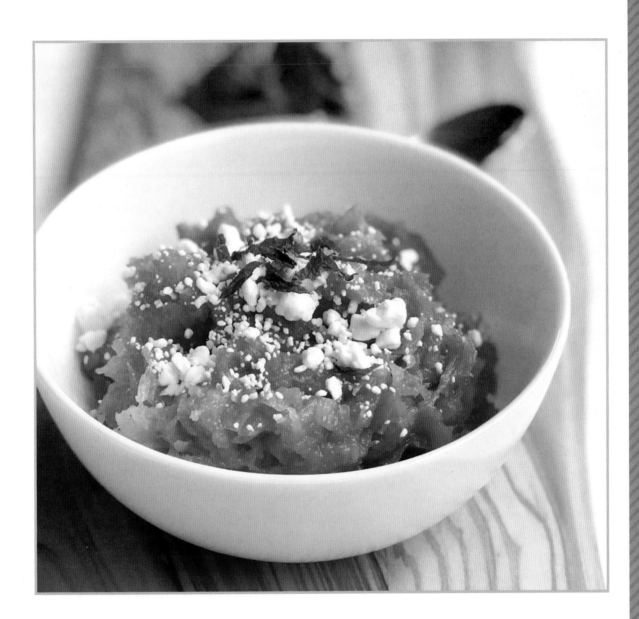

 **Dr. Bear Fun Fact!** Butternut squash and pumpkins belong to the same family! Try substituting pumpkin in this recipe for a slightly different flavor.

*Nutritional data reflects one serving, based on a 6-serving yield.*

**PER SERVING** Calories: 220; Total Fat: 11.4g; Saturated Fat: 1.6g; Cholesterol: 0mg; Sodium: 599.7mg; Total Carbohydrates: 30.3g; Dietary Fiber: 5.3g; Sugars: 14.6g; Protein: 1.7g

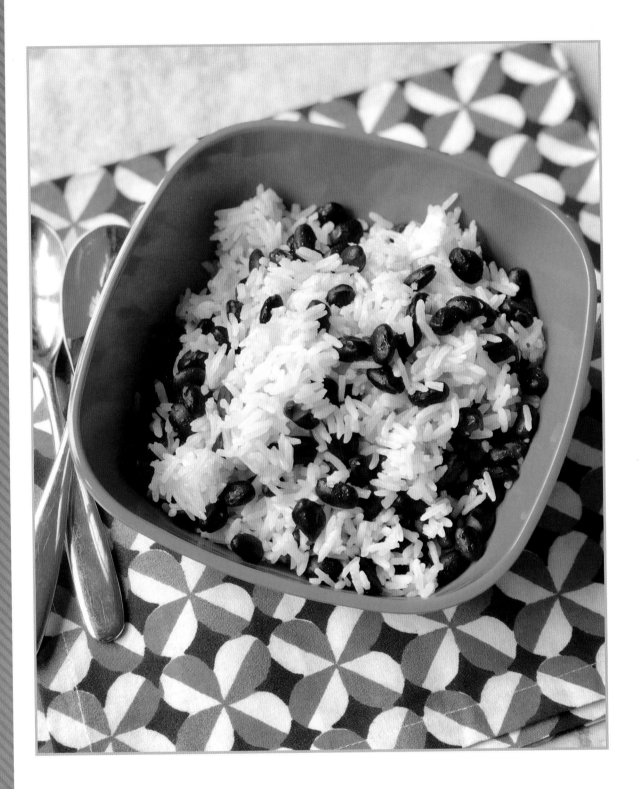

# Garlic Rice & Black Beans

*A simple side dish for any meal!*

**YIELD: 6 SERVINGS**
Prep Time: 10 minutes
Total Time: 30 minutes

1½ cups jasmine rice

3 tablespoons butter

2 tablespoons coconut oil

½ cup finely chopped sweet yellow onion, skin removed

4 cloves garlic, peeled and finely minced

1 (15-ounce can) black beans, drained and rinsed

2 teaspoons garlic salt

¼ cup finely chopped fresh cilantro leaves, rinsed and patted dry

**1.** Cook the rice according to package instructions. Set aside.

**2.** In a large sauté pan, heat butter and coconut oil over medium heat. Add the chopped onion and minced garlic, and cook, stirring frequently, until the onions are soft and translucent and the garlic is fragrant, about 5 minutes.

**3.** Add the cooked rice and, using a spatula, break up the rice and coat with the oil in the pan. Cook and stir until the rice is well coated.

**4.** Add the black beans and garlic salt and toss to combine. Taste the rice and add additional garlic salt, if desired.

**5.** Remove from heat and toss in the chopped fresh cilantro leaves.

 **Dr. Bear Fun Fact!** Versions of rice and beans are very popular in the Caribbean, and Central and South America! The dish provides many nutritional and caloric values, so this is a great side dish or snack for anyone—especially those who play sports!

*Nutritional data reflects one serving, based on a 6-serving yield.*

**PER SERVING** Calories: 353; Total Fat: 11.1g; Saturated Fat: 7.5g; Cholesterol: 15.3mg; Sodium: 599.2mg; Total Carbohydrates: 53.8g; Dietary Fiber: 8g; Sugars: 1g; Protein: 9.4g

# Cheesy Mexican Street Corn

*You'll see this dish often served while still on the cob. Meal time with young kids can be a messy affair at best, so taking the cob out of the equation can drastically cut down on the number of napkins I use to wipe mouths! It also means that I can mix the mayonnaise, queso fresco, lime juice, and paprika better throughout the dish so that every bite is uniformly flavor-filled!*

**YIELD: 6 SERVINGS**
Prep Time: 5 minutes
Total Time: 15 minutes

---

2 tablespoons olive oil

1 (16-ounce) package frozen sweet corn (I mix white and yellow corn)

3 tablespoons mayonnaise

1 cup crumbled queso fresco

Juice of 1 lime

½ teaspoon paprika

½ teaspoon salt

Chopped cilantro leaves for garnish

**1.** In a large skillet, heat olive oil over medium-high heat. Add the corn and cook, stirring frequently, until the corn begins to turn brown, about 7 to 9 minutes.

**2.** Remove pan from heat and toss in mayonnaise, crumbled queso fresco, lime juice, paprika, and salt. Garnish with chopped cilantro and serve immediately.

 **Dr. Bear Fun Fact!** In Mexico, this dish is called "elotes." If you want even more cheesy flavor, try adding some cotija cheese!

*Nutritional data reflects one serving, based on a 6-serving yield.*

**PER SERVING**  Calories: 223; Total Fat: 15.6g; Saturated Fat: 4.4g; Cholesterol: 18.4mg; Sodium: 411.8mg; Total Carbohydrates: 17.1g; Dietary Fiber: 1.7g; Sugars: 2.6g; Protein: 6.5g

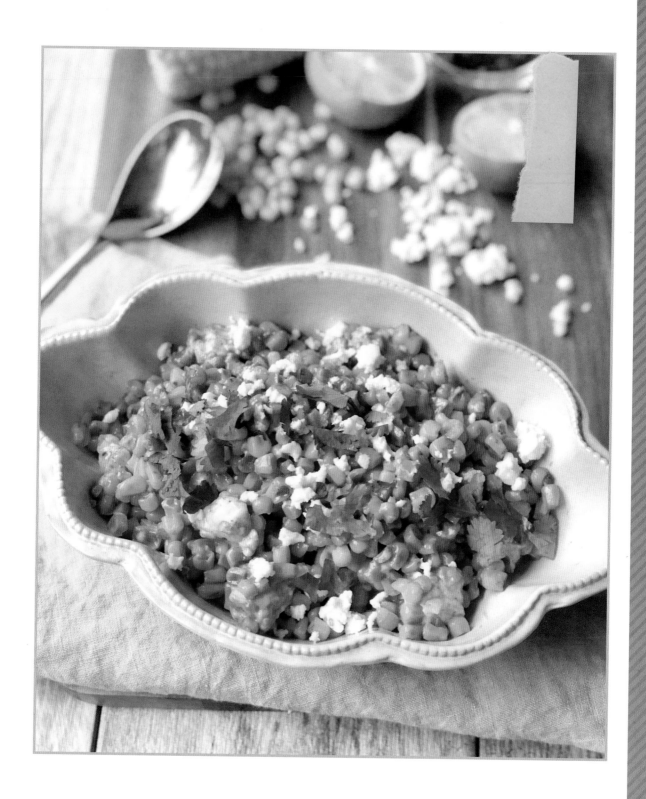

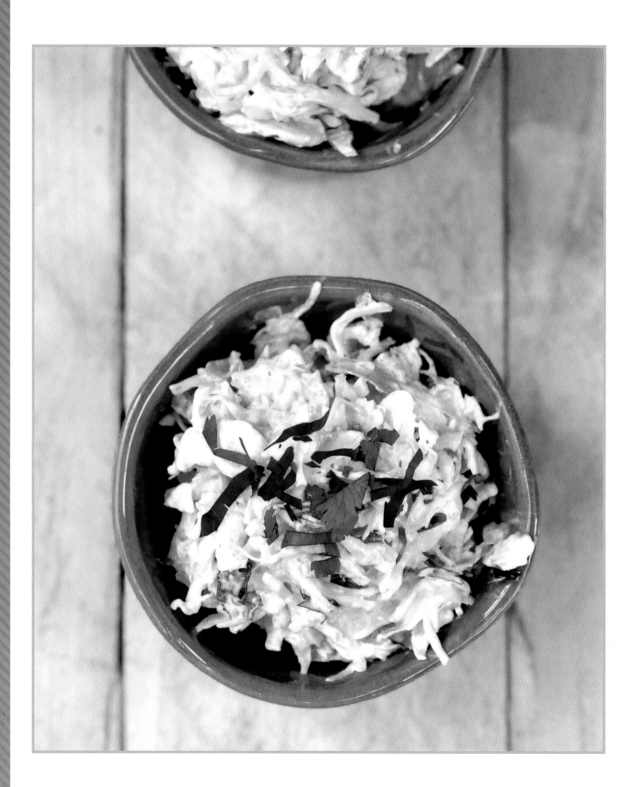

# Jalapeño Lime Coleslaw

*This slaw has just enough spice. If you like your food super spicy, double the jalapeños.*

**YIELD: 4 SERVINGS**
Prep Time: 5 minutes
Total Time: 10 minutes

---

¾ cup sour cream

Juice of 1 lime

2 teaspoons water

½ teaspoon garlic powder

½ teaspoon salt

1 teaspoon finely minced jalapeño, stem and seeds removed

½ cup finely chopped cilantro leaves, rinsed and patted dry

1 (14-ounce) package shredded cabbage coleslaw mix

**1.** In a large mixing bowl, whisk together the sour cream, lime juice, water, garlic powder, and salt. Add the minced jalapeño and mix well.

**2.** Add the chopped cilantro and coleslaw mix and toss together until well combined. Refrigerate until ready to serve.

**Dr. Bear Fun Fact!** Jalapeño peppers are picked before they are fully ripened! The longer they stay on the vine, the redder and spicier they become.

*Nutritional data reflects one serving, based on a 4-serving yield.*

**PER SERVING** Calories: 120; Total Fat: 8.4g; Saturated Fat: 4.4g; Cholesterol: 25.4mg; Sodium: 332.9mg; Total Carbohydrates: 9.3g; Dietary Fiber: 2.6g; Sugars: 5.3g; Protein: 2.4g

# Roasted Brussels Sprouts with Tamari Glaze & Crushed Peanuts

*These Brussels sprouts are excellent in the oven and even better in the air fryer.*

**YIELD: 6 SERVINGS**
Prep Time: 10 minutes
Total Time: 40 minutes

---

1 pound shredded Brussels sprouts

1 pound quartered Brussels sprouts

3 tablespoons olive oil

1 teaspoon garlic powder

1 teaspoon salt

¼ cup gluten-free tamari

2 tablespoons honey

1 tablespoon sesame oil

1 tablespoon rice vinegar

1 tablespoon creamy peanut butter

½ cup crushed, roasted and lightly salted peanuts

1. Preheat oven to 400°F. Line two baking sheets with foil or parchment paper and set aside.

2. In a large mixing bowl, toss together the shredded and quartered Brussels sprouts. Drizzle the olive oil, garlic powder, and salt over the sprouts and toss to combine.

3. Evenly distribute the Brussels sprouts on the two prepared baking sheets and roast for 25 to 30 minutes until browned to your liking. Stir the sprouts at least twice during roasting.

4. While the Brussels sprouts are roasting, in a small mixing bowl, whisk together the gluten-free tamari, honey, sesame oil, rice vinegar, and peanut butter. Set aside.

5. Remove the Brussels sprouts from the oven and transfer to a large mixing bowl. Drizzle the tamari glaze over the sprouts and toss to combine. Serve topped with crushed peanuts.

 **Dr. Bear Fun Fact!** Tamari is a good substitute for soy sauce. Soy sauce is usually fermented with wheat, but tamari is usually made as a byproduct of miso paste and is fermented without wheat. Tamari has a darker color and is richer in flavor but contains a similar amount of sodium as soy sauce. If you're watching your sodium intake, try a reduced-sodium version of tamari.

*Nutritional data reflects one serving, based on a 6-serving yield.*

**PER SERVING** Calories: 263; Total Fat: 16.9g; Saturated Fat: 2.5g; Cholesterol: 0mg; Sodium: 1163.3mg; Total Carbohydrates: 23.7g; Dietary Fiber: 7.1g; Sugars: 10.2g; Protein: 10g

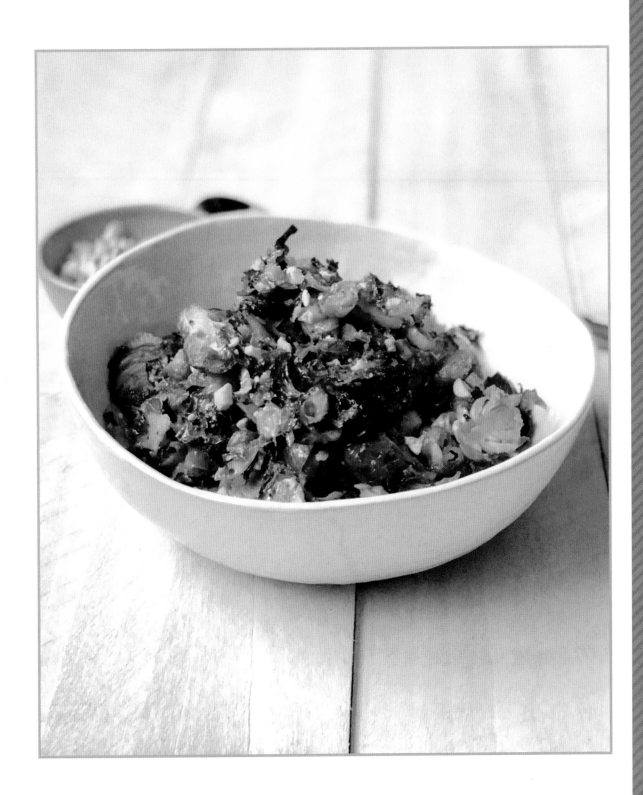

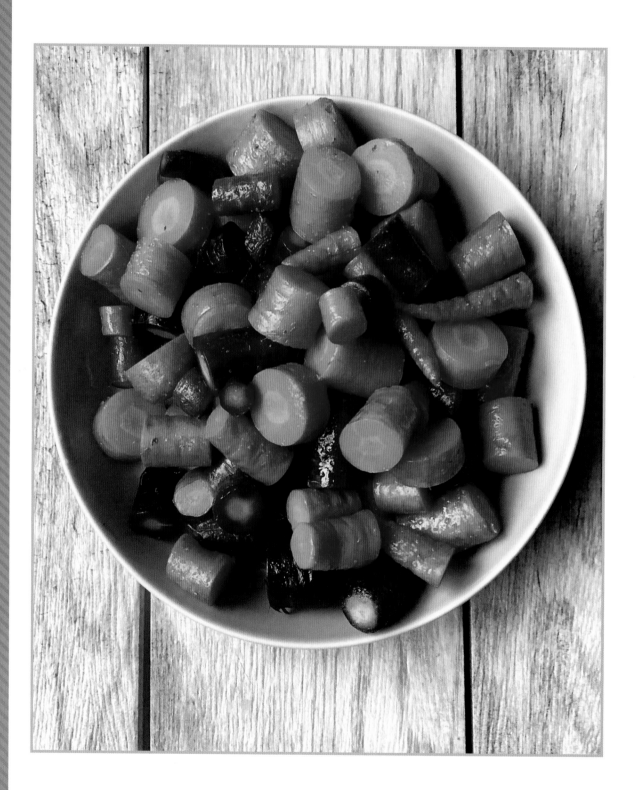

# Balsamic Glazed Carrots

*The balsamic glaze gives a lovely, tart sweetness to the carrots.*

**YIELD: 6 SERVINGS**
Prep Time: 10 minutes
Total Time: 40 minutes

———————

10 carrots, cleaned and sliced into
   1-inch thick pieces

3 tablespoons olive oil

1 teaspoon garlic powder

1 teaspoon salt

¼ cup balsamic glaze

**1.** Preheat oven to 400°F. Line two baking sheets with foil or parchment paper and set aside.

**2.** In a large mixing bowl, toss together the chopped carrots, olive oil, garlic powder, and salt.

**3.** Evenly distribute the coated carrots on the two baking sheets and roast for 25 to 30 minutes until soft and golden.

**4.** Remove carrots from oven and transfer to a serving bowl. Drizzle balsamic glaze over the carrots and toss to combine before serving.

 **Dr. Bear Fun Fact!** Balsamic glaze is just concentrated balsamic vinegar and sugar! Want to make your own? It's easy! Combine equal parts balsamic vinegar and sugar in a saucepan over medium heat. When all of the sugar has dissolved, bring the mixture to a boil. Immediately turn the heat down to low and let the mixture simmer for about twenty minutes or until the mixture has been reduced by half. It should be able to coat the back of a spoon. Let cool and serve!

*Nutritional data reflects one serving, based on a 6-serving yield.*

**PER SERVING** Calories: 120; Total Fat: 7g; Saturated Fat: 1g; Cholesterol: 0mg; Sodium: 463.6mg; Total Carbohydrates: 14.8g; Dietary Fiber: 2.9; Sugars: 9.5g; Protein: 1g

# Sweet Chili Lime Glazed Roasted Broccoli

*If I put large pieces of broccoli on the table, my kids will curl up their noses. But, if the pieces are nice and small and just the "leaves" part, they will eat them. So, I chop the florets extra small for the kids and leave them a little bigger for the grown-ups.*

**YIELD: 6 SERVINGS**
Prep Time: 10 minutes
Total Time: 40 minutes

---

2 pounds broccoli florets, rinsed and patted dry

3 tablespoons olive oil

1 teaspoon garlic powder

1 teaspoon salt

3 tablespoons sweet chili sauce

1 tablespoon gluten-free soy sauce

Juice of 1 lime

1 teaspoon garlic paste

2 tablespoons finely chopped cilantro leaves, rinsed and patted dry

2 tablespoons finely chopped mint leaves, rinsed and patted dry

**1.** Preheat oven to 400°F. Line two baking sheets with foil or parchment paper and set aside.

**2.** In a large mixing bowl, toss together the broccoli florets, olive oil, garlic powder, and salt.

**3.** Evenly distribute the coated broccoli on the two baking sheets and roast for 25 to 30 minutes until starting to brown.

**4.** While the broccoli is roasting, whisk together the sweet chili sauce, gluten-free soy sauce, lime juice, and garlic paste in a small mixing bowl. Set aside.

**5.** Remove the roasted broccoli from the oven and transfer to a large mixing bowl. Drizzle the sweet chili lime sauce over the broccoli and toss to combine. Add the chopped cilantro and mint and toss to combine. Serve immediately.

 **Dr. Bear Fun Facts!** Broccoli was eaten over 2,000 years ago in what is now Italy. It was considered to be very valuable in Mediterranean cultures. We can see why—broccoli is packed with nutrients!

*Nutritional data reflects one serving, based on a 6-serving yield.*

**PER SERVING** Calories: 140; Total Fat: 7.7g; Saturated Fat: 1g; Cholesterol: 0mg; Sodium: 712mg; Total Carbohydrates: 14.4g; Dietary Fiber: 4g; Sugars: 5.7g; Protein: 4.7g

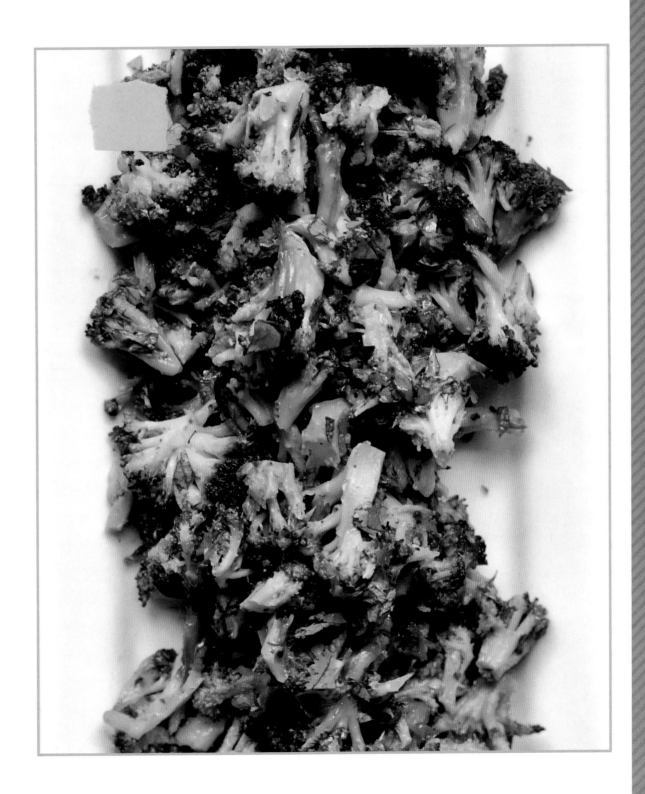

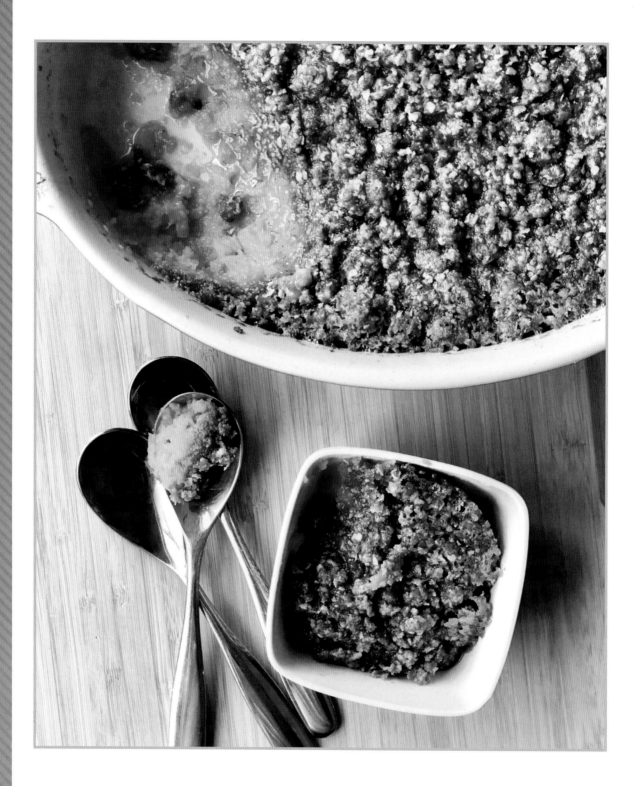

# Baked Mashed Sweet Potatoes with Crispy Oatmeal Coconut Topping

*Soft and creamy inside and crispy on top. This is the perfect side dish for a holiday meal.*

**YIELD: 8–10 SERVINGS**
Prep Time: 60 minutes
Total Time: 95 minutes

---

4 large sweet potatoes
1 cup granulated sugar
1 cup coconut milk
2 eggs
2 teaspoons vanilla extract
1 teaspoon sea salt
1 cup brown sugar
1 cup gluten-free quick cook oats
½ cup shredded coconut
½ cup cornstarch
1 teaspoon ground cinnamon
½ cup coconut butter/oil

1. Preheat oven to 400°F. Line a baking sheet with foil and place sweet potatoes on the lined tray. Using a fork, pierce several places on the surface of each potato. Bake for 45 to 55 minutes until the potatoes are very soft and easily pierced with a fork. Cool for 15 minutes or until cool enough to handle.

2. Preheat oven to 375°F. Spray a 9-by-13-inch baking dish with nonstick spray and set aside.

3. Peel potatoes and transfer soft filling to a large mixing bowl.

4. In a separate bowl, whisk together the granulated sugar, coconut milk, eggs, vanilla extract, and salt. Pour this mixture into the bowl with the potatoes, and mash together until smooth. Pour this mixture into the prepared baking dish. Set aside.

5. To make the crispy topping, combine the brown sugar, gluten-free oats, shredded coconut, cornstarch, cinnamon, and coconut butter in the bowl of a food processor. Pulse until the mixture is crumbly.

6. Sprinkle the crumbly topping over the sweet potato mixture and bake for 35 to 40 minutes until the center is set and topping is golden.

 **Dr. Bear Fun Fact!** Sensitive to oats? Try substituting quinoa flakes. They look and taste similar to oats, and you'll also get the health benefits of quinoa!

*Nutritional data reflects one serving, based on a 9-serving yield.*

**PER SERVING** Calories: 427; Total Fat: 17g; Saturated Fat: 13.4g; Cholesterol: 36.5mg; Sodium: 319.1mg; Total Carbohydrates: 65.8g; Dietary Fiber: 3.9g; Sugars: 41.4g; Protein: 3.9g

# Roasted Sweet Potatoes with Lemon Parsley Salsa Verde

*This dish looks as good as it tastes. If you get frustrated with arranging the sweet potatoes in the baking dish, don't worry about it. Just get them all in the pan. It will taste great no matter how they are arranged.*

**YIELD: 8 SERVINGS**
Prep Time: 20 minutes
Total Time: 70 minutes

---

### For the Sweet Potatoes

5 tablespoons coconut oil

5 medium-sized sweet potatoes, washed and thinly sliced into rounds

2 shallots, skin removed and very thinly sliced

1 teaspoon sea salt

### For the Lemon Parsley Salsa Verde

1 tomatillo, cut into quarters

1 cup flat-leaf parsley leaves, rinsed and patted dry

1 tablespoon fresh rosemary leaves, rinsed and patted dry

1 teaspoon fresh thyme leaves, rinsed and patted dry

1 garlic clove, peeled

Zest of 1 lemon

1 teaspoon lemon juice

½ cup olive oil

Sea salt, to taste

**1.** Preheat oven to 375°F. In a small bowl, melt coconut oil. Pour 2 tablespoons of the oil into the bottom of a 12-inch cast-iron baking dish and brush to evenly coat the pan. Set remaining mixture aside. If you don't have a cast-iron pan, use a 9-by-13-inch glass baking dish.

**2.** Arrange potato slices vertically in the dish and add slices of shallots between every few slices of potatoes.

**3.** Brush the tops of the potatoes with remaining coconut oil and sprinkle with sea salt.

**4.** Cover the potatoes with foil and bake for 40 to 45 minutes until the potatoes are tender. Remove foil and roast an additional 10 minutes or until the tops of the potatoes are lightly browned.

**5.** While the potatoes are cooking, make the salsa. In the bowl of a food processor, combine the tomatillo, parsley, rosemary, thyme, garlic, lemon zest, lemon juice, and olive oil. Purée until the mixture is well chopped and reaches the desired consistency.

**6.** Taste and add salt, as desired. Serve the salsa verde drizzled over the roasted sweet potatoes.

 **Dr. Bear Fun Fact!** Sweet potatoes are more closely related to tomatoes than to the common potato!

*Nutritional data reflects one serving, based on an 8-serving yield.*

**PER SERVING** Calories: 371; Total Fat: 29.5g; Saturated Fat: 11.9g; Cholesterol: 0mg; Sodium: 486.3mg; Total Carbohydrates: 25.6g; Dietary Fiber: 4.3g; Sugars: 6g; Protein: 2.5g

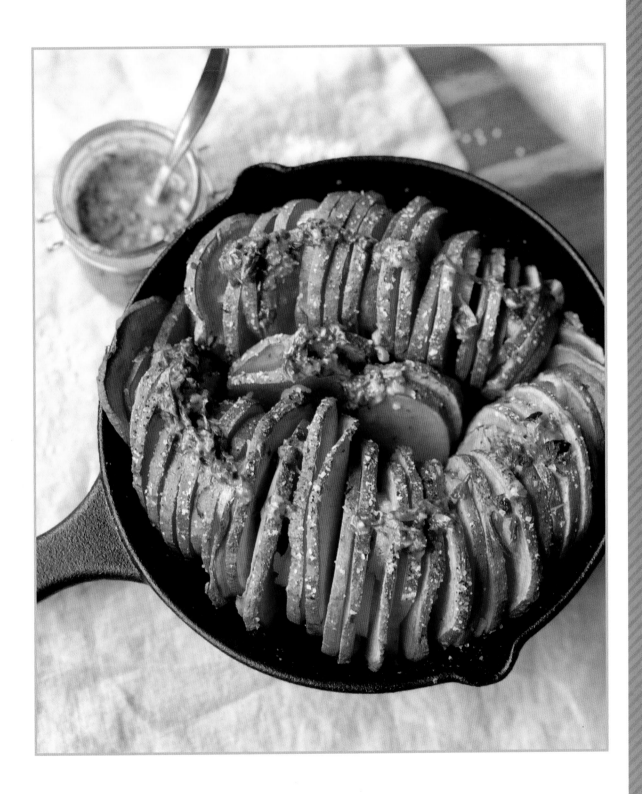

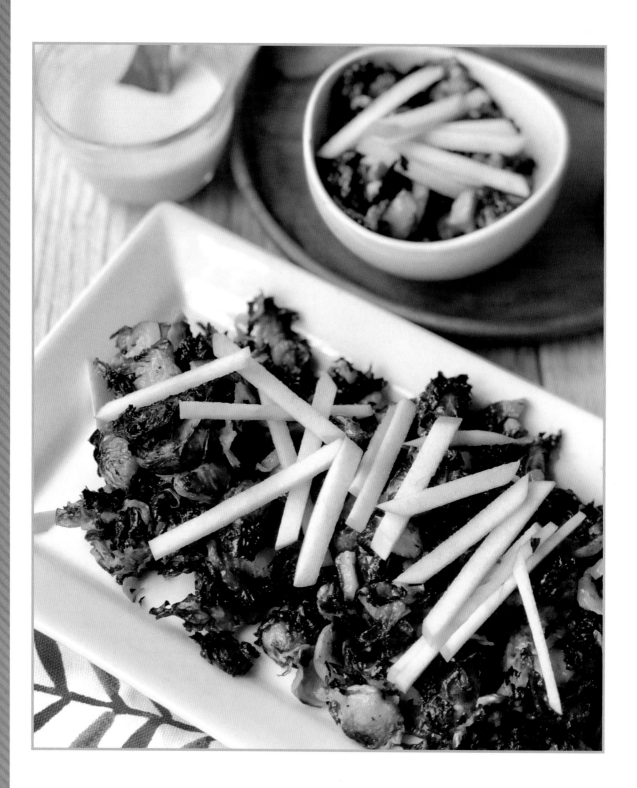

# Charred Brussels Sprouts & Green Apples

*This recipe is inspired by Paul at the Diplomat Resort in Hollywood, Florida. They serve the most wonderful Brussels sprouts I've ever had in a restaurant, and I was determined to figure out my own version of the recipe. Paul, this one's for you.*

**YIELD: 4 SERVINGS**
Prep Time: 10 minutes
Total Time: 30 minutes

---

1 (12-ounce) package shredded Brussels sprouts

1 (12-ounce) package quartered Brussels sprouts

3 tablespoons olive oil

1 teaspoon salt

1/3 cup crème fraîche

2 teaspoons honey

1 teaspoon Dijon mustard

1 teaspoon apple cider vinegar

1 Granny Smith apple, core removed and very thinly sliced

*Nutritional data reflects one serving, based on a 4-serving yield.*

**PER SERVING** Calories: 321; Total Fat: 21g; Saturated Fat: 8g; Cholesterol: 33mg; Sodium: 684.7mg; Total Carbohydrates: 30g; Dietary Fiber: 10g; Sugars: 13g; Protein: 9g

1. Prepare air fryer according to equipment instructions. If you don't have an air fryer, preheat oven to 450°F. Line a baking sheet with foil and set aside.

2. In a large mixing bowl, toss together the shredded and quartered Brussels sprouts, olive oil, and salt. Spread the coated Brussels sprouts on the prepared baking sheet or place in air fryer.

3. If using an air fryer, air fry at 400 for 10 minutes. Carefully remove from fryer and toss the Brussels sprouts. Air fry for an additional 10 minutes.

4. If using the oven, bake for 10 minutes. Carefully remove from the oven and toss the Brussels sprouts. Bake for an additional 10 minutes.

5. While the Brussels sprouts are cooking, whisk together the crème fraîche, Dijon mustard, honey, and apple cider vinegar in a small glass bowl. Cover and refrigerate until ready to serve.

6. Remove the Brussels sprouts from the air fryer or oven and place in a large bowl. Drizzle the Dijon sauce over the sprouts and toss to combine.

7. Serve the Brussels sprouts topped with the sliced Granny Smith apple.

 **Dr. Bear Fun Fact!** Crème fraîche and sour cream are made similarly, but are not exactly the same. Sour cream has less fat than crème fraîche but has a tangier taste!

# Carrot Soufflés

*These soufflés are a recipe from Jackie Kestler, and I love how beautifully bright orange they are!*
*They are a sweet delight to serve alongside grilled chicken and veggies.*

**YIELD: 6 SERVINGS**
Prep Time: 15 minutes
Total Time: 75 minutes

---

2 pounds carrots, ends removed, peeled, and roughly chopped

½ cup butter, room temperature

3 eggs

2 tablespoons gluten-free all-purpose flour

2 tablespoons sugar

2 tablespoons maple syrup

2 teaspoons baking powder

1 teaspoon vanilla extract

Powdered sugar, for garnish

**1.** Preheat oven to 350°F. Spray 6 (8-ounce) ramekins with nonstick spray and place on a baking sheet. Set aside.

**2.** Place chopped carrots in a microwave safe bowl. Pour enough water over carrots to cover them about halfway. Place a paper towel over the top of the bowl and place in the microwave. Microwave on high heat for 5 minutes. Drain the carrots completely and let cool for 5 minutes.

**3.** Place the steamed carrots in the bowl of a food processor. Pulse until smooth. Add the butter, eggs, gluten-free all-purpose flour, sugar, maple syrup, baking powder, and vanilla extract and purée until smooth.

**4.** Fill each of the prepared ramekins about ¾ of the way full. Bake for 60 to 65 minutes until the center of the soufflés are set.

**5.** Cool completely and dust with powdered sugar before serving.

 **Dr. Bear Fun Fact!** Soufflés were created in the eighteenth century in France. The name comes from the French verb "souffler," which means "to breathe" or "to inflate."

*Nutritional data reflects one serving, based on a 6-serving yield.*

**PER SERVING** Calories: 279; Total Fat: 18.1g; Saturated Fat: 10.3g; Cholesterol: 122.7mg; Sodium: 297.3mg; Total Carbohydrates: 26.5g; Dietary Fiber: 4.3g; Sugars: 16.3g; Protein: 4.5g

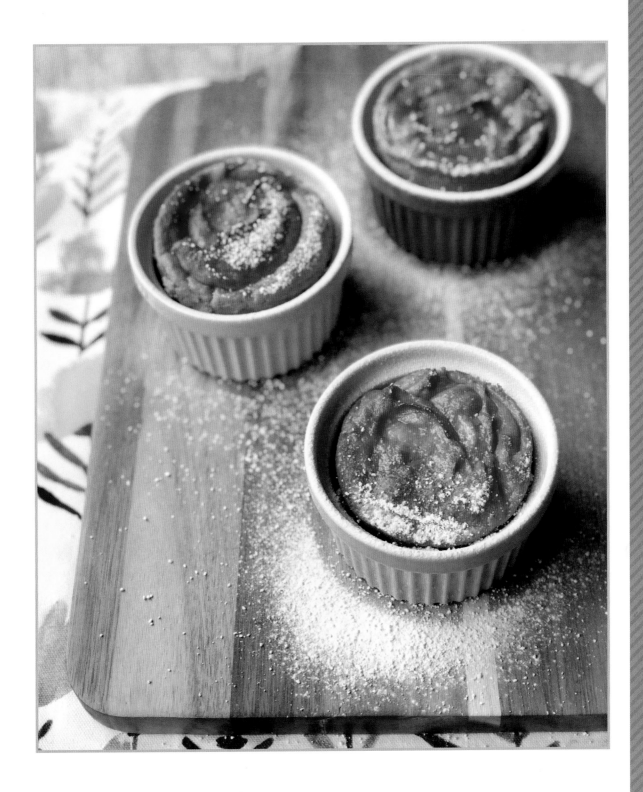

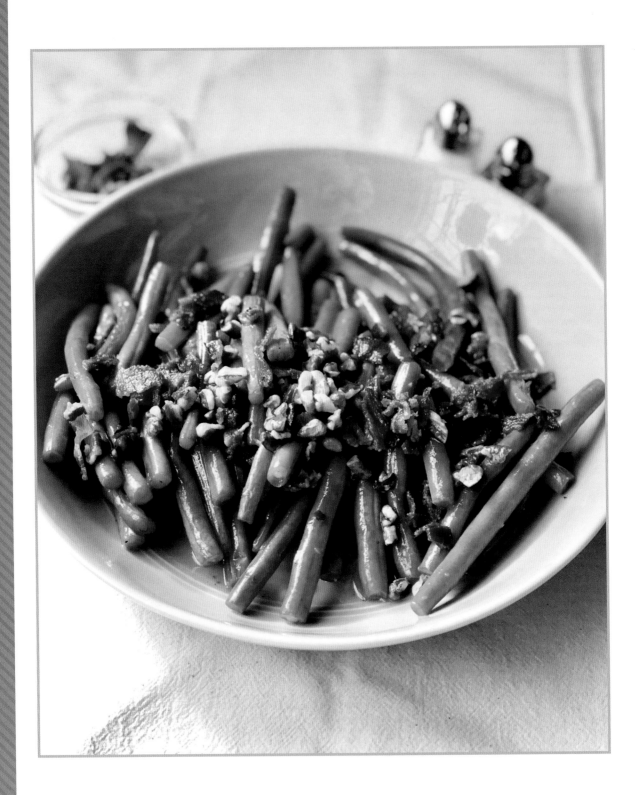

# Maple Dijon Green Beans with Ripped Bacon & Pecans

*These are Jackie's famous green beans. The maple Dijon dressing is a divine addition to the salty bacon and crisp beans.*

**YIELD: 4 SERVINGS**
Prep Time: 25 minutes
Total Time: 35 minutes

——————

6 slices bacon
1 garlic clove
3 tablespoons maple syrup
3 tablespoons olive oil, divided
1 tablespoon red wine vinegar
1 teaspoon Dijon mustard
1 pound fresh green beans, ends trimmed
¼ teaspoon salt
¼ cup chopped pecans

**1.** Preheat oven to 400°F. Line a baking sheet with foil, and lay out slices of bacon. Cook for 15 to 20 minutes until the bacon is crispy. Remove from oven and set aside. Once the bacon is cooled, chop into small pieces.

**2.** In the bowl of a small food processor, combine the garlic, maple syrup, 2 tablespoons olive oil, red wine vinegar, and Dijon mustard and pulse until a smooth mixture forms. Set aside until ready to serve.

**3.** In a large skillet, heat remaining 1 tablespoon olive oil over medium-high heat. Add the green beans and cook, stirring frequently until slightly softened, for about 3 to 5 minutes.

**4.** Transfer the green beans to a serving bowl and toss with the Maple Dijon Dressing. Top with the chopped bacon and pecans.

 **Dr. Bear Fun Fact!** Dijon mustard was named after the city of Dijon, France, as it was the center of mustard production in the Middle Ages!

*Nutritional data reflects one serving, based on a 4-serving yield.*

**PER SERVING** Calories: 210; Total Fat: 12.8g; Saturated Fat: 2.4g; Cholesterol: 11.9mg; Sodium: 388.5mg; Total Carbohydrates: 19.3g; Dietary Fiber: 3.8g; Sugars: 13g; Protein: 6.9g

# Smashed Potatoes with Sea Salt & Vinegar

*My friend Jackie is my side dish superstar. With just a few simple ingredients she taught me to make these awesome salty potatoes.*

**YIELD: 4 SERVINGS**
Prep Time: 20 minutes
Total Time: 60 minutes

---

2 pounds Yukon Gold baby potatoes, rinsed and patted dry

2 teaspoons coarse sea salt, divided

2 tablespoons coconut oil

2 tablespoons olive oil

2 tablespoons white vinegar

**1.** Preheat oven to 450°F. Line a large baking sheet with parchment paper and set aside.

**2.** In a medium-sized sauce pot, place the potatoes and 1 teaspoon sea salt. Add enough water to the pot to fully submerge the potatoes. Bring the mixture to a simmer over medium heat. Cover and let the potatoes cook for about 15 to 20 minutes until tender.

**3.** Drain the potatoes and return to warm pot. Add the coconut oil and toss to coat the potatoes with the oil.

**4.** Transfer the potatoes to the prepared baking sheet, and set them out evenly across the pan. Using a heavy glass or mallet, smash each potato to about ½-inch thickness. Bake for 20 minutes.

**5.** Remove the potatoes from the oven and, using a spatula, flip the potatoes over. Drizzle olive oil over the potatoes and bake for an additional 20 minutes.

**6.** Remove potatoes from the oven and drizzle the white vinegar and remaining sea salt over the tops of the potatoes. Serve immediately.

 **Dr. Bear Fun Fact!** No type of salt is more or less nutritious than another—it's just a matter of personal taste!

*Nutritional data reflects one serving, based on a 4-serving yield.*
**PER SERVING** Calories: 285; Total Fat: 13.5g; Saturated Fat: 6.6g; Cholesterol: 0mg; Sodium: 1241mg; Total Carbohydrates: 41.2g; Dietary Fiber: 4.1g; Sugars: 2.1g; Protein: 4.1g

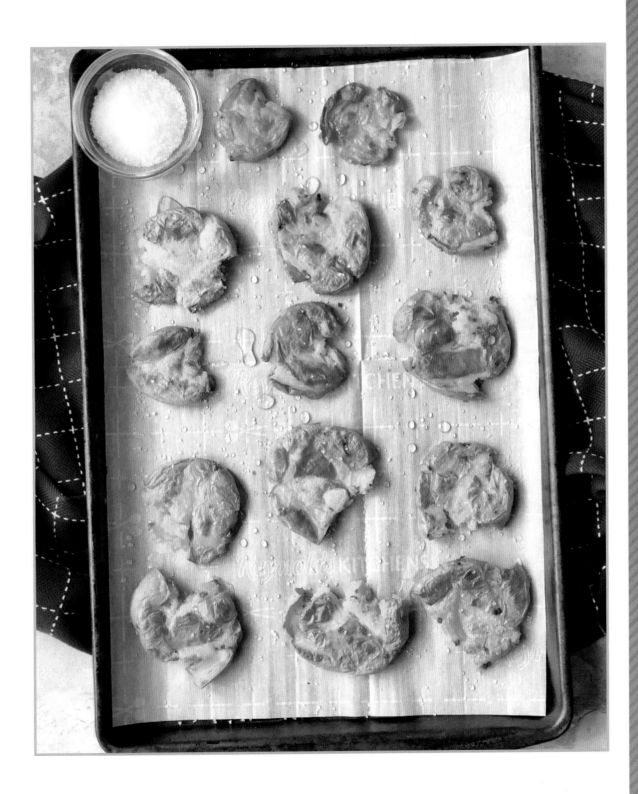

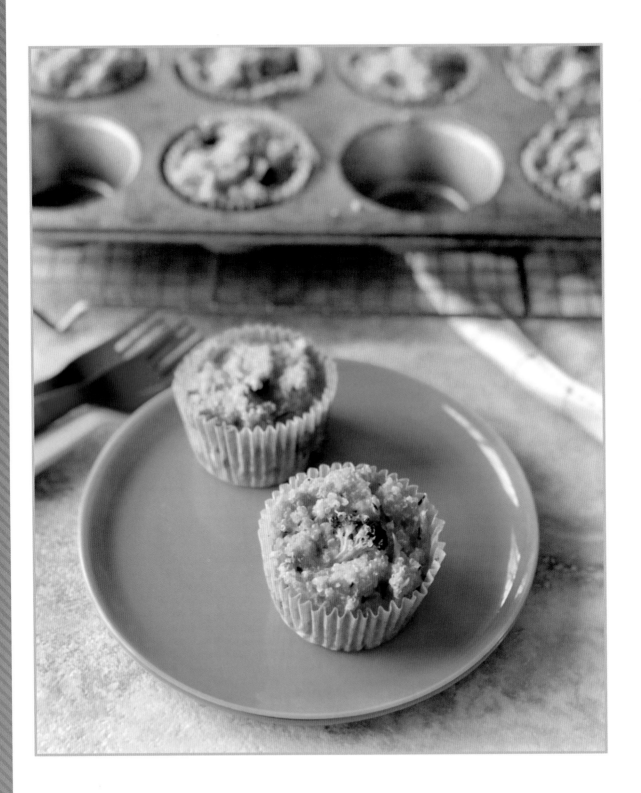

# Cheesy Quinoa Cakes

*The recipe calls for broccoli, carrots, and zucchini, but any veggies can be tossed into these cheesy quinoa cakes. If dairy is an issue in your house, try substituting the coconut-based cheddar shreds. They melt and taste great in these cakes.*

**YIELD: 12 QUINOA CAKES**
Prep Time: 20 minutes
Total Time: 75 minutes

---

2 tablespoons olive oil

2 cloves garlic, peeled and finely minced

1 cup grated zucchini, ends removed

1 cup chopped broccoli, rinsed and patted dry

1 cup grated carrots, ends removed and peeled

½ teaspoon salt

½ teaspoon pepper

2½ cups cooked and cooled quinoa

1½ cups shredded cheddar cheese

2 eggs, beaten

**1.** Preheat oven to 350°F. Line a 12-cup muffin tin with cupcake liners or spray with nonstick spray. Set aside.

**2.** In a large, high-sided sauté pan, heat olive oil over medium heat. Add the garlic and cook for about 2 minutes, stirring frequently until the garlic is soft and fragrant. Add the zucchini, broccoli, and carrots and cook, stirring occasionally, until the vegetables are soft and most of the liquid is evaporated, about 5 minutes. Add the salt and pepper and toss to combine. Remove the pan from heat and set aside to cool completely.

**3.** In a large mixing bowl, mix together the cooled quinoa, vegetables, cheddar cheese, and beaten eggs. Mix until thoroughly combined.

**4.** Divide the mixture evenly among the 12 prepared muffin cups and bake for 20 to 25 minutes until golden. Serve immediately or cool and store in an airtight container in the refrigerator.

 **Dr. Bear Fun Fact!** The Andean people in South America first domesticated quinoa around 3,000 to 4,000 years ago!

*Nutritional data reflects one cake, based on a 12-serving yield.*

**PER SERVING** Calories: 146; Total Fat: 8.6g; Saturated Fat: 3.3g; Cholesterol: 41.3mg; Sodium: 214.8mg; Total Carbohydrates: 11.1g; Dietary Fiber: 1.8g; Sugars: 1.5g; Protein: 6.4g

# Crispy French Fries

*I'm pretty certain that every child loves French fries! My kids equally love traditional russet potato fries and sweet potato fries, so I usually buy two of each type and mix them up!*

**YIELD: 4 SERVINGS**
Prep Time: 10 minutes
Total Time: 30 minutes

---

2 large sweet potatoes, rinsed, patted dry, and cut into ¼-inch matchsticks

2 large russet potatoes, rinsed, patted dry, and cut into ¼-inch matchsticks

3 tablespoons canola oil

1 teaspoon sea salt

For garnish: ketchup or honey mustard dipping sauce

1. Preheat oven to 450°F. Line two baking sheets with parchment paper and set aside.

2. In a large mixing bowl, toss together the cut sweet potatoes, russet potatoes, oil, and sea salt.

3. Transfer the coated potatoes to the baking sheets, making sure to spread them out evenly.

4. Bake for 25 to 35 minutes until the potatoes are golden and crispy. You will want to remove the pan from the oven and toss the fries at least twice during baking to ensure the fries cook evenly.

5. Remove from oven and serve with ketchup or honey mustard dipping sauce.

 **Dr. Bear Fun Fact!** American soldiers stationed in Belgium were first introduced to French fries during World War I. Since the language of Belgians was French, soldiers called the delicious fried potatoes "French fries." The name stuck, and decades later we're still giving credit to the wrong country.

*Nutritional data reflects one serving without garnishes, based on a 4-serving yield.*

**PER SERVING** Calories: 302; Total Fat: 10.4g; Saturated Fat: 0.8g; Cholesterol: 0mg; Sodium: 640.5mg; Total Carbohydrates: 48.6g; Dietary Fiber: 4.7g; Sugars: 4.3g; Protein: 5.1g

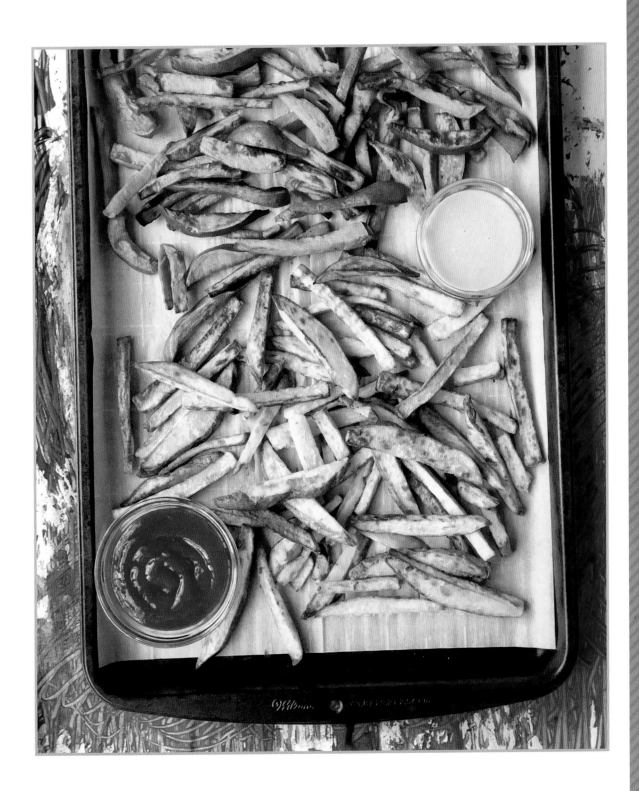

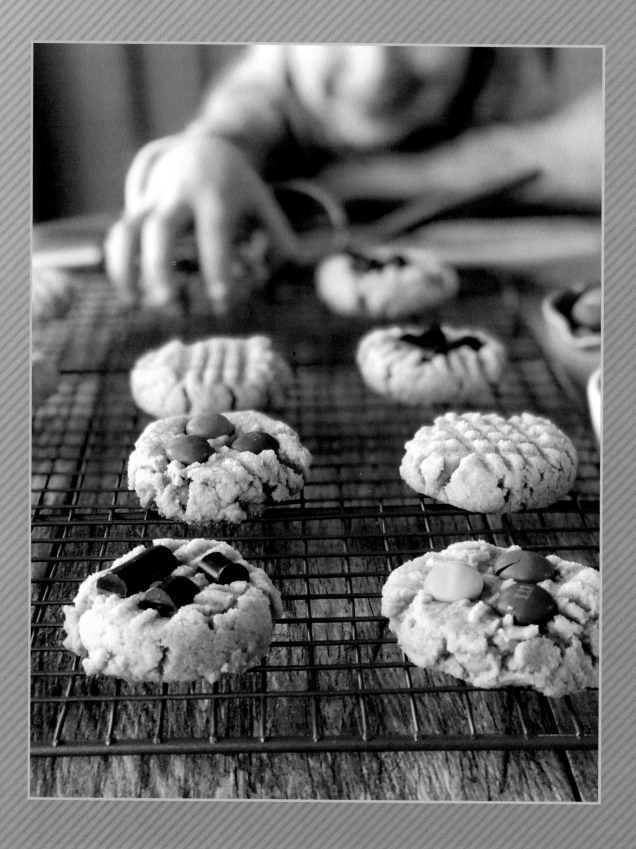

# 10

# Sensibly Sensational Desserts

Kid-friendly participation steps are printed in **ORANGE**

# Delightfully Dairy-Free Caramel Sauce

*This caramel sauce is a huge hit, even if you can eat the traditional dairy-based caramel sauce.*
*Serve it over ice cream or as a dipping sauce for strawberries, bananas, or pineapple.*

**YIELD: APPROXIMATELY 1 CUP**
**(2-TABLESPOON SERVINGS)**
Prep Time: 5 minutes
Total Time: 10 minutes

---

20 pitted dates
⅔ cup plus 2 tablespoons hot water
⅓ cup warmed coconut oil
2 teaspoons vanilla extract
1 teaspoon salt

**1.** In the bowl of a food processor, combine the dates and hot water. Let them sit for 5 minutes to soften.

**2.** Add the coconut oil, vanilla extract, and salt and purée until a very smooth and creamy sauce forms. Serve immediately over ice cream or store in an airtight container until ready to serve.

**3.** Gently warm the sauce before serving or eat at room temperature.

 **Dr. Bear Fun Facts!** This recipe is great for anyone who eats dairy-free and loves natural foods. Coconut oil provides dozens of health benefits, and dates are a great naturally sweet addition.

*Nutritional data reflects one serving size of 2 tablespoons.*

**PER SERVING** Calories: 250; Total Fat: 9.1g; Saturated Fat: 7.5g; Cholesterol: 0mg; Sodium: 295.4mg; Total Carbohydrates: 45.1g; Dietary Fiber: 4g; Sugars: 40g; Protein: 1.1g

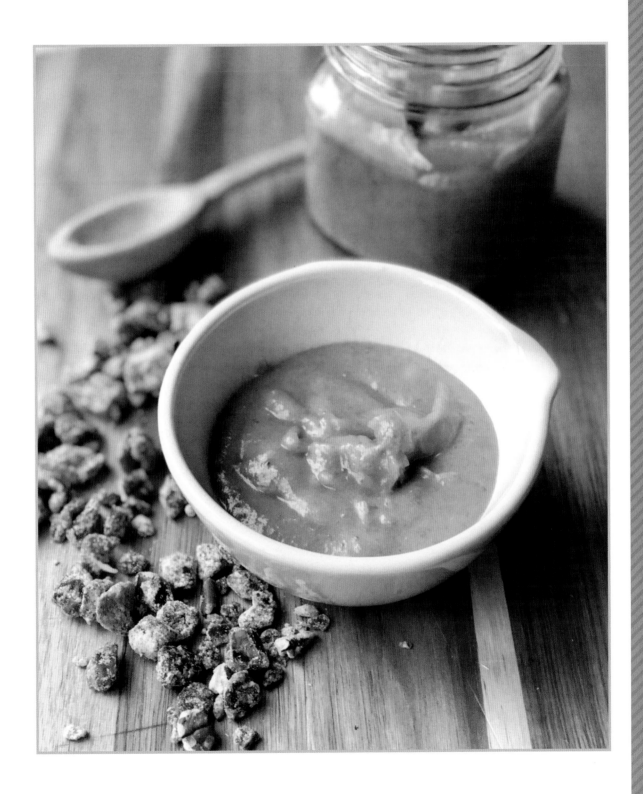

# Chocolate Oatmeal Bars with "Caramel" Date Purée

*I make these bars using dairy-free chocolate chips so everyone in the house can eat them. If you're able to eat dairy, I would recommend trying them using white chocolate. It pairs so well with the caramel date sauce. Also, while the recipe lists butter as an ingredient, the recipe in this photo was made using ¾ cup Smart Balance Butter plus ½ cup solid coconut oil for a dairy-free dessert.*

**YIELD: 24 BARS**
Prep Time: 15 minutes
Total Time: 45 minutes

---

### For the Crust
1½ cups packed dark brown sugar
1¼ cups butter, softened
1 teaspoon vanilla extract
2½ cups gluten-free all-purpose flour
1 teaspoon baking powder
½ teaspoon salt
2 cups gluten-free quick cook oats

### For the Filling
20 pitted dates
⅔ cup plus 2 tablespoons hot water
⅓ cup warmed coconut oil
2 teaspoons vanilla extract
1 teaspoon salt
1 (10-ounce) package dairy-free chocolate chips

**1.** Preheat oven to 350°F. Spray a 9-by-13-inch glass baking dish with nonstick spray and set aside.

**2.** For the crust, beat together the brown sugar, butter, and vanilla extract in the bowl of a stand mixer using the paddle attachment.

**3.** In a separate bowl, whisk together the gluten-free all-purpose flour, baking powder, and salt.

**4.** Add the dry ingredients slowly into the wet ingredients, mixing well after each addition.

**5.** Once fully incorporated, slowly add the gluten-free oats. Mix together on medium speed until well combined.

**6.** Press half of the dough into the bottom of the prepared pan. Bake for 10 minutes. Remove from oven and cool for 5 minutes.

**7.** While the dough is baking, make the filling. In the bowl of a food processor, combine the dates and hot water. Let sit for 5 minutes until softened. Once soft, purée the dates, hot water, coconut oil, vanilla extract, and salt until a very smooth mixture forms. Set aside.

**8.** When the bottom layer of dough is slightly cooled, sprinkle all of the chocolate chips evenly over the surface of the semi-baked dough. Drizzle the date purée mixture over the chocolate chips, and use a spatula to spread the mixture evenly.

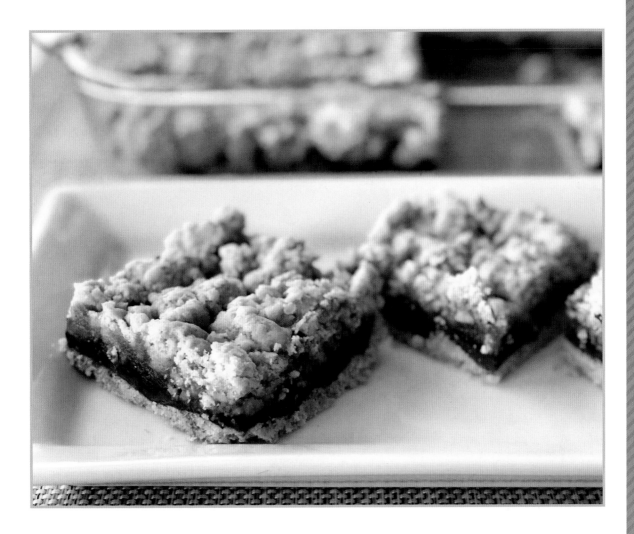

**9.** Crumble the remaining dough over the top of the filling. Make sure the filling is completely covered with dough.

**10.** Bake for 25 to 30 minutes until golden brown. Cool completely on a wire rack before slicing into bars.

*Nutritional data reflects one bar, based on a 24-bar yield.*

**PER SERVING** Calories: 316; Total Fat: 17g; Saturated Fat: 11g; Cholesterol: 25mg; Sodium: 174mg; Total Carbohydrates: 40g; Dietary Fiber: 2g; Sugars: 23g; Protein: 3g

 **Dr. Bear Fun Fact!** Putting oats in sweets is a great way to increase the nutritional value of desserts! They are great sources of fiber, manganese, magnesium, phosphorus, copper, iron, and zinc.

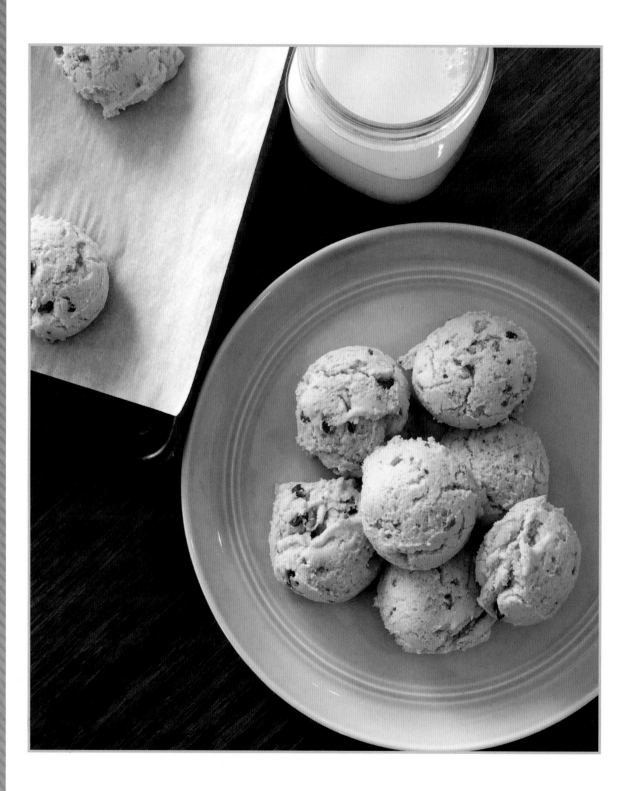

# Coconut Chocolate Chip Sprinkle Cookies

*Sprinkle cookies are a favorite of most kids, so I had to make a gluten-free version! This recipe uses naturally gluten-free whole grain flours and a touch of coconut milk for sweetness. Be sure to double-check labels of confetti candies and sprinkles, as some are made with wheat.*

**YIELD: 24 COOKIES**
Prep Time: 10 minutes
Total Time: 25 minutes

---

½ cup sorghum flour
½ cup coconut flour
½ cup brown rice flour
½ teaspoon xanthan gum
1 teaspoon baking powder
½ teaspoon sea salt
½ cup butter, softened
½ cup granulated sugar
½ cup brown sugar
1 egg
1 tablespoon coconut milk
1 teaspoon vanilla extract
½ cup mini chocolate chips
½ cup gluten-free rainbow confetti candies or sprinkles

**1.** Preheat the oven to 350°F. Line two baking sheets with parchment paper and set aside.

**2.** In a medium-sized mixing bowl, whisk together the sorghum flour, coconut flour, brown rice flour, xanthan gum, baking powder, and salt. Set aside.

**3.** In the bowl of a stand mixer, using the paddle attachment, cream together the butter, granulated sugar, and brown sugar. Add in the egg, milk, and vanilla extract and mix until a smooth batter forms.

**4.** Slowly add the dry ingredients, mixing well after each addition.

**5.** Gently fold in the mini chocolate chips and sprinkles.

**6.** Drop the cookies by rounded tablespoonfuls onto prepared baking sheets, 12 cookies per sheet. Bake for 12 to 14 minutes, until the cookies start to turn slightly golden.

 **Dr. Bear Fun Fact!** Sorghum is an ancient grain with high levels of protein, fiber, phosphorus, anti-oxidants, and potassium!

*Nutritional data reflects one cookie, based on a 24-cookie yield.*
**PER SERVING** Calories: 137; Total Fat: 6.7g; Saturated Fat: 3.5g; Cholesterol: 17.9mg; Sodium: 82.1mg; Total Carbohydrates: 18.3g; Dietary Fiber: 1.3g; Sugars: 11.3g; Protein: 1.4g

# Chocolate Chip Oatmeal Cookies

*I love this recipe because it makes a huge batch, making it perfect for school functions. Since this makes such a big batch, you can make some chewy and some crunchy. Life is beautiful!*

**YIELD: 36 COOKIES**
Prep Time: 10 minutes
Total Time: 25 minutes

---

2 cups gluten-free all-purpose flour

2 cups gluten-free quick cook oats

2 teaspoons baking powder

½ teaspoon salt

1 cup butter or butter replacement, softened

1 cup brown sugar, lightly packed

1 cup granulated sugar

2 eggs

1½ teaspoons vanilla extract

1 cup chocolate chips

1. Preheat oven to 350°F. Line three baking sheets with parchment paper and set aside.

2. In a medium-sized mixing bowl, whisk together the gluten-free all-purpose flour, gluten-free oats, baking powder and salt. Set aside.

3. In the bowl of a stand mixer using the paddle attachment, beat together the butter, the brown sugar and granulated sugar until light and creamy. Add the eggs one at a time, mixing well after each addition. Add the vanilla extract and mix well.

4. Slowly add the dry ingredients into the wet ingredients, mixing well after each addition.

5. Gently fold in the chocolate chips.

6. Drop the cookies by heaping tablespoonfuls onto prepared baking sheets. Bake for 13 to 18 minutes until slightly golden. If you like your cookies on the chewier side, bake for 13 minutes and remove from oven (my kids like them this way). If you like them crispier, bake for 16 to 18 minutes.

 **Dr. Bear Fun Fact!** Many people with celiac disease can't tolerate oats—not because they aren't gluten-free but because they are actually intolerant to oats.

*Nutritional data reflects one cookie, based on a 36-cookie yield.*

**PER SERVING** Calories: 162; Total Fat: 7.3g; Saturated Fat: 4.3g; Cholesterol: 23.8mg; Sodium: 70mg; Total Carbohydrates: 23.1g; Dietary Fiber: 0.8g; Sugars: 14.2g; Protein: 1.7g

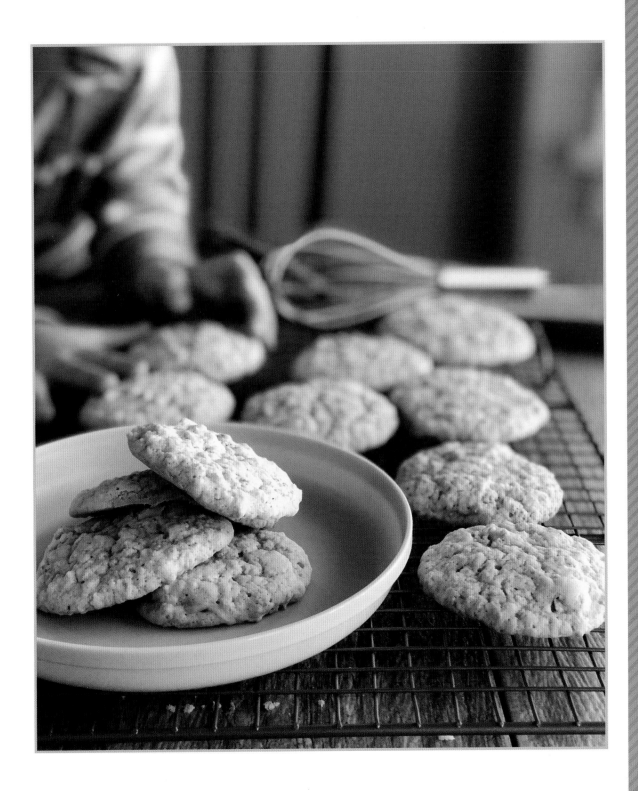

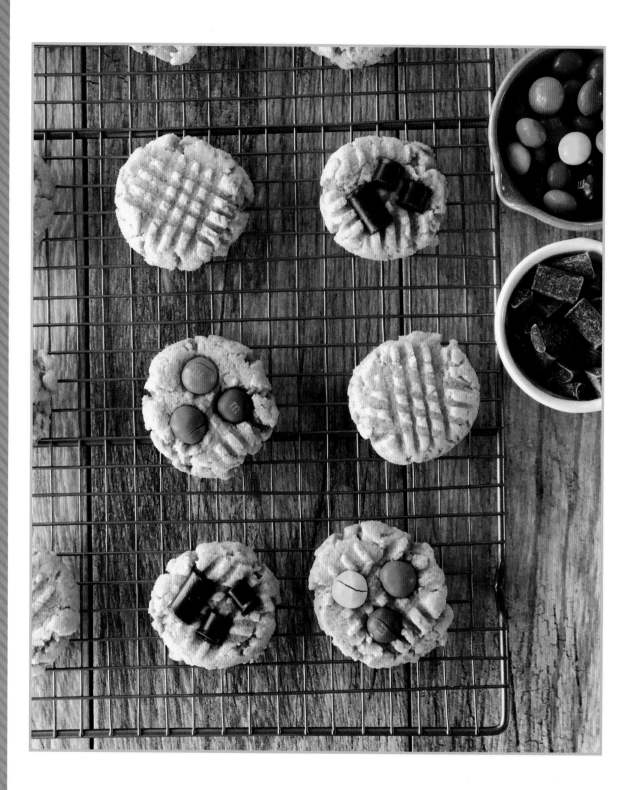

# Peanut Butter Oatmeal Sugar Cookies

*I'm definitely a soccer mom, so I love to make big batches of cookies! If you're making these for a school event, replace the peanut butter with Sunbutter for an allergy-free treat.*

**YIELD: 36 COOKIES**
Prep Time: 10 minutes
Total Time: 20 minutes

---

1 cup gluten-free all-purpose flour

1 cup gluten-free quick cook oats

2 teaspoons baking powder

½ teaspoon salt

1 cup butter or solid coconut oil, softened (solid coconut oil used in the cookie photo)

1 cup granulated sugar plus extra ¼ cup for rolling

1 cup brown sugar

2 eggs

1½ teaspoons vanilla extract

1 cup creamy peanut butter

Optional toppings: M&Ms, chocolate chips, Reese's peanut butter cups

**1.** Preheat oven to 350°F. Line three baking sheets with parchment paper and set side.

**2.** In a mixing bowl, whisk together the gluten-free all-purpose flour, gluten-free oats, baking powder, and salt. Set aside.

**3.** In the bowl of a stand mixer, using the paddle attachment, beat together the butter, 1 cup granulated sugar, and brown sugar until light and creamy. Add the eggs one at a time, mixing well after each addition. Add the vanilla extract and mix well. Add the peanut butter and mix until smooth and fully combined.

**4.** Slowly add the dry ingredients into the wet ingredients, mixing well after each addition.

**5.** Drop the cookies by heaping tablespoonful onto prepared baking sheets.

**6.** Roll each cookie in the remaining sugar and make a crisscross pattern over the top with a fork. Press candies of choice into the cookies, if desired, before baking.

**7.** Bake for 8 to 15 minutes, depending on desired level of crispiness. If you like chewy cookies, bake them for 8 to 10 minutes. If you like them crispy, bake for 13 to 15 minutes.

 **Dr. Bear Fun Fact!** Peanut butter is high in protein, good fat, and fiber, making this a great dessert that keeps you fuller longer!

*Nutritional data reflects one cookie without toppings, based on a 36-cookie yield.*

**PER SERVING** Calories: 155; Total Fat: 9.1g; Saturated Fat: 3.9g; Cholesterol: 22.7mg; Sodium: 95.1mg; Total Carbohydrates: 17g; Dietary Fiber: 0.8g; Sugars: 11.6g; Protein: 2.4g

# Mimi's Chocolate Peppermint Crinkle Cookies

*My mom made these for me all the time as a kid, and now she makes them with Brandon and Leo. The kids love trying to figure out how the crinkles came to be and licking the powdered sugar off first. It's adorable to watch how carefully they eat these cookies! Also, if dairy is a concern, replace the chocolate with a dairy-free chocolate and the butter with coconut oil.*

**YIELD: 24–28 COOKIES**
Prep Time: 2 hours, 15 minutes
  (includes dough chilling)
Total Time: 2 hours, 25 minutes

---

4 ounces unsweetened chocolate, chopped

½ cup butter

2 cups gluten-free all-purpose flour

2 teaspoons baking powder

¼ teaspoon salt

3 eggs

2 cups granulated sugar

1 teaspoon vanilla extract

1 teaspoon peppermint extract

1 cup powdered sugar

1. In a small sauce pot set over low heat, melt together the chocolate and butter, stirring frequently to prevent burning. Once melted and smooth, remove from heat and let cool for about 10 minutes.

2. In a mixing bowl, whisk together gluten-free all-purpose flour, baking powder, and salt. Set aside.

3. In the bowl of a stand mixer, using the paddle attachment, beat together the eggs, sugar, vanilla extract, and peppermint extract until smooth. Add the melted chocolate and butter mixture and mix until smooth.

4. Slowly add the dry ingredients into the wet ingredients, mixing well after each addition. Scrape down the sides of the bowl and mix again.

5. Cover the dough and refrigerate for 2 hours until firm enough to roll into balls.

6. Preheat oven to 375°F. Line two baking sheets with parchment paper.

7. Place the powdered sugar in a small bowl. Form the cookie dough into tablespoon-sized balls and then roll in the powdered sugar.

8. Place dough balls about 2 inches apart on the prepared baking sheets and bake for 10 minutes. Cool before serving. Store in an airtight container.

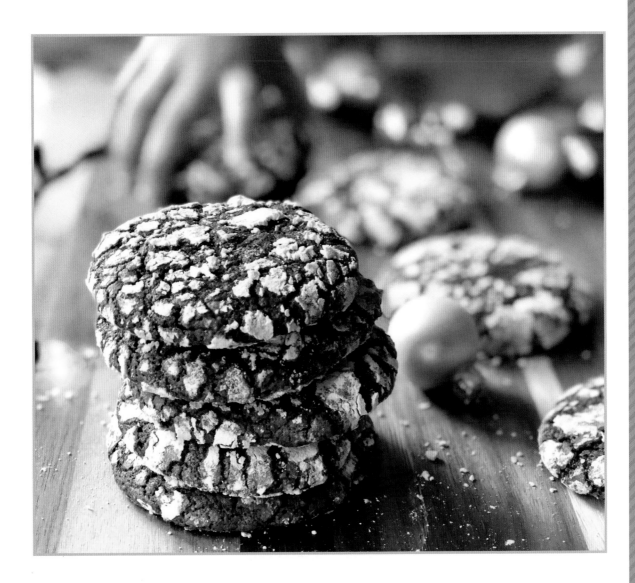

 **Dr. Bear Fun Fact!** Peppermint is actually a mixture of two plants—watermint and spearmint. Morocco grows about 92 percent of the world's peppermint, and the United States grows just a small amount for things like toothpaste and oils.

*Nutritional data reflects one cookie, based on a 26-cookie yield.*

**PER SERVING**  Calories: 173; Total Fat: 6.6g; Saturated Fat: 3.8g; Cholesterol: 28.3mg; Sodium: 68.5mg; Total Carbohydrates: 29g; Dietary Fiber: 0.9g; Sugars: 20g; Protein: 1.6g

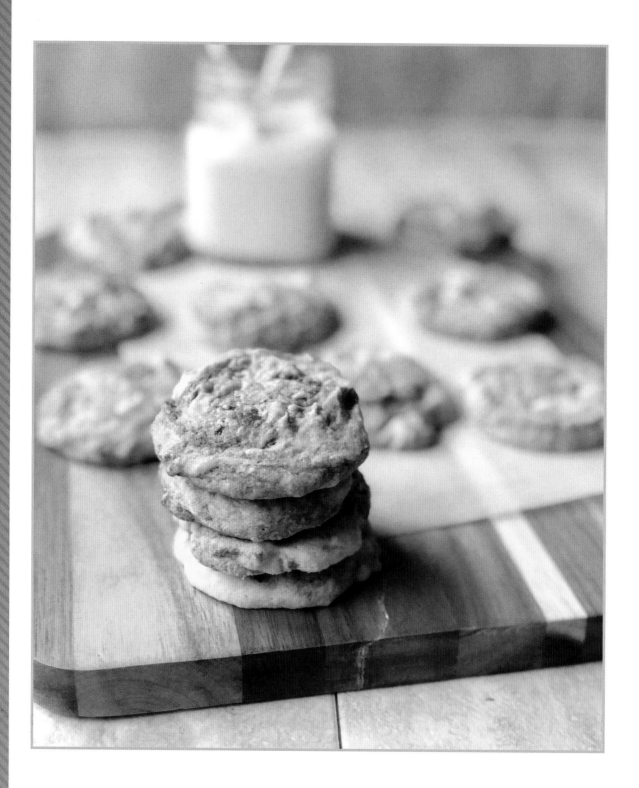

# White Chocolate Hazelnut Cookies

*I intended to make peanut butter cookies for this recipe, but I opened the cabinet and the jar was empty! Oh no!! Thankfully, I had a jar of Nutella. I swirled it into the cookie batter, and I'm really glad I did. If you're making these for a school event, replace the Nutella with Sunbutter for a nut-free treat.*

**YIELD: 36 TO 40 COOKIES**
Prep Time: 10 minutes
Total Time: 25 minutes

---

2¼ cups gluten-free
   all-purpose flour
1 teaspoon baking powder
1 teaspoon salt
1 cup butter, softened
¾ cup brown sugar
½ cup granulated sugar
1 teaspoon vanilla extract
2 eggs
1 cup white chocolate chips
½ cup Nutella

**1.** Preheat oven to 350°F. Line two baking sheets with parchment paper and set aside.

**2.** In a mixing bowl, whisk together the gluten-free all-purpose flour, baking powder, and salt. Set aside.

**3.** In the bowl of a stand mixer, using the paddle attachment, beat together the butter, brown sugar, and granulated sugar until light and creamy. Add the vanilla extract and eggs and mix until well combined.

**4.** Slowly add the dry ingredients into the wet ingredients, mixing well after each addition. Gently mix in the white chocolate chips.

**5.** Turn off the mixer and use a spoon to drop the Nutella in globs into the dough. Turn the mixer on and let it spin about 3 times, just long enough to swirl in the Nutella. Do not over mix. You want the swirls.

**6.** Drop the dough by rounded tablespoonfuls onto prepared baking pans. Bake for 15 minutes. Allow to cool before serving.

 **Dr. Bear Fun Fact!** Nutella production uses a whopping 25 percent of the world's hazelnuts each year to create their famous spread!

*Nutritional data reflects one cookie, based on a 38-cookie yield.*
**PER SERVING** Calories: 138; Total Fat: 7.7g; Saturated Fat: 4.3g; Cholesterol: 21.7mg; Sodium: 92.5mg; Total Carbohydrates: 16.5g; Dietary Fiber: 0.4g; Sugars: 10.3g; Protein: 1.3g

# Blueberry & Strawberry Coconut Ice Cream

*When my son Leo was diagnosed with a dairy allergy, I wanted to jump on the nice cream train and have my kids love 100 percent frozen fruit instead of adding in sugar and cream. Unfortunately, they were not the biggest fans, so I kept trying until I found a mixture that they actually loved. Here's what I came up with. In the photo, you will see the result of making one batch of this recipe with blueberries and one batch with strawberries.*

**YIELD: 2–4 SERVINGS**
Prep Time: 5 minutes
Total Time: 6–8 hours, depending on
    freezing time

---

2 cups frozen fruit (strawberries,
    blueberries, blackberries, etc.)
1 ripe banana, peeled
½ cup coconut milk
2 tablespoons honey
½ teaspoon salt

1. Combine the frozen fruit, banana, coconut milk, honey, and salt in the bowl of a food processor. Purée until smooth.

2. Transfer to a freezer-safe container and freeze until desired consistency is reached.

3. Serve with sprinkles or any toppings of your choosing.

 **Dr. Bear Fun Fact!** Salt in ice cream? It's actually a crucial ingredient! Salt helps to lower the freezing point of the milk, allowing it to be creamy instead of filled with ice crystals!

*Nutritional data reflects one serving, based on a 4-serving yield.*

**PER SERVING**  Calories: 99; Total Fat: 0.7g; Saturated Fat: 0.5g; Cholesterol: 0mg; Sodium: 295.7mg; Total Carbohydrates: 24.1g; Dietary Fiber: 3.3g; Sugars: 17.9g; Protein: 0.4g

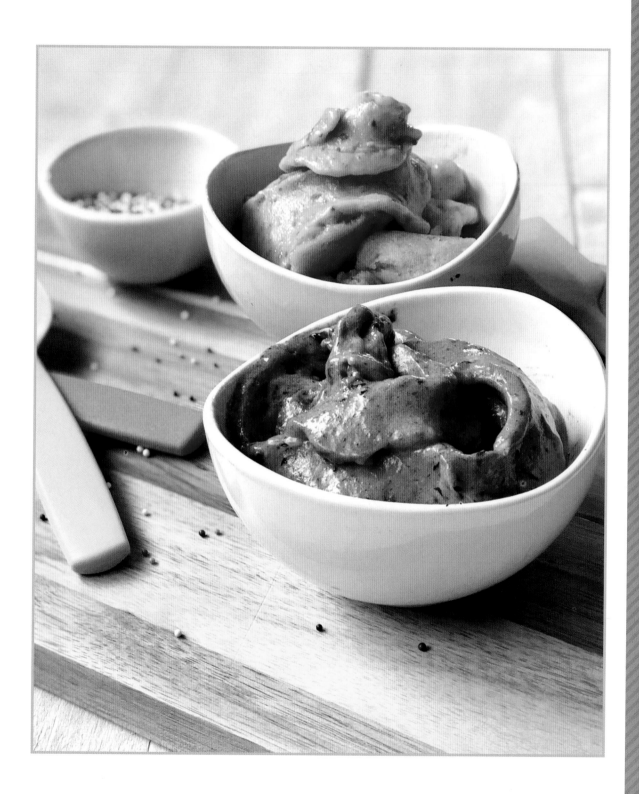

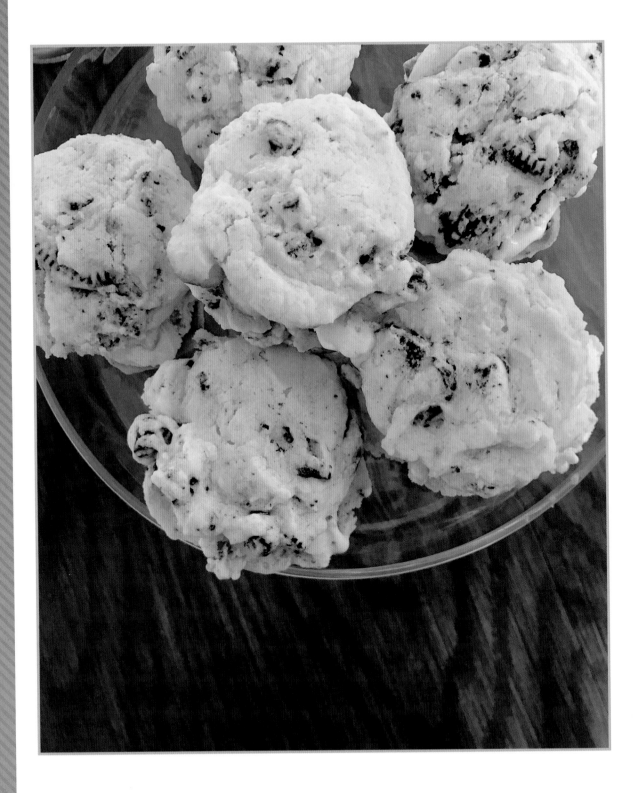

# Ice Cream Cookie Sandwiches with Strawberry Ice Cream

*Ice cream sandwiches are a childhood favorite, and I've kicked it up a notch by adding a cookie in a cookie. I filled the sandwiches with strawberry ice cream, but go ahead and pick your child's favorite flavor! Let your kids crush the Oreo-style cookies. They'll have a blast!*

**YIELD: 12 COOKIE SANDWICHES**
Prep Time: 15 minutes
Total Time: 75 minutes

---

2 cups gluten-free all-purpose flour

1 teaspoon baking powder

½ teaspoon salt

8 ounces cream cheese, softened

1 cup unsalted butter, softened

1½ cups sugar

2 eggs

1 teaspoon vanilla extract

20 gluten-free, Oreo-style cookies, crushed

1½ cups strawberry ice cream, softened

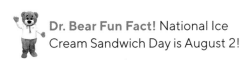 **Dr. Bear Fun Fact!** National Ice Cream Sandwich Day is August 2!

*Nutritional data reflects one sandwich, based on a 12-sandwich yield.*

**PER SERVING** Calories: 516; Total Fat: 26g; Saturated Fat: 15g; Cholesterol: 96mg; Sodium: 303mg; Total Carbohydrates: 66g; Dietary Fiber: 1g; Sugars: 43g; Protein: 6g

1. Preheat oven to 350°F. Line two baking sheets with parchment paper and set aside.

2. In a mixing bowl, whisk together gluten-free all-purpose flour, baking powder, and salt. Set aside.

3. In the bowl of a stand mixer, using the paddle attachment, beat together the cream cheese, butter, and sugar. Add the eggs, one at a time, mixing well after each addition. Add in the vanilla extract.

4. Slowly add the dry ingredients into the wet ingredients, mixing well after each addition.

5. Gently fold the crushed cookies into the batter.

6. Cover the bowl with plastic wrap and refrigerate the dough for 30 minutes.

7. Once chilled, scoop the dough by heaping tablespoonfuls onto the prepared baking sheets. Using your fingers, press down gently on each cookie to flatten.

8. Bake for 11 to 13 minutes until the bottoms of the cookies turn slightly golden. Do not overcook; you want them soft.

9. Remove cookies from the oven and cool completely.

10. To make ice cream sandwiches, spread approximately ⅛ cup of the softened strawberry ice cream onto each of 12 cookies. Top with a second cookie and press together gently. Eat immediately, or wrap the ice cream cookie sandwiches in plastic wrap and freeze until ready to enjoy. Repeat with remaining cookies.

# Spiced Pear & Blackberry Oatmeal Cookie Cobbler

*This cobbler combines the best parts of two desserts: cobbler and cookies! In this tasty dish, I've tossed together pears and blackberries for the cobbler base and topped it with a giant white chocolate oatmeal cookie. If you don't have pears or blackberries on hand, replace with any fruit in your refrigerator. Try plums and apples or even mango and pineapple!*

**YIELD: 12 SERVINGS**
Prep Time: 15 minutes
Total Time: 80 minutes

---

1½ cups gluten-free oats

1 cup gluten-free all-purpose flour

1 cup white chocolate chips

2 teaspoons baking powder

1 teaspoon salt

1 cup brown sugar

¾ cup coconut oil, melted

2 teaspoons vanilla extract

5 pears, cored and chopped into bite-sized pieces

2 cups roughly chopped blackberries

3 tablespoons granulated sugar

2 tablespoons cornstarch

1 tablespoon lemon juice

1 teaspoon cinnamon

Optional garnish: vanilla ice cream

**1.** Preheat oven to 350°F. Spray a 9-by-13-inch baking dish with nonstick spray and set aside.

**2.** In a mixing bowl, mix together the gluten-free oats, gluten-free all-purpose flour, white chocolate chips, baking powder, and salt. Set aside.

**3.** In a larger mixing bowl, mix together the brown sugar and coconut oil until well combined. Add the vanilla extract and mix well.

**4.** Add the dry ingredients into the wet ingredients and mix until a smooth dough forms. Set dough aside.

**5.** Place the chopped pears and blackberries into the prepared baking dish. Sprinkle with sugar, cornstarch, lemon juice, and cinnamon. Gently mix the fruit together until well coated.

**6.** Crumble the cookie dough over the top of the fruit in an even layer.

**7.** Bake for 45 to 50 minutes until bubbly and golden. Serve hot, topped with vanilla ice cream, if desired.

 **Dr. Bear Fun Fact!** Did you know that white chocolate doesn't technically fall under the "chocolate" definition? To be considered chocolate, the product must have cocoa solids in it—white chocolate only has cocoa butter!

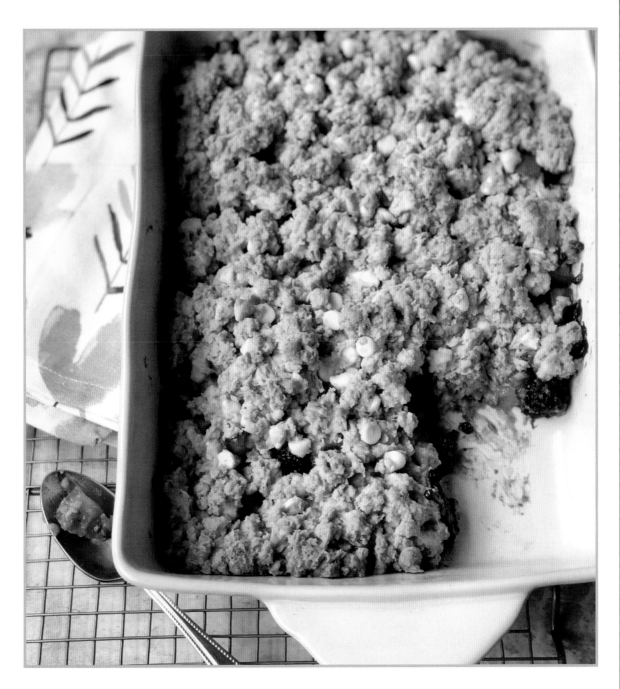

*Nutritional data reflects one serving without ice cream, based on an 8-serving yield.*

**PER SERVING** Calories: 390; Total Fat: 18.6g; Saturated Fat: 14.7g; Cholesterol: 0.6mg; Sodium: 319mg; Total Carbohydrates: 54.4g; Dietary Fiber: 5.1g; Sugars: 32.2g; Protein: 3.6g

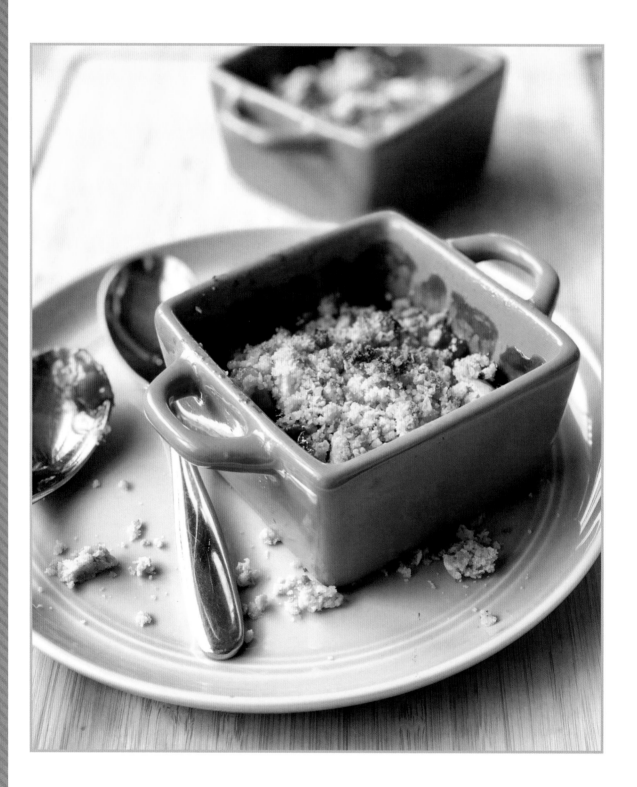

# Strawberry Apple Crisp

*This dessert is a childhood favorite. My sister and I would beg my mom to make her famous fruity crisps for dessert, and we would rush to eat it before our ice cream melted too much. Pictured using 10 small (8-ounce) ramekins, but if you don't have ramekins, bake in a 9-by-13-inch glass baking dish for 50 to 55 minutes.*

**YIELD: 10 SERVINGS**
Prep Time: 15 minutes
Total Time: 55 minutes

---

### For the Filling
¾ cup granulated sugar
½ cup orange juice
1 tablespoon cornstarch
Zest of 1 orange
    (about 1 tablespoon)
4 cups fresh strawberries,
    rinsed, stems removed and
    cut into quarters
4 apples, cores removed and
    chopped into bite-sized pieces

### For the Crispy Topping
1 cup gluten-free all-purpose flour
1 cup gluten-free rolled oats
1 cup brown sugar
½ teaspoon salt
¾ cup coconut butter

1. Preheat oven to 350°F. Spray 10 (8-ounce) ramekins with nonstick spray and set on top of a baking sheet. Set aside.

2. To make the filling, mix together the sugar, orange juice, cornstarch, and orange zest in a large mixing bowl until well combined.

3. Add the chopped fruit into the mixing bowl and toss with the sugar mixture until well combined. Evenly divide the coated fruit among the prepared ramekins.

4. To make the topping, combine the gluten-free all-purpose flour, gluten-free oats, brown sugar, salt, and coconut butter in the bowl of a food processor. Pulse until the mixture is crumbly.

5. Evenly distribute the topping mixture over the fruit in the ramekins and bake for 30 to 35 minutes until the fruit is bubbling and the topping is golden.

6. Serve topped with vanilla ice cream, if desired.

 **Dr. Bear Fun Fact!** This is a great treat to serve in the spring! Strawberries are usually the first fruit to ripen when the weather gets warmer.

*Nutritional data reflects one serving without ice cream, based on a 10-serving yield.*

**PER SERVING** Calories: 362; Total Fat: 11.9g; Saturated Fat: 9.8g; Cholesterol: 0mg; Sodium: 130.9mg; Total Carbohydrates: 65.4g; Dietary Fiber: 6.7g; Sugars: 42g; Protein: 3.5g

# Banana Ice Cream Cake with Chocolate Swirl & Graham Cracker Crust

*I was thrilled to find sweetened condensed milk made from coconut milk! This is a game changer for managing a dairy-free lifestyle. If dairy fits into your diet, you can use regular sweetened condensed milk as a replacement.*

**YIELD: 1 LOAF CAKE (10 SERVINGS)**
Prep Time: 20 minutes
Total Time: 6 hours 20 minutes
 (including freezing)

3 ripe bananas, peeled

1 (11.25-ounce) can sweetened condensed coconut milk

1 (13.5-ounce) can coconut milk

2 teaspoons vanilla extract

½ cup dairy-free chocolate chips

1 tablespoon coconut oil

15 gluten-free graham-style crackers, crushed

**1.** Prepare an ice-cream maker according to manufacturer's instructions. If you don't have an ice-cream maker, don't worry! You can freeze the ice cream in the baking pan. Line an 8-by-4-inch loaf pan with plastic wrap and set aside.

**2.** In the bowl of a food processor, combine bananas, sweetened condensed coconut milk, coconut milk, and vanilla extract. Purée until no lumps remain.

**3.** Pour the mixture into the prepared ice-cream maker and churn according to manufacturer's instructions. It takes my Cuisinart ice-cream maker about 20 minutes to churn the mixture.

**4.** While the ice cream is churning, add the chocolate chips and coconut oil to a small sauce pot. Heat over medium-low heat, whisking constantly, until the chocolate is melted. Remove from heat and set aside.

**5.** Sprinkle half of the crushed gluten-free graham-style crackers into the bottom of the prepared loaf pan. Spread about half of the ice-cream mixture on top of the graham crackers, then drizzle the melted chocolate across the surface of the ice cream.

**6.** Top the chocolate mixture with remaining ice cream and then sprinkle remaining graham-style crackers on top. Gently press the graham-style crackers into the ice cream.

**7.** Freeze the ice cream cake for 4 to 6 hours until completely firm.

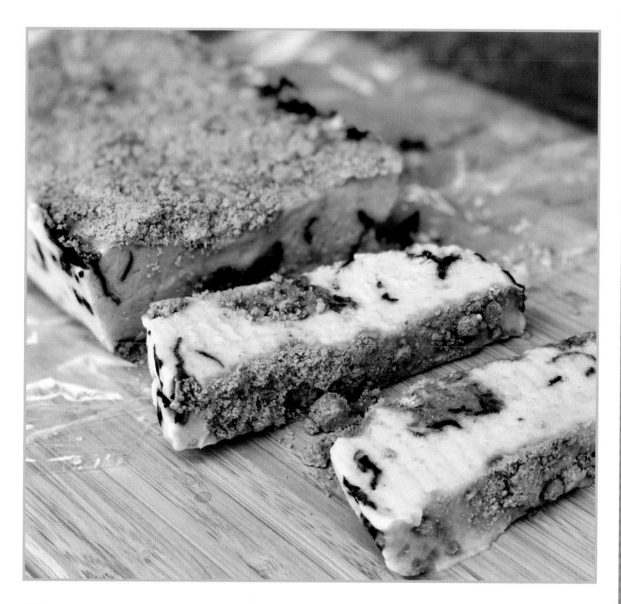

 **Dr. Bear Fun Fact!** Bananas aren't just a yummy fruit! They provide excellent levels of potassium, pectin, magnesium, and Vitamins B$_6$ and C.

*Nutritional data reflects one serving, based on a 10-serving yield.*

**PER SERVING** Calories: 627; Total Fat: 31.9g; Saturated Fat: 20.4g; Cholesterol: 41.7mg; Sodium: 262mg; Total Carbohydrates: 82.1g; Dietary Fiber: 3.8g; Sugars: 41.3g; Protein: 5.6g

# Glazed Donut Holes

*When I was a little girl, my dad would take me on Sunday mornings to Happy Donuts in San Mateo, California. I will never forget biting into the sweet and moist donuts and how happy it made me. Now my dad comes to my house for homemade gluten-free donuts! They taste just as great, minus the gluten.*

**YIELD: 24 DONUT HOLES**
Prep Time: 10 minutes
Total Time: 30 minutes

### For the Donut Holes
2 cups gluten-free
    all-purpose flour
3 tablespoons sugar
4 teaspoons baking powder
½ teaspoon salt
¼ cup vegetable oil plus more
    for frying
1 cup milk
1 egg
1 teaspoon vanilla extract

### For the Glaze
3 tablespoons milk
2 teaspoons vanilla extract
Approximately 1½–1¾ cups
    powdered sugar

**1.** Line a baking sheet with paper towels or parchment paper. Set a cooling rack on top of paper towels or parchment and set aside.

**2.** In a medium-sized mixing bowl, whisk together the gluten-free all-purpose flour, sugar, baking powder, and salt. Set aside.

**3.** In a second mixing bowl, whisk together the vegetable oil, milk, egg, and vanilla extract until well combined.

**4.** Slowly mix the dry ingredients into the wet ingredients until a smooth dough forms.

**5.** Pour about 3 inches of oil into a high sided pot. Heat over medium heat until the oil reaches 350°F. If you don't have a thermometer, test the oil's readiness by dropping a small piece of dough into the oil. If it sizzles immediately, you're ready to fry the donuts.

**6.** Using a small cookie scoop, dip the dough out. Take the dough in your hand and roll into a ball. Repeat with remaining dough.

**7.** Drop the dough balls into the heated oil and cook for about 4 to 6 minutes until toasty and golden all around. You'll want to use a slotted spoon to toss the dough balls for even frying.

**8.** Transfer the fried donuts to the prepared cooling rack. Repeat until all donuts are fried.

**9.** While the donuts cool, make the glaze by whisking together the milk and vanilla extract. Slowly add the powdered sugar, whisking constantly. Continue adding powdered sugar until the glaze easily coats a spoon.

**10.** Gently roll each donut hole into the glaze to cover completely. Serve immediately!

**Dr. Bear Fun Fact!** Nobody really knows why donut holes were created! Some think it was a sailor who needed a free hand on deck, so he made a hole in his pastry and speared it on the spoke of his ship's wheel, thereby creating the donut hole! However, culinary historians generally think donut holes were invented because they cook faster than ringed donuts.

*Nutritional data reflects one donut hole, based on a 24-donut hole yield. It does not account for frying oil, as data will vary.*

**PER SERVING** Calories: 104; Total Fat: 3g; Saturated Fat: 1g; Cholesterol: 8mg; Sodium: 139mg; Total Carbohydrates: 18g; Dietary Fiber: 1g; Sugars: 10g; Protein: 1g

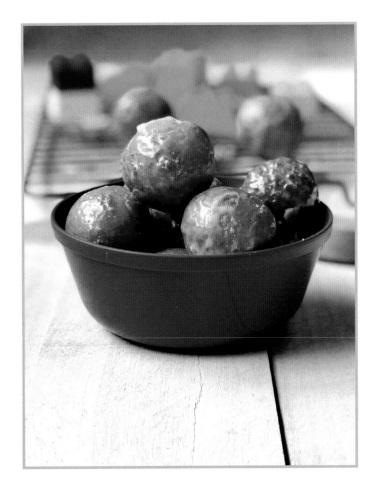

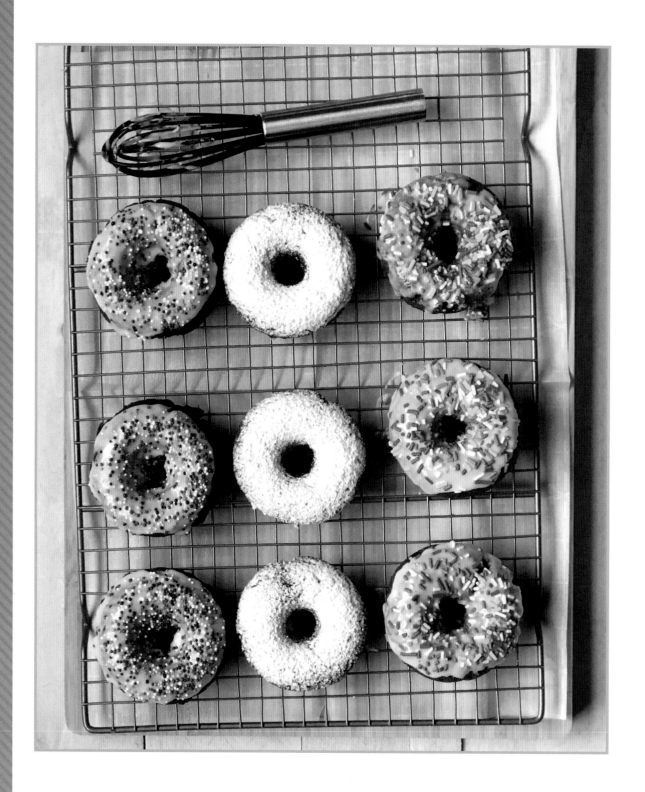

# Chocolate Glazed Donuts

*I make these regularly to eat at home and also for special occasions at school. They're very moist and not overly sweet. For dairy-free donuts, replace the milk with coconut milk, the sour cream with SO Delicious Plain coconut yogurt, and pick a gluten-free flour without dry milk powder.*

**YIELD: 18–20 DONUTS**
Prep Time: 10 minutes
Total Time: 30 minutes

———————

### For the Donuts
2½ cups gluten-free all-purpose flour

1¼ cups sugar

⅔ cup cocoa powder

2 teaspoons baking powder

½ teaspoon salt

½ cup mini chocolate chips

1 cup plus 2 tablespoons sour cream

¾ cup milk

¾ cup vegetable oil

2 eggs

2 teaspoons vanilla extract

### For the Glaze
3 tablespoons milk

2 teaspoons vanilla extract

Approximately 1½–1¾ cups
    powdered sugar

**1.** Preheat oven to 375°F. Spray two donut pans with nonstick spray and set aside.

**2.** In a medium-sized mixing bowl, whisk together gluten-free all-purpose flour, sugar, cocoa powder, baking powder, salt, and chocolate chips. Set aside.

**3.** In a second large mixing bowl, whisk together the sour cream, milk, vegetable oil, eggs, and vanilla extract.

**4.** Slowly add the dry ingredients into the wet ingredients and mix until well combined.

**5.** Using a spoon, evenly distribute the dough into prepared donut pan wells.

**6.** Bake for 16 to 18 minutes until a toothpick inserted into the donuts comes out clean. Cool in pan before glazing.

**7.** While the donuts cool, make the glaze by whisking together the milk and vanilla extract. Slowly add the powdered sugar and whisk constantly. Continue adding powdered sugar until the glaze easily coats a spoon.

**8.** Gently dip each donut into the glaze to cover about ½ of the donut. Enjoy immediately or store in an airtight container.

 **Dr. Bear Fun Fact!** Donuts were first popularized in the United States by veterans of World War I. The Salvation Army served them to soldiers on the front lines of battle, but when they returned home, the veterans continued to ask for them!

*Nutritional data reflects one donut, based on a 20-donut yield.*

**PER SERVING** Calories: 286; Total Fat: 14g; Saturated Fat: 4g; Cholesterol: 25mg; Sodium: 124mg;
Total Carbohydrates: 41g; Dietary Fiber: 2g; Sugars: 26g; Protein: 3g

# Pumpkin Spice Donuts

*I love experimenting with different blends of gluten-free flour, and this recipe boasts one of my favorites. If you don't have almond flour, cornstarch, brown rice flour, and sorghum flour on hand, just replace those ingredients with 1½ cups of gluten-free all-purpose flour.*

**YIELD: 12 DONUTS**
Prep Time: 10 minutes
Total Time: 35 minutes

---

½ cup finely ground almond flour

½ cup cornstarch

¼ cup brown rice flour

¼ cup sorghum flour

3 teaspoons baking powder

1 teaspoon pumpkin pie spice

½ teaspoon salt

¼ teaspoon freshly ground nutmeg

1 cup granulated sugar

1 cup pumpkin purée

¼ cup butter, melted and slightly cooled

2 tablespoon maple syrup

2 eggs, room temperature

1 teaspoon vanilla extract

Powdered sugar for dusting

**1.** Preheat oven to 350°F and lightly grease two 6-hole donut pans with cooking spray or oil. Set aside.

**2.** To make the batter, whisk together the almond flour, cornstarch, brown rice flour, sorghum flour, baking powder, pumpkin pie spice, salt and nutmeg in a large bowl.

**3.** In the bowl of stand mixer, using the paddle attachment, combine the sugar, pumpkin purée, butter, maple syrup, eggs, and vanilla extract. Mix until thoroughly combined.

**4.** Slowly add the dry ingredients into wet ingredients, mixing well after each addition.

**5.** Fill each donut well about three-quarters full with batter. Bake for 22 to 25 minutes until a toothpick inserted into the center of the donuts comes out clean.

**6.** Let the donuts cool for 10 minutes. Remove from pan and transfer to a wire rack.

**7.** Dust with powdered sugar before serving.

 **Dr. Bear Fun Fact!** These deliciously soft donuts are bursting with flavor and good-for-you ingredients! Almond and sorghum flours are naturally gluten-free ingredients that are packed with protein and fiber and add a great subtle sweetness to baked goods.

*Nutritional data reflects one donut, based on a 12-donut yield.*

**PER SERVING** Calories: 205; Total Fat: 7.3g; Saturated Fat: 2.9g; Cholesterol: 37.5mg; Sodium: 232.8mg; Total Carbohydrates: 33.8g; Dietary Fiber: 1.5g; Sugars: 22.2g; Protein: 2.6g

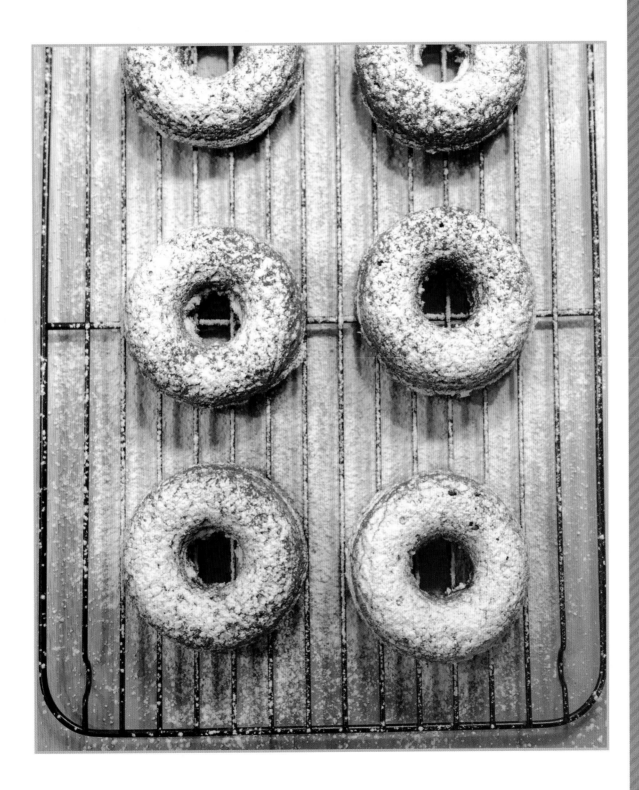

# Colorful Cupcakes with Vanilla Frosting

*This is my favorite photo in the book, and it happened completely organically. Leo was patiently waiting for me to finish taking the photos so he could take a cupcake. He knew how important the photo was and promised not to mess it up. The look in his eyes the moment I finished was priceless, and he immediately dug right in! I made this recipe dairy-free to accommodate Leo's dairy allergy, but you can use regular milk as well.*

**YIELD: 18 REGULAR-SIZED CUPCAKES OR 36 MINI CUPCAKES**
Prep Time: 15 minutes
Total Time: 40 minutes

---

**For the Cupcakes**

2 cups gluten-free all-purpose flour

1 tablespoon baking powder

1 teaspoon salt

1 cup vegetable or coconut oil

2 cups sugar

2 eggs, yolks and whites separated

3 teaspoons vanilla extract

1 cup coconut milk

½ cup rainbow confetti candies

**For the Frosting**

1 (16-ounce) box powdered sugar

½ cup coconut butter

1 teaspoon vanilla extract

3 to 4 tablespoons coconut milk

Sprinkles, or other edible decorating items

**1.** Preheat oven to 350°F. Place cupcake liners in desired cupcake pans and set aside.

**2.** In a mixing bowl, whisk together the gluten-free all-purpose flour, baking powder and salt. Set aside.

**3.** In the bowl of a stand mixer, using the paddle attachment, beat together the oil, sugar, egg yolks, and vanilla extract. Slowly add the coconut milk and mix until well combined.

**4.** Slowly add the dry ingredients into the wet ingredients, mixing well after each addition.

**5.** In a separate mixing bowl, add the egg whites. Using a hand mixer, beat the egg whites until stiff peaks form. Using a spatula, gently fold the stiff egg whites into the cake batter, until combined. Gently stir in the confetti candies.

**6.** Pour the batter into the prepared cupcake pans, and fill the cups about ⅔ full. Bake for 22 to 27 minutes for regular-sized cupcakes or 15 to 17 minutes for mini cupcakes. Check the doneness by inserting a toothpick into the center of the cupcakes. If it comes out clean, the cupcakes are done baking.

**7.** Let the cupcakes cool for 10 minutes in the pans, then transfer to a cooling rack to cool completely.

**8.** To make the frosting, combine the powdered sugar, coconut butter, and vanilla extract in a food processor. Pulse the mixture as you add the coconut milk. Continue adding coconut milk until desired consistency is reached. The frosting should heavily coat a spoon.

**9.** Frost the cupcakes with a generous portion of frosting and top with sprinkles, as desired.

 **Dr. Bear Fun Fact!** The inventor of sprinkles called them "jimmies," claiming he named them after an employee!

*Nutritional data reflects one regular-sized cupcake, based on an 18-cupcake yield.*

**PER SERVING** Calories: 417; Total Fat: 19g; Saturated Fat: 6g; Cholesterol: 18mg; Sodium: 222mg; Total Carbohydrates: 64g; Dietary Fiber: 1g; Sugars: 50g; Protein: 1.7g

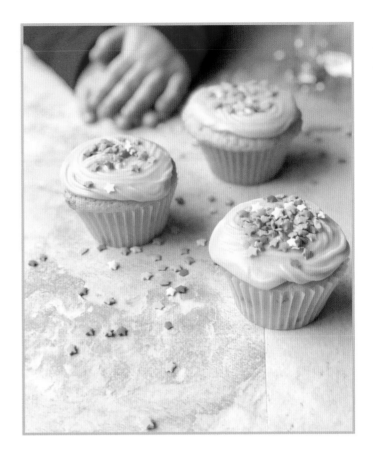

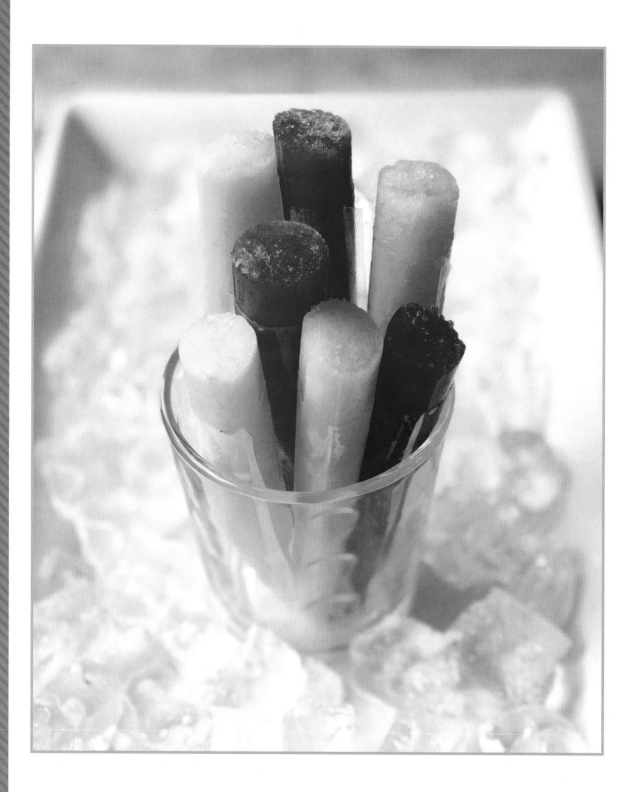

# Strawberry & Mango Fruity Ice Pops

*Below are the ingredients used for strawberry ice pops and mango ice pops. Follow the instructions below for each type of ice pop you want to make. Purchase the zip-top ice-pop bags on Amazon. You can get hundreds of them for just a few dollars. Keep them around for summer freezing fun!*

**YIELD: 14–16 ICE POPS PER RECIPE**
Prep Time: 10 minutes
Total Time: 4 hours (includes freezing)

**Strawberry Ice Pops**

4 cups lemonade
1 (10-ounce) bag frozen strawberries
2 tablespoons honey

**Mango Ice Pops**

3 cups lemonade
1 cup orange juice
1 (10-ounce) bag frozen mango
2 tablespoons honey

**1.** In a blender combine the juice(s), frozen fruit, and honey. Blend until a smooth mixture forms.

**2.** Using a funnel, fill each of the ice pop mold bags about ¾ full. Do not overfill. You need to leave room for expansion during freezing or the bags will burst in the freezer.

**3.** Freeze for about 4 hours until the ice pops are solid.

 **Dr. Bear Fun Fact!** Mangoes come in all shapes, sizes, and colors! Don't be surprised if you find red, orange, or green mangoes in addition to the popular yellow ones!

*Nutritional data reflects one strawberry ice pop, based on a 15-pop yield.*

**PER SERVING** Calories: 42; Total Fat: 0.1g; Saturated Fat: 0g; Cholesterol: 0mg; Sodium: 3.1mg; Total Carbohydrates: 10.9g; Dietary Fiber: 0.4g; Sugars: 9.8g; Protein: 0.1g

*Nutritional data reflects one mango ice pop, based on a 15-pop yield.*

**PER SERVING** Calories: 48; Total Fat: 0.1g; Saturated Fat: 0g; Cholesterol: 0mg; Sodium: 2.3mg; Total Carbohydrates: 12.5g; Dietary Fiber: 0.3g; Sugars: 11.5g; Protein: 0.2g

# Fudgy Nutella Fudge Brownies with Sea Salt

*Rich, fudgy, and delectable, as my friend Dr. Jocelyn Silvester says! These are great with a big glass of milk or a cup of piping hot coffee.*

**YIELD: 16–20 BROWNIES**
Prep Time: 15 minutes
Total Time: 60 minutes

---

1½ cups Nutella

¾ cup butter, cut into pieces

4 ounces semisweet chocolate chips

¾ cup gluten-free all-purpose flour

¼ cup cocoa powder

4 eggs

½ cup granulated sugar

½ cup brown sugar

1 teaspoon vanilla extract

1 teaspoon coarse sea salt

1. Preheat oven to 350°F. Line an 8-by-8-inch glass baking dish with parchment paper and set aside.

2. In a small pot over medium-low heat, whisk together the Nutella, butter, and chocolate chips until melted and smooth. Remove from heat and let cool, about 10 minutes.

3. In a mixing bowl, whisk together the gluten-free all-purpose flour and cocoa powder. Set aside.

4. In the bowl of stand mixer, using the paddle attachment, beat together the eggs, sugars, and vanilla extract until well combined. Add the cooled Nutella mixture and mix together well.

5. Slowly add the dry ingredients into the wet ingredients, mixing well after each addition.

6. Pour the batter into the prepared baking pan and sprinkle coarse sea salt across the top. Bake for 35 to 40 minutes until set. You'll know the brownies are done when a toothpick inserted into the center comes out with a few wet crumbs still attached.

7. Cool to room temperature before slicing.

 **Dr. Bear Fun Fact!** Why does adding salt to sweet foods taste so good? Our bodies are hardwired to love it! Sugar signals the body that there is energy coming its way (in the form of calories), and salt is a necessary mineral for bodily function. Mix the two together and your brain wants more!

*Nutritional data reflects one brownie, based on an 18-brownie yield.*

**PER SERVING** Calories: 245; Total Fat: 14.8g; Saturated Fat: 7.7g; Cholesterol: 56.8mg; Sodium: 151.9mg; Total Carbohydrates: 25.6g; Dietary Fiber: 1g; Sugars: 20g; Protein: 2.9g

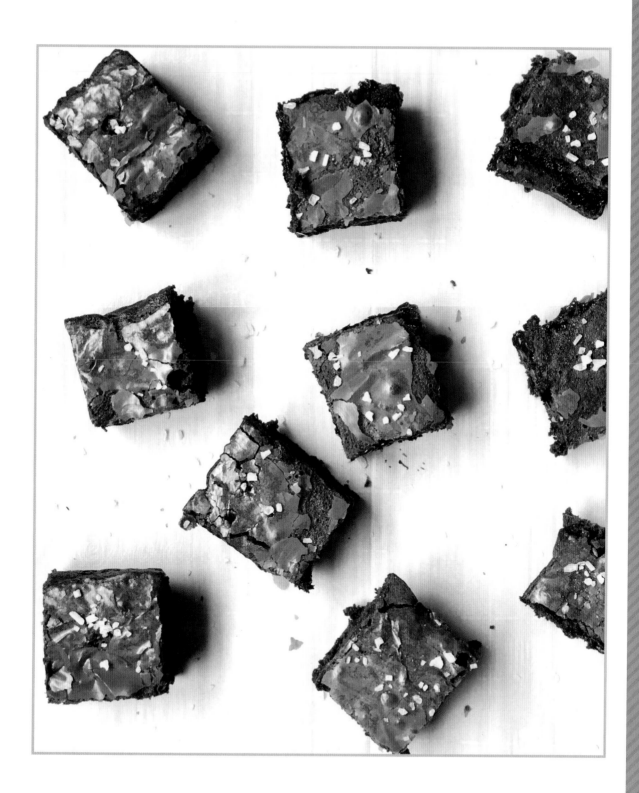

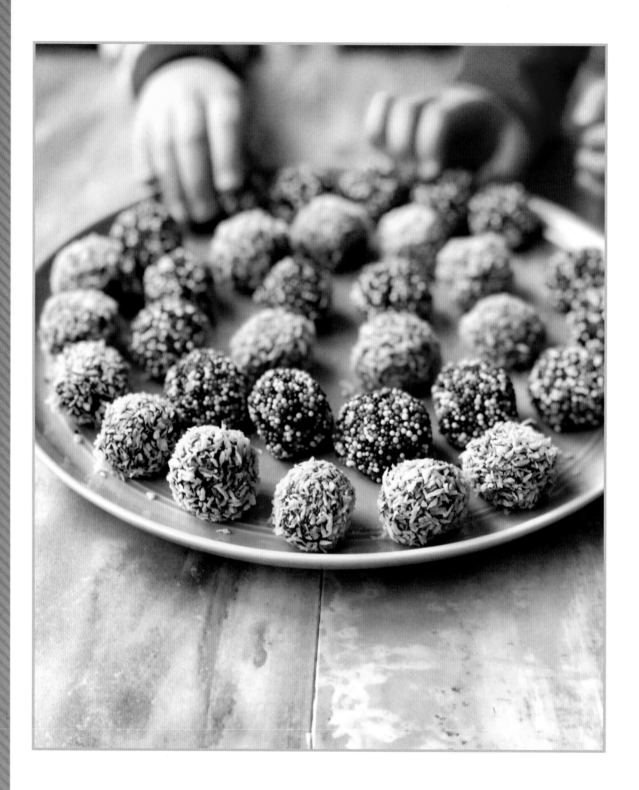

# Brazilian Brigadeiro Truffles

*These incredible truffles come from our amazing au pair, Brenda Cota, from Brazil. She made these for a holiday dinner, and everyone around the table agreed they are sensational. In the photo the truffles are rolled in sprinkles and grated coconut, but you can roll them in any chopped toppings you'd like. Try chopped pecans or walnuts or even crushed candy canes.*

**YIELD: 40–48 TRUFFLES**
Prep Time: 10 minutes
Total Time: 40 minutes

¼ cup butter
2 (14-ounce) cans sweetened
  condensed milk
4 tablespoons cocoa powder
Sprinkles or grated coconut for rolling

**1.** Grease an 8-by-8-inch glass baking dish with nonstick spray. Set aside.

**2.** In a medium-sized pot, melt the butter over low heat.

**3.** Add the condensed milk and stir to combine. Add the cocoa powder, one tablespoon at a time, mixing well after each addition.

**4.** Cook, stirring constantly, until the mixture loosens and pulls away from the sides of the pan, about 5 to 7 minutes. Remove from heat and pour the mixture into the prepared baking dish. Cool completely.

**5.** Grease your hands with butter or nonstick spray, and roll the truffle mixture into small balls about 1 inch in diameter. Roll the balls in sprinkles or grated coconut and transfer to a serving plate.

 **Dr. Bear Fun Fact!** Brigadeiro truffles are a sentimental dessert for Brazilians. They are often eaten at birthday parties or family reunions.

*Nutritional data reflects one truffle without toppings, based on a 44-truffle yield.*

**PER SERVING**  Calories: 66; Total Fat: 2.4g; Saturated Fat: 1.5g; Cholesterol: 8.2mg; Sodium: 23.1mg; Total Carbohydrates: 10.1g; Dietary Fiber: 0.2g; Sugars: 9.8g; Protein: 1.5g

# Crispy Ooey & Gooey Baked Apples

*After a trip to our local orchard, we have hundreds of apples to eat and cook with. These baked apples are such a simple and comforting dessert. Serve them topped with vanilla ice cream.*

**YIELD: 8 SERVINGS**
Prep Time: 20 minutes
Total Time: 50 minutes

---

4 Golden Delicious apples
1 cup brown sugar
1 cup gluten-free quick cook oats
½ cup shredded coconut
½ cup cornstarch
1 teaspoon ground cinnamon
½ teaspoon salt
½ cup solid coconut oil
Vanilla ice cream, for serving

**1.** Preheat oven to 375°F. Spray a 9-by-13-inch baking dish with nonstick spray and set aside.

**2.** Slice the apples in half and, using a melon baller or apple corer, scrape out the core and about ¾-inch of apple flesh to make room for the topping to sink in. Place the apples cut side up in the prepared baking dish.

**3.** To make the topping, combine the brown sugar, gluten-free oats, shredded coconut, cornstarch, cinnamon, salt, and coconut oil in the bowl of a food processor. Pulse until the mixture is crumbly.

**4.** Evenly distribute the topping between the 8 apple halves. Bake for 15 to 20 minutes until the apples are soft and the topping is golden and crispy.

**5.** Place one apple half on each serving plate and top with a heaping scoop of ice cream.

 **Dr. Bear Fun Fact!** Baking apples has been one of the most popular methods of eating apples in history! Researchers discovered charred remains of wild apples from a lake in southern Germany that were thousands of years old!

*Nutritional data reflects one serving without ice cream, based on an 8-serving yield.*
**PER SERVING** Calories: 310; Total Fat: 13g; Saturated Fat: 11g; Cholesterol: 0mg; Sodium: 162.3mg; Total Carbohydrates: 48.4g; Dietary Fiber: 6g; Sugars: 27.5g; Protein: 3g

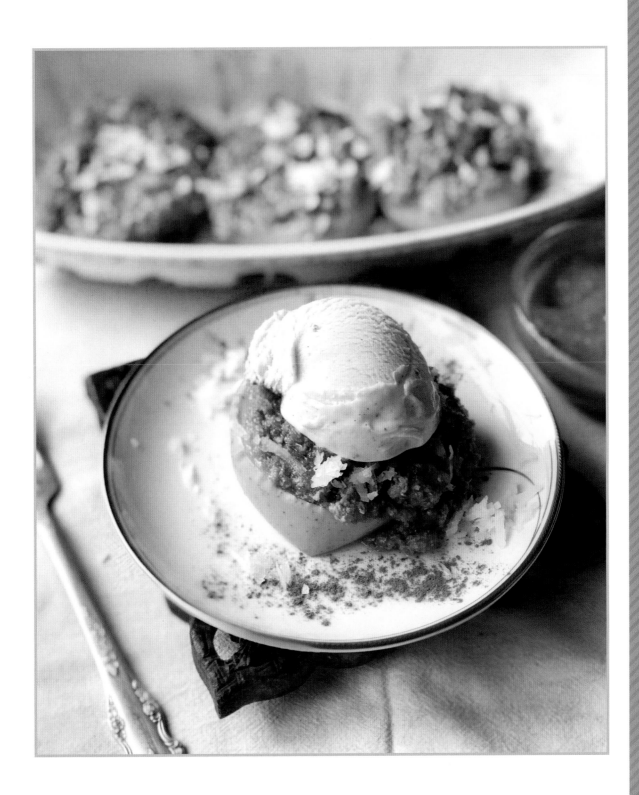

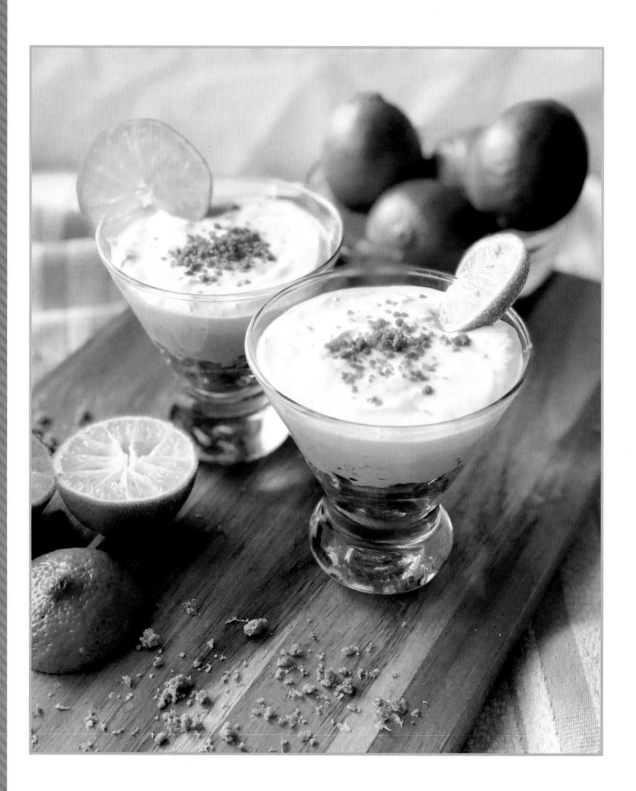

# Key Lime Pudding Parfaits with Sweet Cream

*My mother-in-law's favorite dessert is key lime pie, so this recipe is dedicated to Marcia Weisbrod. It's just the perfect amount of sweetness with a touch of crispy graham-style crumbs.*

**YIELD: 8 SERVINGS**

Prep Time: 30 minutes
Total Time: 2 hours, 30 minutes
  (includes chilling time)

---

2 (14-ounce cans) sweetened condensed milk

2 eggs

1 cup key lime juice

Zest of 2 limes, divided

1 (10.5-ounce) package gluten-free graham cracker crumbs (pictured is Kinnikinnick brand)

3 tablespoons butter, melted

¼ cup sugar

1 cup sour cream

3 tablespoons powdered sugar

Optional garnishes: additional lime zest or graham cracker crumbs

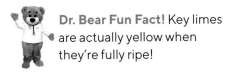 **Dr. Bear Fun Fact!** Key limes are actually yellow when they're fully ripe!

*Nutritional data reflects one serving, based on an 8-serving yield.*

**PER SERVING** Calories: 652; Total Fat: 28g; Saturated Fat: 16g; Cholesterol: 124mg; Sodium: 283mg; Total Carbohydrates: 91g; Dietary Fiber: 1g; Sugars: 73g; Protein: 11g

**1.** Preheat oven to 375°F. Spray an 8-by-8-inch glass baking dish with nonstick spray and set aside. Line a baking sheet with foil and set aside.

**2.** In a large mixing bowl, whisk together the sweetened condensed milk, eggs, key lime juice, and zest of 1 lime until a smooth mixture forms.

**3.** Pour this mixture into the prepared baking dish and bake for 20 to 25 minutes until the center is set. Remove from oven and cool completely. Refrigerate for 2 hours before assembling parfaits.

**4.** In a clean mixing bowl, mix together the gluten-free graham cracker crumbs, melted butter, and sugar. Spread this mixture evenly across the prepared baking sheet. Bake for 10 minutes until crispy. Remove from oven and cool completely.

**5.** While the pudding and crumbs are cooling, whisk together the sour cream, powdered sugar, and remaining zest of 1 lime in a small glass mixing bowl. Cover and refrigerate until ready to serve.

**6.** To assemble the parfaits, spoon about 3 teaspoons of graham cracker crumbs into the bottom of each parfait dish. Top with about 3 tablespoons of the key lime pudding and then about 2 teaspoons of the sweet cream. Repeat to form a second layer. Keep layering until no more ingredients are left.

**7.** Garnish with lime zest and a sprinkle of gluten-free graham cracker crumbs.

# Chocolate Cupcakes with Chocolate Frosting

*These cupcakes are a classic childhood favorite. I make these in big batches and freeze them, so I always have a cupcake to send with my kids for a birthday party.*

**YIELD: 18 CUPCAKES**
Prep Time: 15 minutes
Total Time: 40 minutes

---

### For the Chocolate Cake

2 cups gluten-free all-purpose flour
1 cup granulated sugar
¾ cup cocoa powder
½ cup brown sugar
2 teaspoons baking powder
1 teaspoon salt
2 eggs
1½ cups coconut milk
½ cup vegetable oil
2 teaspoons vanilla extract
½ cup boiling water

### For the Chocolate Frosting

3 cups powdered sugar
⅔ cup cocoa powder
½ cup coconut oil
1 teaspoon vanilla extract
2 to 5 tablespoons coconut milk

*Nutritional data reflects one cupcake, based on an 18-cupcake yield.*

**PER SERVING** Calories: 321; Total Fat: 14g; Saturated Fat: 7g; Cholesterol: 18mg; Sodium: 195mg; Total Carbohydrates: 50g; Dietary Fiber: 3g; Sugars: 35g; Protein: 3g

1. Preheat oven to 350°F, and lightly grease two 12-cup cupcake pans with nonstick spray or cupcake liners. Set aside.

2. To make the cupcake batter, in a mixing bowl, whisk together the gluten-free all-purpose flour, granulated sugar, cocoa powder, brown sugar, baking powder and salt. Set aside.

3. In the bowl of a stand mixer, using the paddle attachment, beat together the eggs, coconut milk, oil, and vanilla extract.

4. Slowly add the dry ingredients into the wet ingredients, mixing well after each addition. Slowly add the boiling water and mix well until a smooth batter forms.

5. Divide the batter evenly among the prepared baking cups and bake for 15 to 18 minutes until a toothpick inserted into the center comes out clean. Let cool completely on a cooling rack.

6. While the cupcakes are cooling, make the frosting. Combine the powdered sugar, cocoa powder, coconut oil, and vanilla extract in a food processor. Pulse the mixture as you add the coconut milk. Add coconut milk until desired consistency is reached. The frosting should heavily coat a spoon.

7. Once cooled, frost each cupcake and decorate with sprinkles, if desired.

**Dr. Bear Fun Fact!** The concept of a "cupcake" dates back to 1796 where the intention was to bake cakes in small cups.

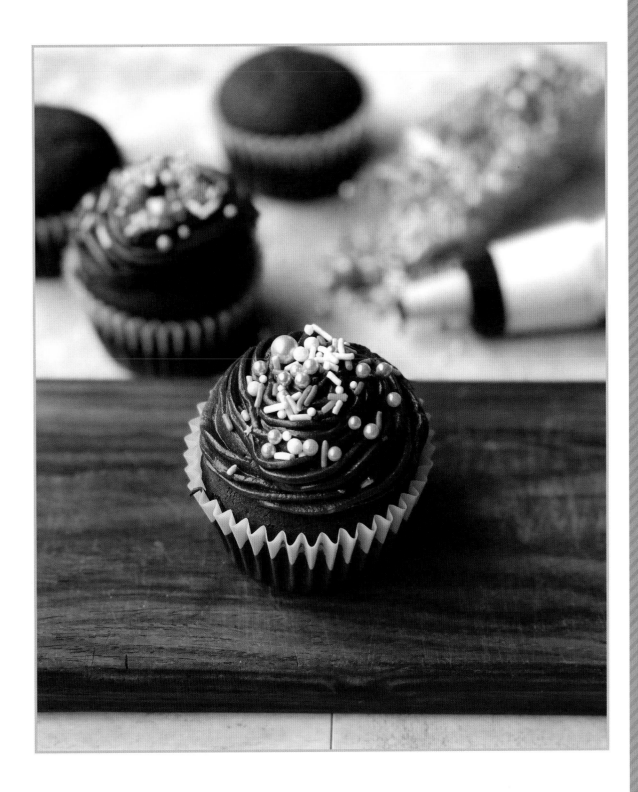

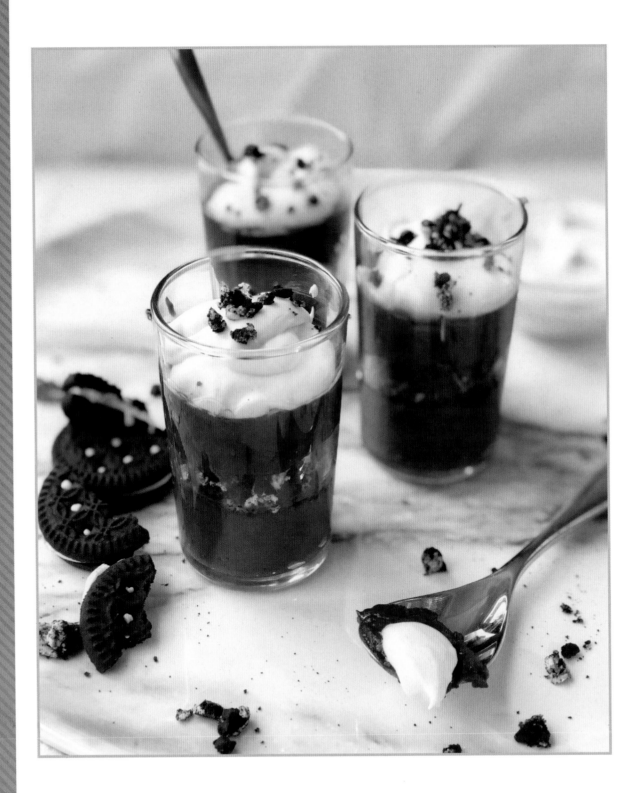

# Cookies & Cream Chocolate Pudding Cups

*This is a dairy-free delight that my family eats for dessert. But we also eat the pudding topped with granola and sliced berries for breakfast!*

**YIELD: 8 SERVINGS**
Prep Time: 10 minutes
Total Time: 20 minutes

---

20 pitted dates
½ cup hot water
⅓ cup coconut oil, warmed
1 teaspoon vanilla extract
1 teaspoon salt
2 ripe avocados, skin and pit removed
1 banana, peeled
¾ cup peanut butter
½ cup cocoa powder
½ cup coconut milk
2 tablespoons honey
1 (14-ounce) can coconut milk, refrigerated overnight
½ cup powdered sugar
1 teaspoon vanilla extract
15 gluten-free Oreo-style cookies, crushed

**1.** In the bowl of a food processor, combine the dates and hot water. Let sit for about 5 minutes to soften. Once softened, pulse together the dates, hot water, coconut oil, vanilla extract, and salt. Purée until smooth.

**2.** Add the avocados, banana, peanut butter, cocoa powder, coconut milk, and honey and pulse until a smooth pudding forms. Cover and refrigerate until ready to serve.

**3.** To make the coconut whipped cream, carefully open the chilled can of coconut milk. Scrape off just the solid portion at the top of the can and place in a glass bowl. Add the powdered sugar and vanilla extract and beat with a hand mixer for about 30 seconds. The cream will not be as stiff as whipped cream, but that's OK. You want it softer for this recipe!

**4.** To assemble the pudding cups, place a scoop of pudding in the bottom of each serving dish. Top with crushed gluten-free Oreo-style cookies. Repeat with a second layer of pudding and crushed cookies. Top with a dollop of coconut whipped cream and garnish with a sprinkle of crushed cookies.

 **Dr. Bear Fun Fact!** Dates were a superfood in antiquity! Because they are packed with vitamins, minerals, and energy, nomadic tribes in the Middle East and North Africa relied on these naturally dry fruits to survive in the desert.

*Nutritional data reflects one serving, based on an 8-serving yield.*
**PER SERVING** Calories: 546; Total Fat: 33.2g; Saturated Fat: 13.8g; Cholesterol: 0mg; Sodium: 476.9mg; Total Carbohydrates: 61.9g; Dietary Fiber: 8.4g; Sugars: 40.9g; Protein: 8.3g

# Cut-Out Sugar Cookies

*I use this recipe almost every time there is a snow day at school. Making the cookie dough, watching them bake, and then decorating with colorful frosting and sprinkles provides at least an hour's worth of entertainment for my boys.*

**YIELD: 18–24 COOKIES (DEPENDS ON SIZE OF COOKIE CUTTERS)**
Prep Time: 10 minutes
Total Time: 30 minutes

1½ cups gluten-free all-purpose flour, plus more for dusting
1 teaspoon baking powder
½ teaspoon salt
½ cup coconut oil
½ cup sugar
1 egg
½ teaspoon vanilla extract
½ teaspoon almond extract
Garnishes: frosting, sprinkles, decor of your choice.

**1. In a mixing bowl, whisk together the gluten-free all-purpose flour, baking powder, and salt. Set aside.**

**2.** In the bowl of a stand mixer, using the paddle attachment, beat together the coconut oil, sugar, egg, vanilla extract, and almond extract.

**3.** Slowly add the dry ingredients into the wet ingredients, mixing well after each addition.

**4.** Cover and chill the dough for 30 to 60 minutes until firm enough to roll out.

**5.** Preheat oven to 325°F. Line two baking sheets with parchment paper and set aside.

**6.** Dust a work surface with gluten-free all-purpose flour. Roll the dough out to about ½ inch thick.

**7.** Cut out the dough in desired shapes with cookie cutters and transfer to the parchment lined baking sheets.

**8.** Bake for 10 to 13 minutes until set. Do not overcook. It's very important to cool completely before moving the cookies to a plate for decorating.

 **Dr. Bear Fun Fact!** What does it mean when you have vanilla or almond extract? An "extract" is a very concentrated liquid that gives flavor to food. This way, you can add a dash of it into recipes to pack in more flavor!

*Nutritional data reflects one cookie without toppings, based on a 20-cookie yield.*
**PER SERVING** Calories: 105; Total Fat: 5.8g; Saturated Fat: 4.6g; Cholesterol: 8.2mg; Sodium: 86.7mg; Total Carbohydrates: 12.4g; Dietary Fiber: 0.3g; Sugars: 5.1g; Protein: 0.7g

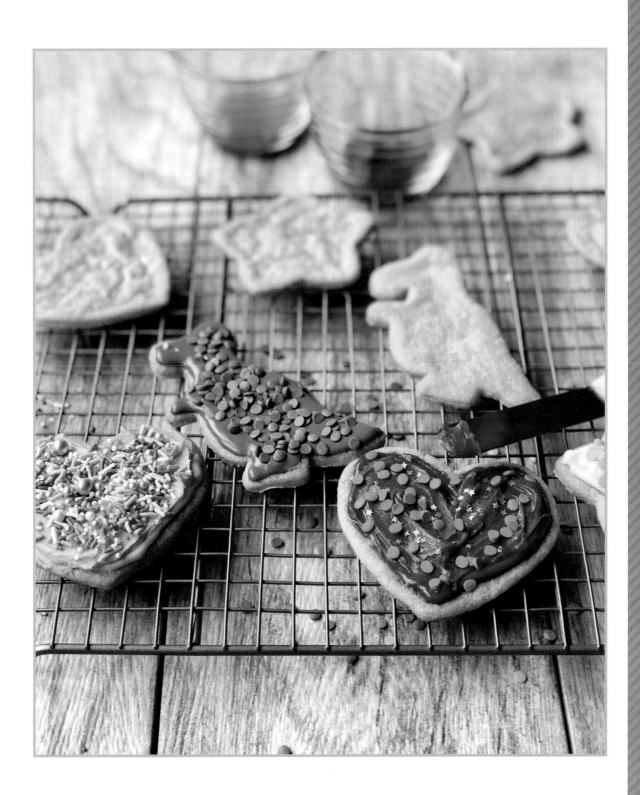

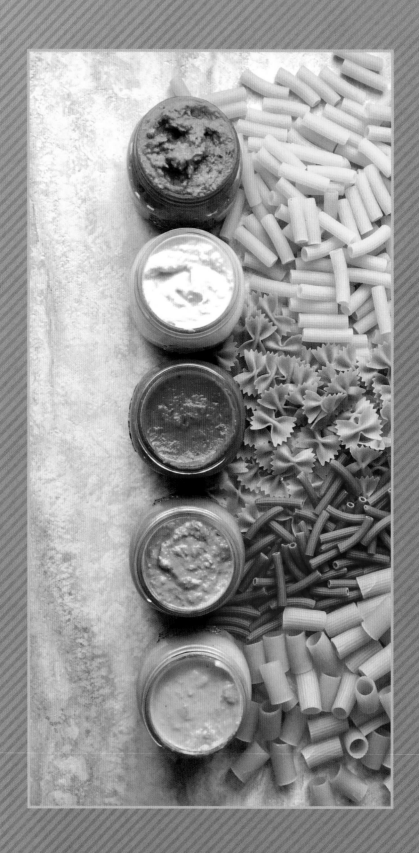

# 11

# Dressings, Butters, & Sauces

Kid-friendly participation steps are printed in **ORANGE**

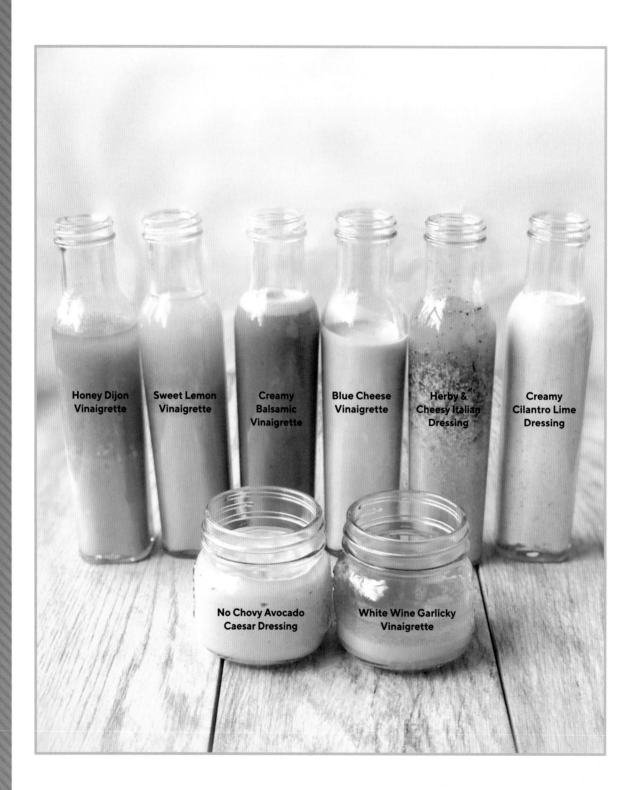

Honey Dijon
Vinaigrette

Sweet Lemon
Vinaigrette

Creamy
Balsamic
Vinaigrette

Blue Cheese
Vinaigrette

Herby &
Cheesy Italian
Dressing

Creamy
Cilantro Lime
Dressing

No Chovy Avocado
Caesar Dressing

White Wine Garlicky
Vinaigrette

# Herby & Cheesy Italian Dressing

*I've tried a lot of store-bought Italian dressings and just never found one I really liked. I started working on creating my own after eating at Calabria in Livingston, New Jersey. They toss their salads in the most divine Italian dressing. This recipe is my attempt at replicating it!*

**YIELD: 1 CUP**
**(2-TABLESPOON SERVINGS)**
Prep Time: 5 minutes
Total Time: 10 minutes

---

½ cup olive oil
¼ cup red wine vinegar
¼ cup grated Romano cheese
Juice of 2 lemons
2 teaspoons Dijon mustard
2 teaspoons sugar
2 teaspoons Italian seasoning blend
½ teaspoon garlic powder
½ teaspoon salt

1. In a glass mixing bowl or mason jar, whisk together all of the ingredients.

2. Cover and refrigerate until ready to use.

*Nutritional data reflects one serving size of 2 tablespoons.*
**PER SERVING** Calories: 143; Total Fat: 14.5g; Saturated Fat: 2.4g; Cholesterol: 2.7mg; Sodium: 234.9mg; Total Carbohydrates: 2.7g; Dietary Fiber: 0.2g; Sugars: 1.4g; Protein: 1.1g

# Creamy Balsamic Vinaigrette

*I had so much fun creating this recipe. It started out as a delicious Balsamic Vinaigrette from my mom pal Jackie and morphed into something a little different when my two-year-old son came to help me in the kitchen. He stuck his finger in the bowl of dressing, tasted it, squeezed his eyes shut, and said "eeewww." But then he went back in and got more. So, I knew he liked it, but something wasn't sitting right. I immediately got out more ingredients and started over. This time I removed the garlic clove and the oregano. Not only did he love it, but he now insists on dipping his tomatoes and cucumbers in this dressing. The lesson is that with a few simple modifications, the dressing became something our entire family enjoys.*

**YIELD: 1⅔ CUPS**
**(2-TABLESPOON SERVINGS)**
Prep Time: 5 minutes
Total Time: 10 minutes

---

¾ cup olive oil

½ cup balsamic vinegar

3 fresh basil leaves, rinsed, patted dry, and roughly chopped

3 tablespoons mayonnaise

2 tablespoons lemon juice

1 tablespoon Dijon mustard

1 tablespoon sugar

1 teaspoon salt

**1.** In a small blender or food processor, combine all the ingredients together and pulse until a smooth mixture forms.

**2.** Cover and refrigerate until ready to serve with the salad.

*Nutritional data reflects one serving size of 2 tablespoons.*

**PER SERVING** Calories: 146; Total Fat: 14.9g; Saturated Fat: 2.1g; Cholesterol: 1.3mg; Sodium: 232.3mg; Total Carbohydrates: 2.9g; Dietary Fiber: 0.1g; Sugars: 2.5g; Protein: 0.2g

# Sweet Lemon Vinaigrette

*This is by far my favorite salad dressing. It's light, simple, and tastes great with any salad fixings. My favorite though, is to toss this dressing together with chopped butter lettuce, cucumbers, and avocado.*

**YIELD: 1¼ CUPS (2-TABLESPOON SERVINGS)**
Prep Time: 5 minutes
Total Time: 10 minutes

---

½ cup olive oil
Zest of 2 lemons
½ cup lemon juice
4 teaspoons sugar
2 teaspoons Dijon mustard
½ teaspoon sea salt

1. In a glass mixing bowl or mason jar, whisk together all of the ingredients.
2. Cover and refrigerate until ready to serve.

*Nutritional data reflects one serving size of 2 tablespoons.*
**PER SERVING** Calories: 105; Total Fat: 10.9g; Saturated Fat: 1.5g; Cholesterol: 0mg; Sodium: 144mg; Total Carbohydrates: 2.4g; Dietary Fiber: 0.1g; Sugars: 1.9g; Protein: 0.1g

# Blue Cheese Vinaigrette

*My friend Julianne is the inspiration behind this salad dressing. She threw a gender-reveal party for a pregnant friend and made a salad using a blue cheese and red wine vinegar dressing with candied pecans. It was divine. I tried my own version at dinner with my parents a few weeks later, but my dad has a thing about chunky blue cheese and raw onions, so I puréed all of the ingredients together into a very smooth dressing. Needless to say, he loved it.*

**YIELD: 1 CUP
(2-TABLESPOON SERVINGS)**
Prep Time: 5 minutes
Total Time: 10 minutes

---

½ cup olive oil

½ cup blue cheese crumbles

¼ cup red wine vinegar

1 shallot, skin removed and finely minced

½ teaspoon salt

**1.** In small food processor, combine all of the ingredients. Pulse until a smooth mixture forms. If you like a chunkier blue cheese dressing, you can skip the food processor and whisk the ingredients together in a mixing bowl.

**2.** Cover and refrigerate until ready to serve.

*Nutritional data reflects one serving size of 2 tablespoons.*

**PER SERVING** Calories: 153; Total Fat: 15.9g; Saturated Fat: 3.4g; Cholesterol: 6.3mg; Sodium: 245.4mg; Total Carbohydrates: 0.9g; Dietary Fiber: 0.1g; Sugars: 0.3g; Protein: 1.9g

# Honey Dijon Vinaigrette

*This is one of the easiest dressings to make. Be sure to make it far enough in advance to allow it to chill in the refrigerator for about 30 minutes before serving. The flavors really brighten after giving it time to rest.*

**YIELD: 1 CUP (2-TABLESPOON SERVINGS)**

Prep Time: 5 minutes

Total Time: 40 minutes
  (including chill time)

---

½ cup olive oil

3 tablespoons apple cider vinegar

1 shallot, skin removed and
  finely chopped

1 tablespoon Dijon mustard

2 teaspoons honey

Juice of 1 lemon

½ teaspoon salt

1. In a small glass mixing bowl or mason jar, whisk together all of the ingredients.

2. Cover and refrigerate until ready to serve.

*Nutritional data reflects one serving size of 2 tablespoons.*

**PER SERVING** Calories: 132; Total Fat: 13.6g; Saturated Fat: 1.9g; Cholesterol: 0mg; Sodium: 193.4mg; Total Carbohydrates: 2.7g; Dietary Fiber: 0.2g; Sugars: 1.9g; Protein: 0.2g

# Honey Poppy Seed Vinaigrette

*This dressing is sweet and pairs well with salads that have citrus in them like oranges or grapefruits.*

**YIELD: 1 CUP
(2-TABLESPOON SERVINGS)**
Prep Time: 5 minutes
Total Time: 10 minutes

---

½ cup olive oil

¼ cup honey

2 tablespoons white vinegar

1 tablespoon Dijon mustard

1 small shallot, skin removed
   and finely minced

2 teaspoons poppy seeds

½ teaspoon salt

1. In a glass bowl or mason jar, whisk together all of the ingredients.

2. Cover and refrigerate until ready to serve.

*Nutritional data reflects one serving size of 2 tablespoons.*

**PER SERVING**  Calories: 160; Total Fat: 13.9g; Saturated Fat: 1.9g; Cholesterol: 0mg; Sodium: 193.3mg; Total Carbohydrates: 9.3g; Dietary Fiber: 0.3g; Sugars: 8.8g; Protein: 0.3g

# White Wine Garlicky Vinaigrette

*A little sweet and a little tart, this goes great with salads that include roasted vegetables.*

**YIELD: ½ CUP**
**(2-TABLESPOON SERVINGS)**
Prep Time: 5 minutes
Total Time: 10 minutes

---

2 tablespoons white wine vinegar

1 garlic clove, peeled and
   finely minced

2 teaspoons lemon juice

1 teaspoon Dijon mustard

1 teaspoon sugar

¼ cup olive oil

1. In a small mixing bowl or mason jar, whisk together all of the ingredients.

2. Cover and refrigerate until ready to serve.

*Nutritional data reflects one serving size of 2 tablespoons.*

**PER SERVING**  Calories: 128; Total Fat: 13.6g; Saturated Fat: 1.9g; Cholesterol: 0mg; Sodium: 30.4mg; Total Carbohydrates: 1.4g; Dietary Fiber: 0.1g; Sugars: 1.1g; Protein: 0.1g

# No-Chovy Avocado Caesar Dressing

*I really don't like the taste of anchovies, but I love Caesar salad. This Caesar-like dressing uses avocado for creaminess and comes pretty close to the real deal.*

**YIELD: 1 CUP
(2-TABLESPOON SERVINGS)**
Prep Time: 5 minutes
Total Time: 10 minutes

---

1 avocado, skin and pit removed
½ cup olive oil
1 garlic clove, peeled
2 tablespoons mayonnaise
2 tablespoons lemon juice
1 tablespoon Dijon mustard
1 tablespoon red wine vinegar
1 tablespoon Worcestershire sauce
½ teaspoon salt

1. In a food processor, combine all ingredients. Purée until smooth.

2. Cover and refrigerate until ready to serve.

*Nutritional data reflects one serving size of 2 tablespoons.*

**PER SERVING** Calories: 235; Total Fat: 25.1g; Saturated Fat: 3.5g; Cholesterol: 1.9mg; Sodium: 316.1mg; Total Carbohydrates: 3.2g; Dietary Fiber: 1.7g; Sugars: 0.5g; Protein: 0.7g

# Creamy Cilantro Lime Dressing

*Taco salad is one of my favorite meals, and I firmly believe that all taco salads need some sort of dressing. This creamy cilantro lime vinaigrette pairs great with shredded lettuce, black beans, cheese, rice, pico de gallo, and any type of grilled meats.*

**YIELD: 1¼ CUPS**
**(2-TABLESPOON SERVINGS)**
Prep Time: 10 minutes
Total Time: 10 minutes

---

¾ cup sour cream

½ cup fresh cilantro leaves, rinsed and patted dry

2 tablespoons olive oil

2 tablespoons lime juice

Zest of 1 lime

1 teaspoon ground cumin

1 teaspoon sugar

½ teaspoon salt

**1.** In a food processor, combine all ingredients. Purée until smooth.

**2.** Cover and refrigerate until ready to serve.

*Nutritional data reflects one serving size of 2 tablespoons.*

**PER SERVING**  Calories: 102; Total Fat: 10.2g; Saturated Fat: 3.5g; Cholesterol: 17mg; Sodium: 206.8mg; Total Carbohydrates: 2.7g; Dietary Fiber: 0.1g; Sugars: 1.8g; Protein: 0.8g

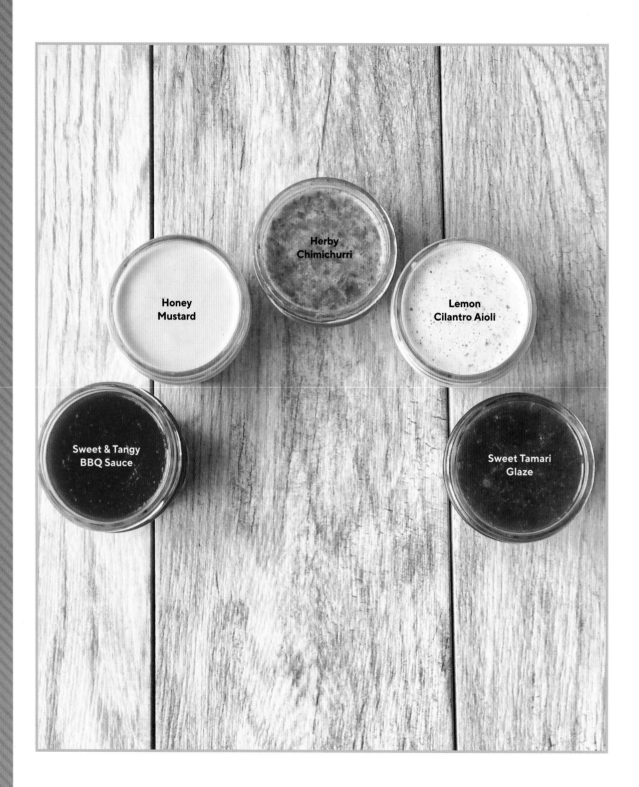

Honey
Mustard

Herby
Chimichurri

Lemon
Cilantro Aioli

Sweet & Tangy
BBQ Sauce

Sweet Tamari
Glaze

# Honey Mustard Dipping Sauce

*This sauce has so many uses for dipping, including homemade chicken tenders and French fries, or spread it on a wrap with your favorite lunch meats.*

**YIELD: ¾ CUP**
**(2-TABLESPOON SERVINGS)**
Prep Time: 5 minutes
Total Time: 5 minutes

---

¼ cup Dijon mustard

¼ cup mayonnaise

¼ cup honey

1 teaspoon red wine vinegar

1. In a small glass bowl or mason jar, whisk together all of the ingredients.

2. Cover and refrigerate until ready to serve.

*Nutritional data reflects one serving size of 2 tablespoons.*

**PER SERVING** Calories: 116; Total Fat: 7.4g; Saturated Fat: 1.1g; Cholesterol: 3.9mg; Sodium: 298.6mg; Total Carbohydrates: 12.3g; Dietary Fiber: 0.4g; Sugars: 11.8g; Protein: 0.6g

# Herby Chimichurri

*Packed with bright herbs, this chimichurri is delightful served on grilled fish and steak.*

**YIELD: 1 CUP
(2-TABLESPOON SERVINGS)**
Prep Time: 5 minutes
Total Time: 10 minutes

---

½ cup olive oil

½ cup fresh cilantro leaves,
   rinsed and patted dry

½ cup fresh parsley leaves,
   rinsed and patted dry

⅓ cup red wine vinegar

1 tablespoon lemon juice

½ teaspoon salt

**1.** Combine all ingredients in a small food processor and pulse until the desired consistency is reached. This chimichurri can be as smooth or chunky as you'd like.

**2.** Cover and refrigerate until ready to serve.

*Nutritional data reflects one serving size of 2 tablespoons.*

**PER SERVING**  Calories: 62; Total Fat: 6.8g; Saturated Fat: 0.9g; Cholesterol: 0mg; Sodium: 75.5mg; Total Carbohydrates: 0.2g; Dietary Fiber: 0.1g; Sugars: 0g; Protein: 0.1g

# Sweet & Tangy BBQ Sauce

*This BBQ sauce works great as a dipping sauce for homemade chicken tenders or slathered on chicken wings.*

**YIELD: 1 CUP**
**(2-TABLESPOON SERVINGS)**
Prep Time: 5 minutes
Total Time: 10 minutes

---

¾ cup ketchup

¼ cup Worcestershire sauce

2 tablespoons apple cider vinegar

2 tablespoons honey

1 tablespoon brown sugar

1 teaspoon lemon juice

½ teaspoon garlic powder

½ teaspoon paprika

¼ teaspoon salt

1. In a small sauce pot set over medium heat, whisk together all of the ingredients.

2. Bring to a simmer and then reduce heat to low. Let simmer for 5 minutes.

3. Serve warm or cool completely before serving.

*Nutritional data reflects one serving size of 2 tablespoons.*

**PER SERVING** Calories: 52; Total Fat: 0g; Saturated Fat: 0g; Cholesterol: 0mg; Sodium: 362.9mg; Total Carbohydrates: 13.6g; Dietary Fiber: 0.2g; Sugars: 11.2g; Protein: 0.3g

# Sweet Tamari Glaze

*This glaze is incredible served over pan-seared salmon or halibut but is also great served over roasted vegetables.*

**YIELD: 1¼ CUPS
(2-TABLESPOON SERVINGS)**
Prep Time: 5 minutes
Total Time: 10 minutes

---

4 tablespoons butter
½ teaspoon garlic paste
¾ cup apricot preserves
⅓ cup gluten-free tamari soy sauce

1. In a small sauce pot set over medium heat, continuously whisk together all ingredients until the butter is melted and a smooth sauce forms, about 5 minutes.

2. Drizzle sauce over desired protein.

*Nutritional data reflects one serving size of 2 tablespoons.*

**PER SERVING** Calories: 53; Total Fat: 2.4g; Saturated Fat: 1.4g; Cholesterol: 6.1mg; Sodium: 141mg; Total Carbohydrates: 7.9g; Dietary Fiber: 0g; Sugars: 5.2g; Protein: 0.4g

# Lemon Cilantro Aioli

*I originally created this aioli to serve with fried shrimp, but it was so good, I started dipping lots of foods in it like carrot and cucumber sticks and even French fries!*

**YIELD: 1¼ CUPS
(2-TABLESPOON SERVINGS)**
Prep Time: 5 minutes
Total Time: 10 minutes

---

½ cup mayonnaise

½ cup fresh cilantro leaves, rinsed
  and patted dry

¼ cup lemon juice

3 scallions, ends removed and
  roughly chopped

½ teaspoon salt

**1.** In a small food processor, combine all ingredients. Purée until a smooth mixture forms.

**2.** Cover and refrigerate until ready to serve.

*Nutritional data reflects one serving size of 2 tablespoons.*

**PER SERVING** Calories: 39; Total Fat: 4.1g; Saturated Fat: 0.7g; Cholesterol: 2.3mg; Sodium: 94.4mg; Total Carbohydrates: 0.4g; Dietary Fiber: 0.1g; Sugars: 0.2g; Protein: 0.1g

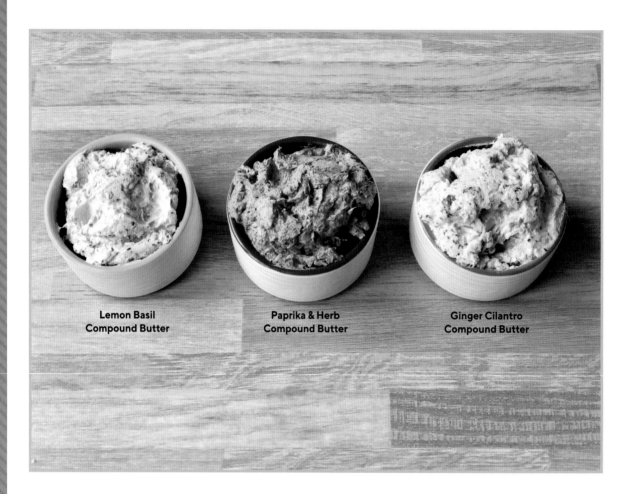

Lemon Basil
Compound Butter

Paprika & Herb
Compound Butter

Ginger Cilantro
Compound Butter

# Lemon Basil Compound Butter

*Use this butter on chicken wings, fish, or veggies. It's packed with flavor that will leave you licking your fingers!*

**YIELD: ⅔ CUP
(1-TABLESPOON SERVINGS)**
Prep Time: 5 minutes
Total Time: 10 minutes

---

½ cup butter

10 fresh basil leaves, rinsed
   and patted dry

2 tablespoons fresh oregano leaves,
   rinsed and patted dry

Zest of 2 lemons

½ teaspoon salt

**1.** In the bowl of a food processor, combine all ingredients, and pulse until a smooth butter forms.

**2.** Transfer to a covered container and refrigerate until ready to serve.

*Nutritional data reflects one serving size of 1 tablespoon.*

**PER SERVING** Calories: 83; Total Fat: 9.2g; Saturated Fat: 5.7g; Cholesterol: 24.4mg; Sodium: 119.3mg; Total Carbohydrates: 0.4g; Dietary Fiber: 0.3g; Sugars: 0g; Protein: 0.2g

# Paprika & Herb Compound Butter

*My favorite serving suggestion for this butter is on steaks and roasted vegetables, but it really goes with anything. I had about 2 tablespoons left over last night, so I tossed it into a plain risotto. My risotto instantly perked up with wonderful flavors. I also love it spread on a toasted gluten-free baguette.*

**YIELD: ⅔ CUP
(1-TABLESPOON SERVINGS)**

Prep Time: 5 minutes
Total Time: 10 minutes

---

½ cup butter, room temperature

2 cloves garlic, peeled and finely minced

1 teaspoon paprika

¼ cup finely chopped fresh cilantro leaves, rinsed and patted dry

¼ cup finely chopped fresh parsley, rinsed and patted dry

½ teaspoon salt

1. In a small food processor, combine all of the ingredients. Pulse until a smooth butter forms. If you like a slightly chunkier butter, combine the ingredients in a glass bowl and use a fork to mash together.

2. Cover and refrigerate until ready to serve.

*Nutritional data reflects one serving size of 1 tablespoon.*

**PER SERVING** Calories: 84; Total Fat: 9.3g; Saturated Fat: 5.8g; Cholesterol: 24.4mg; Sodium: 192.2mg; Total Carbohydrates: 0.4g; Dietary Fiber: 0.2g; Sugars: 0.1g; Protein: 0.2g

# Ginger Cilantro Compound Butter

*I typically serve this butter with fish or shrimp, but you could really put it on anything! Try making fried rice with this butter instead of oil.*

**YIELD: ⅔ CUP**
**(1-TABLESPOON SERVINGS)**
Prep Time: 5 minutes
Total Time: 10 minutes

---

½ cup butter

½ cup fresh cilantro leaves, rinsed and patted dry

Zest of 1 lemon

2 scallions, ends removed and roughly chopped

1 tablespoon minced fresh ginger, peeled

1 clove garlic, peeled

2 teaspoons sesame oil

½ teaspoon salt

1. In the bowl of a food processor, combine all ingredients and purée until smooth.

2. Cover and refrigerate until ready to serve.

*Nutritional data reflects one serving size of 1 tablespoon.*

**PER SERVING** Calories: 91; Total Fat: 10.1g; Saturated Fat: 5.9g; Cholesterol: 24.4mg; Sodium: 120mg; Total Carbohydrates: 0.4g; Dietary Fiber: 0.1g; Sugars: 0.1g; Protein: 0.2g

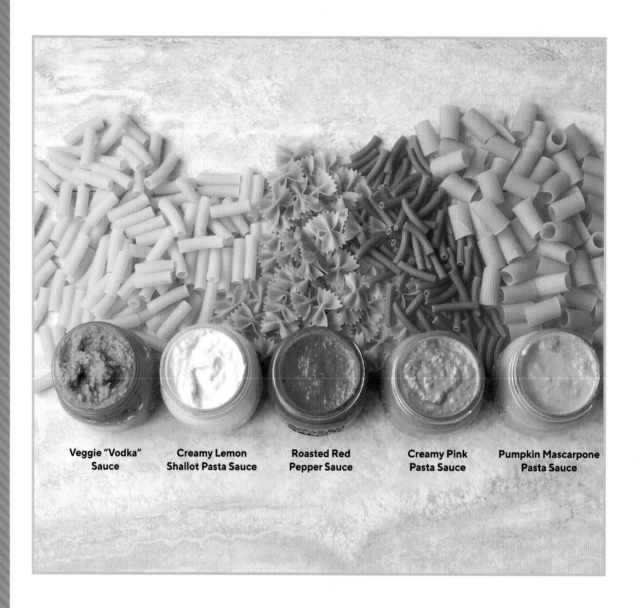

Veggie "Vodka" Sauce

Creamy Lemon Shallot Pasta Sauce

Roasted Red Pepper Sauce

Creamy Pink Pasta Sauce

Pumpkin Mascarpone Pasta Sauce

# Creamy Pink Pasta Sauce

*This is my go-to pasta sauce. It's so easy to make and is bursting with bright flavors. If your house is dairy-free, simply leave out the mascarpone. Or, if you want the sauce creamy with no dairy, roast 1 cup of chopped eggplant alongside the tomatoes and purée with the sauce.*

**YIELD: 1½ CUPS**
**(6-TABLESPOON SERVINGS)**
Prep Time: 5 minutes
Total Time: 40 minutes

1 pint grape tomatoes

3 tablespoons olive oil, divided

2 cloves garlic, peeled

½ teaspoon salt

2 shallots, skin removed and roughly chopped

12 basil leaves, rinsed and patted dry

Zest of 1 lemon

Juice of 1 lemon

1 teaspoon sugar

3 tablespoons mascarpone cheese

1. Preheat oven to 400°F. Line a baking sheet with foil and evenly spread the grape tomatoes across the baking sheet. Drizzle the tomatoes with 2½ tablespoons olive oil and salt and toss to evenly coat all of the tomatoes.

2. Place the garlic cloves on a small, separate piece of foil, drizzle with remaining olive oil, wrap it up, and place on same baking tray with tomatoes. Roast for 15 to 20 minutes until the tomatoes are soft and beginning to brown. Remove from oven and cool completely.

3. Once the tomatoes are cooled, combine the tomatoes, garlic, and all remaining liquids from the cooking juices in a food processor or blender. Add the shallots, basil leaves, lemon zest, lemon juice, sugar, and mascarpone and purée until a smooth sauce forms.

4. Taste and season with salt, if desired.

5. Cover and refrigerate until ready to use.

*Nutritional data reflects one serving size of 6 tablespoons.*

**PER SERVING** Calories: 189; Total Fat: 15.3g; Saturated Fat: 4.6g; Cholesterol: 14mg; Sodium: 306.3mg; Total Carbohydrates: 9.4g; Dietary Fiber: 1.8g; Sugars: 6g; Protein: 1.9g

# Roasted Red Pepper Sauce

*Roasting veggies brings out so many wonderful flavors. This recipe utilizes a red pepper, but if you don't have one, swap in any type of veggies, particularly tomatoes, squash, or carrots.*

**YIELD: 1½ CUPS
(6-TABLESPOON SERVINGS)**
Prep Time: 5 minutes
Total Time: 40 minutes

---

1 red pepper

1 tablespoon olive oil

¼ teaspoon salt

1 shallot, skin removed and
    roughly chopped

12 basil leaves, rinsed and
    patted dry

Zest of 1 lemon

Juice of 1 lemon

**1.** Preheat oven to 400°F. Line a baking sheet with foil and place the red pepper on the baking sheet. Drizzle the red pepper with olive oil and salt and rub with your fingers to fully coat the pepper.

**2.** Roast for 20 to 25 minutes until the pepper is soft and beginning to brown. Remove from oven and cool completely.

**3.** Once the red pepper is cooled, discard the stem and seeds. Place remaining pepper flesh in a food processor or blender. Add the shallots, basil leaves, lemon zest, and lemon juice and purée until a smooth sauce forms.

**4.** Taste and season with salt, if desired.

**5.** Cover and refrigerate until ready to use.

*Nutritional data reflects one serving size of 6 tablespoons.*

**PER SERVING**  Calories: 51; Total Fat: 3.5g; Saturated Fat: 0.5g; Cholesterol: 0mg; Sodium: 150.2mg; Total Carbohydrates: 4.6g; Dietary Fiber: 1.2g; Sugars: 2.6g; Protein: 0.7g

# Pumpkin Mascarpone Pasta Sauce

*This recipe is inspired by Jackie Kestler. She invited our crew of four families over for a dinner party and made the most amazing stuffed shells with a butternut squash sauce. Of course, she made a point of ordering the jumbo-sized, gluten-free stuffed shells because, well, she's awesome like that. The following weekend, my parents and sister were coming over for dinner, and I wanted to make something similar, but I had no butternut squash. I did have a leftover can of pumpkin purée, so I mixed it into the sauce, and it was outstanding! So, if you have pumpkin, use pumpkin. If not, roast 2 pounds of butternut squash in place of the pumpkin purée.*

**YIELD: 4 CUPS**
**(½-CUP SERVINGS)**
Prep Time: 10 minutes
Total Time: 30 minutes

2 tablespoons olive oil

3 shallots, skin removed and roughly chopped

1 apple, core removed and chopped into bite-sized pieces

2 cups chicken broth

1 (15-ounce) can pumpkin purée

1 (8-ounce) container mascarpone

Zest of 1 lemon

3 tablespoons maple syrup

½ teaspoon salt

**1.** In a high-sided sauté pan or pot, heat olive oil over medium heat. Add the shallots and cook for about 5 minutes, stirring frequently, until softened. Add the apples and cook for 2 to 3 minutes, just until soft. Add the chicken broth and stir until the mixture comes to a simmer.

**2.** Stir in the pumpkin purée, mascarpone, lemon zest, maple syrup, and salt and mix until well combined.

**3.** Remove the pot from the heat. Using an immersion blender, purée the mixture until smooth. If you don't have an immersion blender, transfer the mixture to a blender or food processor and pulse until smooth.

**4.** Cover and refrigerate until ready to use.

*Nutritional data reflects one serving size of ½ cup.*

**PER SERVING** Calories: 218; Total Fat: 16.8g; Saturated Fat: 8.8g; Cholesterol: 36.6mg; Sodium: 182.8mg; Total Carbohydrates: 16.1g; Dietary Fiber: 2.5g; Sugars: 10.7g; Protein: 3.1g

# Veggie "Vodka" Sauce

*My two-and-a-half-year-old son loves vodka sauce, but when he was diagnosed with a dairy allergy, I had to find a new way for him to still enjoy the creamy sauce. After lots of tries, I found that puréeing roasted eggplant gives a tomato sauce an excellent creamy feel, while keeping cream out of it. Plus, this recipe is loaded with veggies, so it's far more nutritious than your traditional vodka sauce.*

**YIELD: 2 CUPS
(⅓-CUP SERVINGS)**
Prep Time: 10 minutes
Total Time: 45 minutes

---

1 pint grape tomatoes

1 eggplant, ends removed, sliced lengthwise and then into half moons

12 baby carrots

1 sweet yellow onion, skin removed and sliced into thick pieces

6 tablespoons olive oil, divided

1½ teaspoons salt plus a pinch

6 cloves garlic, peeled

1 teaspoon Italian seasoning

½ teaspoon paprika

½ cup chicken stock

**1.** Preheat oven to 450°F. Line a baking sheet with parchment paper, and spread the tomatoes, eggplant, carrots, and onion slices evenly across the pan. Drizzle 3 tablespoons olive oil over the vegetables and rub to fully coat. Sprinkle 1½ teaspoons salt over the tops of the vegetables.

**2.** Place the garlic cloves in a small piece of foil. Drizzle 1 teaspoon olive oil and a pinch of salt over the garlic. Wrap the foil up and place on the baking sheet alongside the vegetables. Roast for 18 to 22 minutes until the vegetables are soft and beginning to brown.

**3.** Transfer the vegetables to a food processor. Drizzle remaining olive oil, Italian seasoning, and paprika over the vegetables and purée until a smooth sauce forms.

**4.** Slowly add in the chicken stock to thin out the sauce. You may not need to use all of it.

**5.** Set aside or cover and refrigerate until ready to serve.

*Nutritional data reflects one serving size of ⅓ cup.*

**PER SERVING** Calories: 191; Total Fat: 14g; Saturated Fat: 2g; Cholesterol: 0mg; Sodium: 680.4mg; Total Carbohydrates: 14g; Dietary Fiber: 5.3g; Sugars: 7.8g; Protein: 2.7g

# Creamy Lemon Shallot Pasta Sauce

*If you want to get full flavor out of this sauce, follow the instructions below. But if it's a crazy day and you need a shortcut, skip all of the instructions below and instead, put all of the ingredients in a blender and purée until smooth. Pour the sauce over hot pasta and toss to combine. Dinner's ready!*

**YIELD: 2½ CUPS**
**(½-CUP SERVINGS)**
Prep Time: 5 minutes
Total Time: 15 minutes

---

2 tablespoons olive oil

2 shallots, skin removed and finely minced

3 cloves garlic, peeled and finely minced

½ cup white wine

¾ cup chicken stock

½ cup lemon juice

1 (8-ounce) container mascarpone cheese

2 teaspoons lemon zest

1 teaspoon salt

**1.** In a high-sided sauté pan, heat olive oil over medium heat. Add the minced shallots and cook, stirring frequently, until the shallots are soft and translucent, about 4 to 5 minutes. Add the garlic and cook 1 additional minute until fragrant.

**2.** Add the white wine and cook, stirring occasionally, until the wine reduces by half, about 3 to 4 minutes. Add the chicken stock and lemon juice, and bring to a simmer over medium heat. Simmer for 3 minutes.

**3.** Reduce heat to low and whisk in the mascarpone cheese, lemon zest, and salt.

**4.** Serve immediately with pasta or cool, cover, and refrigerate until ready to use.

*Nutritional data reflects one serving size of ½ cup.*

**PER SERVING** Calories: 280; Total Fat: 26g; Saturated Fat: 13.7g; Cholesterol: 58.5mg; Sodium: 570.9mg; Total Carbohydrates: 6.7g; Dietary Fiber: 0.5g; Sugars: 3.6g; Protein: 2.6g

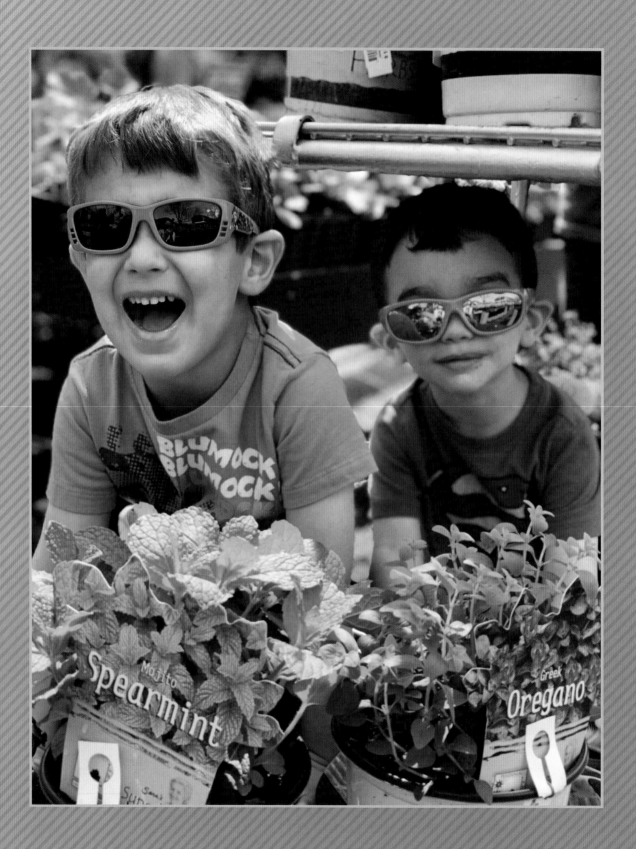

# Gluten-Free Ingredients Glossary

While having a list of safe gluten-free foods is nice, it's even better if you understand what each food really is. This detailed glossary identifies safe gluten-free flours, grains, and additives. Study it carefully to become an expert on gluten-free terminology.

**Acacia Gum:** Acacia gum is a natural gum consisting of the hardened sap of various species of the acacia tree. Also known as gum Arabic, it is soluble in water. It is edible and used primarily in the food industry as a stabilizer.

**Acorn Flour:** Acorn flour is naturally gluten-free and should be mixed with other gluten-free flours. Many recipes combine wheat with acorn flour, but you can mix it with other flours of your choice. Acorn flour can be used to make cakes, cookies, muffins, pancakes, pasta, noodles, flatbreads, pizza crust, and pie crust, and it is also used for thickening sauces and soups. Since acorns are naturally sweet, one needs to be aware of the slight sweetness that will be added to food made with this versatile flour.

**Adipic Acid:** Adipic acid has a tart taste and is used as an additive and gelling agent in jello or gelatins.

**Algin:** Algin, also called alginic acid, is a polysaccharide that is widely distributed in the cell walls of brown algae. When it binds with water, it forms a viscous gum. It is used to make medicine and skincare products.

**Almond Flour:** Almond flour is a naturally gluten-free flour made from blanched whole almonds that have been ground into a fine powder. It's packed with protein and fiber which means using almond flour will help you feel full longer. (Per ¼ cup: 3g fiber and 4g protein). It will also help give your breads and muffins a soft texture. You can use almond flour as a one-to-one replacement in baking, but it's most often used as part of a gluten-free flour blend.

**Amaranth:** Amaranth has been cultivated as a seed for 8,000 years. Studies show that amaranth is an effective way to increase calcium, zinc, and iron which help strengthen your bones, improve circulation, optimize digestion, and boost immunity. Amaranth also lowers your appetite. It can be found in health food stores because it is not widely used yet, but demand for this fiber- and mineral-packed seed is growing. You can use amaranth as a filling breakfast cereal or as a creamy pudding or parfait.

**Annatto:** Annatto is an orange-red condiment and food coloring derived from the seeds of the achiote tree. It is often used to impart a yellow or orange color to foods, but is sometimes used for its flavor and aroma as well. Its scent is described as "slightly peppery with a hint of nutmeg" and its flavor as "slightly nutty, sweet, and peppery."

**Arborio Rice:** Arborio is a traditional Italian rice used often in dishes in which a creamy texture is desired. Risotto is a popular use for Arborio rice.

**Arrowroot:** Arrowroot starch/flour is a wonderful grain-free, paleo-friendly, gluten-free thickener and emulsifier. Use arrowroot starch one-for-one in place of cornstarch in your recipes. Added to baked goods, it creates a softer, lighter texture.

**Aspartame:** Aspartame is an artificial non-saccharide sweetener used as a sugar substitute in some foods and beverages.

**Autolyzed Yeast Extract:** Yeast extract is made from the same type of yeast used in baking or brewing beer. "Autolyzed" just means that this type of yeast is produced by broken-down yeast cells. Ensure the product is labeled "gluten-free" before using it.

**Baker's Yeast:** Baker's yeast is a common baking yeast that is used in breads to make them rise. It is naturally gluten-free.

**Basmati Rice:** Basmati is a fragrant, nutty-tasting variety of long, slender-grained rice which is traditionally from the Indian subcontinent.

**Benzoic Acid:** Benzoic acid is a compound widely used as a food preservative. It can be found in many plants or created in a laboratory.

**Beta-Carotene:** Beta-carotene is one of a group of red, orange, and yellow pigments called carotenoids. Beta-carotene and other carotenoids provide approximately 50 percent of the vitamin A needed in a healthy diet. Beta-carotene can be found in fruits, vegetables, and whole grains. It can also be made in a laboratory.

**BHT:** BHT (butylated hydroxytoluene) is a lab-made chemical that is added to foods as a preservative.

**Brown Rice Flour:** Brown rice flour is a whole grain rice flour. It's rich with protein, iron, fiber, and vitamin B, and also contains healthy rice bran. It is a staple ingredient in gluten-free baked goods.

**Brown Sugar:** Brown sugar is a sugar product with a distinctive brown color due to the presence of molasses. It is either an unrefined or partially refined soft sugar consisting of sugar crystals with some residual molasses content (which is labeled as "natural brown sugar"), or it is produced by the addition of molasses to refined white sugar (which is labeled as "commercial brown sugar").

**Buckwheat:** Despite the word "wheat" in its name, buckwheat is a naturally gluten-free food related to the rhubarb plant. It's a versatile seed that can be steamed and eaten in place of rice. Alternatively, the whole seeds can be ground into a fine flour. Buckwheat has high levels of fiber and is a great source of protein. While most baking recipes will suggest using buckwheat as part of a flour blend with other ingredients like rice flour or almond flour, there are lots of recipes for pancakes that use 100 percent buckwheat flour. Or, try roasting the whole buckwheat groats and using them as an add-in for whole-grain granola.

**Calcium:** Calcium, the most abundant mineral in the body, is found in some foods, added to others, available as a dietary supplement, and is present in some medicines (such as antacids). It is an essential part of bones and teeth. The heart, nerves, and blood-clotting systems also need calcium to work. It is used for treatment and prevention of low calcium levels and resulting bone conditions including osteoporosis (weak bones due to low bone density), rickets (a condition in children involving softening of the bones), and osteomalacia (a softening of bones involving pain). Calcium is also used for premenstrual syndrome (PMS), leg cramps in pregnancy, high blood pressure in pregnancy (pre-eclampsia), and reducing the risk of colon and rectal cancers.

**Calrose Rice:** Grown in California, Calrose rice is the most popular type of rice in the United States and the Pacific. After cooking, Calrose rice grains hold flavor well, are soft and stick together, making it good for use in sushi.

**Canola Oil:** Canola is a crop with plants from three to five feet tall that produce pods from which seeds are harvested and crushed to create canola oil and meal. Canola seeds contain about 45 percent oil.

**Caramel Coloring:** This is the most used food coloring in the world. Made by heating carbohydrates, caramel coloring can be derived from wheat, but if it is, it will be listed on the packaging as "caramel color from wheat." If the label reads "caramel color," it is gluten-free.

**Carboxymethyl Cellulose:** Carboxymethyl cellulose (CMC), also known as "cellulose gum," is used as a thickener and emulsifier in food products.

**Carob Bean Gum:** Carob bean gum, also known as locust bean gum, is a thickening and gelling agent used in food products. It is extracted from the seeds of a carob tree.

**Carrageenan:** Carrageenan is an additive used to thicken, emulsify, and preserve foods and drinks. It's a natural ingredient that comes from red seaweed (also called Irish moss). You'll often find this ingredient in nut milks, meat products, and yogurt.

**Cassava Root and Flour:** Cassava is naturally gluten-free. The most commonly consumed part of cassava is the root, which is very versatile. It can be eaten whole, grated, or ground into flour to make bread and crackers.

**Chestnut:** Chestnuts contain very little fat—mostly unsaturated—and no gluten. They are the only "nuts" that contain vitamin C, with about 40mg per 100g of raw product. That is approximately 65 percent of the US recommended daily intake.

**Chickpea Flour:** The chickpea is a legume. Its different varieties are variously known as gram, garbanzo bean, or the Egyptian pea. They are high in protein and fiber.

**Coconut:** Coconut is naturally gluten-free and packed with nutrients. You can buy coconut as an oil, butter, flour, sugar, and flakes. In gluten-free baking, coconut flour is often blended with other flours, and is made from dried, defatted coconut meat. Packed with fiber yet low in carbohydrates, coconut flour gives baked goods a rich texture and adds natural sweetness, allowing you to cut down on the amount of sugar. Coconut milk can be used in soups, stews, curries, beverages, and baked goods.

**Corn:** Corn is naturally gluten-free and can be used as a gluten-free substitute. Cornstarch can be used as a thickening agent in gravies or sauces. Corn flour can be used as a breading alternative and as a combination with other flours in baked goods. "Masa" is used in many Mexican dishes and is sometimes called "maize." And, of course, corn on the cob can be enjoyed with melted butter!

**Corn Gluten:** Corn gluten meal (CGM) is a gluten-free byproduct of corn ("maize") processing that is historically used as animal feed. The expression "corn gluten" is colloquial jargon that describes corn proteins that are neither gliadin nor glutenin. Only wheat, barley, and rye contain true gluten, formed by the interaction of gliadin and glutenin proteins.

**Corn Syrup:** Corn syrup is a food syrup made from the starch of corn ("maize") and contains varying amounts of maltose and higher oligosaccharides, depending on the grade. Corn syrup, also known as glucose syrup to confectioners, is used in foods to soften texture, add volume, prevent crystallization of sugar, and enhance flavor.

**Cottonseed:** Cottonseed, the seed of the cotton plant, is important commercially for its oil and other products. Cottonseed oil is used in salad and cooking oils and, after hydrogenation, in shortenings and margarine. The cake, or meal, remaining after the oil is extracted is used in poultry and livestock feeds.

**Cream of Tartar:** Cream of Tartar is a white, crystalline, acidic compound obtained as a byproduct of wine fermentation and is used chiefly in baking powder.

**Dal:** Dal is a term used in Indian cooking to describe split peas or lentils. The term is also used to describe soups made from these products.

**Dasheen Flour:** A variety of taro root (also known as taro root flour), dasheen is a starchy edible tuber that can be used as a potato. However, raw dasheen is toxic, so it must be cooked. Boiling the tuber rids it of toxic calcium oxalate. This tuber is cream-colored to white and resembles a water chestnut. It has a mild, nutty flavor when cooked. Dasheen is high in vitamin C, among other nutrients, making it a healthier choice than potatoes or rice. The leaves can be used as greens and the shoots as vegetables.

**Dextrose:** Dextrose is a simple sugar that is made from corn and is therefore gluten-free. Dextrose is commonly found in corn syrup and is used as a sweetener in processed foods and baked goods. Even if it is listed as "wheat dextrose," it is also gluten-free because it is highly processed which removes the gluten.

**Disodium Phosphate:** Disodium phosphate is a food additive. Phosphates like disodium phosphate are derived from the element phosphorus. Disodium phosphate is used as an emulsifier as well as to enhance cooking performance. It's used in packaged foods, including macaroni and pastas. You can also find it in meat products, some cheeses, canned sauces, Jell-O, evaporated milk, and some chocolate.

**Distilled Vinegar:** Distilled vinegar is used in salad dressings and marinades. In the United States, most distilled vinegars are made from corn, grapes, apples, or rice, all of which are gluten-free. Even if a distilled vinegar is made from wheat (usually outside of the USA), it is considered gluten-free since the process of distilling removes the gluten. Many non-distilled vinegars (such as "malt vinegar" which is fermented— not distilled—from wheat barley and/or rye) are not gluten-free, but the label will always tell you what ingredients were used in making the vinegar.

**Enriched Rice:** Enriched rice is white rice that has been coated with nutrients, such as iron, niacin, thiamin, and folic acid, which are lost when the rice is initially processed. Despite replacing some of the vitamins and protein, enriched rice is not as nutritious as whole grain brown rice.

**Ethyl Maltol:** Ethyl maltol is an organic compound that is a common flavorant in some confectioneries. It is white and solid with a sweet smell that can be described as caramelized sugar and cooked fruit.

**Fava Bean Flour:** Fava bean flour is naturally gluten-free. It has a distinctive flavor and is most often used in combination with garbanzo bean flour for gluten-free baking. Fava bean flour is perfect for all kinds of baking including breads, pizza, cakes, and cookies.

**Flaxseed Flour:** Flax is a naturally gluten-free food. Flaxseed flour, also called ground flaxseed, offers some benefits over whole flaxseed. Whole flax passes through your system undigested, causing us to miss out on its health benefits. Flax is full of fiber, which helps to relieve constipation, and the omega-3 fatty acids in flax reduce cholesterol and provide protection against heart disease. You can even replace some of the flour or all of the eggs in a baking recipe by substituting ground flaxseed.

**Fumaric Acid:** Fumaric acid is a common food additive included in many processed foods to keep them stable and add tartness. The substance is more sour than citric acid, another common food additive. Fumaric acid occurs naturally in fumaria, bolete mushrooms, lichen, and Iceland moss. As an additive, fumaric acid is produced synthetically, mainly from the malic acid in apples.

**Garbanzo Beans:** Garbanzo beans (also known as chickpeas) are naturally gluten-free. Flour made from this delicious bean lends a sweet, rich flavor to baked goods. It is also a wonderful ingredient for gluten-free baking. Garbanzo beans are loaded with protein and dietary fiber and are a good source of iron.

**Gelatin:** Gelatin was first used in Medieval Britain to create elaborate desserts and to make certain glues and adhesives. Now, it is mainly used as a colorless and tasteless protein in food, cosmetics, and medicine. In foods, this gluten-free additive is used not only as a dessert component, but also as a thickener. It is made from extracting the collagen from various animal parts.

**Glucose Syrup:** Glucose is made mostly from corn in the US, while Europe often uses wheat to make glucose syrup. Either type is considered safe for people with celiac disease since gluten is removed in the processing. Glucose syrup is used to enhance the volume and flavor of foods. It also prevents sugar from crystallizing, so the candy industry uses it a lot. Since glucose circulates in the bodies of animals as blood sugar, it is best to eat it in moderation.

**Glutinous Rice:** Sticky rice goes by many names—waxy rice, sweet rice, and pearl rice among them—but "glutinous" in its name is a bit confusing. Does glutinous rice actually contain gluten? The answer is no. Glutinous rice is gluten-free. The misleading name simply comes from the fact that glutinous rice gets glue-like and sticky when cooked.

**Gram Flour:** Gram flour is a naturally gluten-free legume flour made from a variety of ground chick-peas. It is often used to make Indian dishes.

**Guar Gum:** Guar gum is made from a seed native to tropical Asia and is used as a thickener in gluten-free recipes. Guar gum is good for cold foods such as ice cream or pastry fillings. It's a wonderful ingredient in gluten-free baking as well, since it provides the gluten-free dough with more elasticity.

**Hominy:** Hominy is made from whole corn kernels that have been soaked in a lye or lime solution to soften the tough outer hulls. It is gluten-free and typically used to make grits, but can also be used as a thickener for stew, to make tortillas or tamales, or as a dish all its own.

**Indian Rice Grass:** A wild grass first used by Native Americans thousands of years ago, Indian rice grass has a very versatile seed. Historic uses included: eating the raw seeds to relieve stomach ache, colic, and aching bones, and eating them cooked as dumplings. The seeds were added to soups and ground into flour and meal for cakes and bread. While they are rarely used as raw seeds anymore, this grass makes a terrific gluten-free flour.

**Instant Rice:** Instant rice is rice that has been precooked. Some types are microwave-ready, while others are dehydrated so that they cook more rapidly. Regular rice requires eighteen to thirty minutes to cook while instant rice needs one to seven minutes. Because it has already been cooked, you can simply microwave it or re-hydrate it with hot water. Be sure to check that gluten-containing flavorings haven't been added.

**Inverted Sugar Syrup:** Inverted sugar syrup, also known as invert syrup, is an edible mixture of two simple sugars (glucose and fructose) that is made by heating table sugar (sucrose) with water.

**Karaya Gum:** Karaya gum (also known as gum karaya or Indian gum tragacanth) is used as a thickener and emulsifier in food products. It is a vegetable gum created from the trees of the Sterculia genus.

**Kasha:** Kasha is organic buckwheat groats that have been hulled and roasted. It is 100 percent whole grain and makes a wonderfully flavorful hot cereal or delicious side dish.

**Lactic Acid:** Lactic acid is primarily found in soured milk products, such as yogurt, kefir, and cottage cheese. It is also used as a food preservative, curing agent, and flavoring agent.

**Lactose:** Lactose is a sugar present in milk and is gluten-free. It is a by-product of the dairy industry and is produced from whey. Lactose has a slightly sweet flavor, so it is a popular filler to bulk up baked goods. It also prevents caking of dry ingredients.

**Lecithin:** Lecithin is an essential fat that is found in many foods, such as soybeans, egg yolks, and in some supplements, as it contains an essential nutrient called choline. It is used in foods as an emulsifier to help ingredients stick together (think of flowing chocolate). Although lecithin is a fat, it is typically added in very small amounts, so the total fat content of any food should not be influenced by the presence of lecithin.

**Lentils:** Lentils are naturally gluten-free legumes that work well in place of noodles in soups and stews. They're rich in fiber and protein, making them a healthy meat substitute for vegetarians and vegans. Lentils are also packed with folate, iron, phosphorus, and potassium.

**Malic Acid:** Malic acid is a naturally occurring acid made by all living organisms. It contributes to the sour taste of fruits and is also used as a food additive to give candies a sour flavor.

**Maltodextrin:** Maltodextrin can be made from a variety of starches like potato, rice, corn, or wheat. In the United States, it is usually made from corn. Regardless, the starch is so highly processed that maltodextrin made from wheat is still gluten-free.

**Maltol:** Maltol is a naturally occurring compound extracted from the bark of larch trees and pine needles. It is used as a flavor enhancer in foods.

**Maltose:** Maltose is a sugar produced during the breaking down of starches and is, therefore, gluten-free.

**Mannitol:** Mannitol is a type of sugar alcohol used as a sweetener. Because it is poorly absorbed by the body, it is a good sweetener for diabetics. It can also be used as a medication to treat glaucoma and elevated intracranial pressure.

**Methylcellulose:** Methylcellulose is derived from cellulose, a common compound found in plants. It is used as a thickener and emulsifier in food products.

**Millet:** Millet is a naturally gluten-free grain that can be used as a whole grain (to replace rice, for example) or ground into a flour to be used for baking. It is a cereal crop that has been grown in India and Africa for hundreds of years, but only recently became popular in the United States. It is rich in minerals and protein, with 3g of fiber and 4g of protein per ¼ cup. Bake with it, try it out as a breakfast porridge, or try it as a replacement for corn-based polenta.

**Modified Corn Starch:** The FDA's Code of Federal Regulations spells out what can be used to modify corn starch, as well as other starches, and none of the allowed substances contain gluten. Modified corn starch sometimes appears on a label as "modified food starch." In that case, it is still gluten-free.

**Modified Tapioca Starch:** Modified tapioca starch is derived from tapioca and it is gluten-free. It is used in foods as a thickener and stabilizer. In baking, it can help improve the appearance and texture of products.

**Monosodium Glutamate:** Monosodium Glutamate, or MSG, is made by fermenting starches and sugars including corn starch, beet sugar, sugar cane, and tapioca starch.

**Nutritional Yeast:** Nutritional yeast is simply deactivated yeast. It has a nutty, cheesy, and creamy taste to it, making it a great ingredient for dairy-free cheese and butter products.

**Papain:** Papain is an enzyme extracted from the raw fruit of the papaya plant. These enzymes break proteins down into smaller fragments. It is a popular ingredient in meat tenderizer.

**Peanut Flour:** Peanut flour is made from crushed peanuts. The peanuts can be partly or fully defatted. Peanut flour, depending on the quantity of fat removed, is highly protein-dense, providing up to 52.2g of protein per 100g of peanuts.

**Pectin:** Pectin is a gelling agent found in jams and jellies. It is made from citrus peel or apples and is, therefore, gluten-free.

**Polysorbates:** Polysorbates are emulsifiers used in food production and pharmaceuticals.

**Potato Starch:** Potatoes and potato starch are naturally gluten-free. The starch is often used as a thickener for sauces, soups, and stews. Potato starch tolerates higher temperatures than cornstarch when used as a thickener. It's a natural way to add moisture to many baked goods.

**Propylene Glycol:** Propylene glycol is a food additive that helps balance the amount of moisture in a food. It is also used as a solvent for food colors and flavors.

**Psyllium:** Psyllium fiber is made from the husk or outer shell of the psyllium plant's seeds. It provides a good source of natural fiber.

**Quinoa:** Quinoa is a naturally gluten-free superfood that contains all nine essential amino acids. Technically, it's a seed, but it is eaten like a grain. It comes in a variety of different colors like red, white, and black. Although quinoa has been consumed for thousands of years in South America, it's only recently that this protein-rich food became popular in the United States. Use whole quinoa as a replacement for rice and quinoa flour in baked goods.

**Red Rice:** Red rice is a variety of rice that is colored red by its anthocyanin content. It is usually eaten unhulled or partially hulled and has a red husk, rather than the more common brown husk. Red rice has a nutty flavor. Compared to polished rice, it has the highest nutritional value of rices eaten with the germ intact.

**Rice:** Rice is a naturally gluten-free grain and comes in many varieties. Rice flour (also rice powder) is made from finely-milled rice. Rice flour is a particularly good substitute for wheat flour. Rice flour is also used as a thickening agent in recipes that are refrigerated or frozen, since it inhibits liquid separation.

**Rice Bran:** The outer layer of the rice grain (bran) and the oil made from the bran are sometimes used for medicine. Rice bran oil is popular as a "healthy oil" in Asia, particularly in India. Be careful not to confuse rice bran with other forms of bran such as oat and wheat bran.

**Sago:** Sago is a gluten-free starch taken from the center of sago palm stems. Sago has similarities to tapioca, including its look, taste, and feel. You can substitute tapioca for sago in many recipes. You can also use sago in the preparation of desserts and some breads. Sago is also sometimes used to make the Asian drink known as bubble tea.

**Sesame Seeds:** Sesame seeds are tiny, flat, oval seeds with a nutty taste and a delicate crunch. They come in a host of different colors depending on the variety, including white, yellow, black, and red. Not only are sesame seeds an excellent source of copper and a very good source of manganese, they are also a good source of calcium, magnesium, iron, phosphorus, vitamin B$_1$, zinc, molybdenum, selenium, and dietary fiber.

**Sodium Benzonate:** Sodium benzoate is used as a food preservative, mostly in acidic products. It occurs naturally in fruits, vegetables, seafood, and dairy products.

**Sodium Metabisulfite:** Sodium metabisulfite (or sodium metabisulphite) is used as a preservative and antioxidant in food.

**Sodium Nitrate:** Sodium nitrate is used to preserve color and shelf life in processed meats. It is gluten-free but can be hard on people with sensitive stomachs.

**Sodium Sulfite:** Sodium sulfite (or sodium sulphite) is used as a preservative in food. Most commonly, it is found in dried fruit and preserved meat.

**Sorbitol:** Sorbitol is a sugar alcohol that the human body metabolizes slowly. Very similar to mannitol, it is usually created from corn syrup but can also be created from fruits like apples, pears, peaches, and prunes.

**Sorghum:** Sorghum is a naturally gluten-free grain that is used for many purposes in the gluten-free food world. The whole grain is ground into a soft flour that can be used for gluten-free baking. The flour has a smooth texture which makes it a perfect substitute in baked goods. Brewers often malt the sorghum grains and then use them to make naturally gluten-free beer. You can also use whole-grain sorghum as a replacement for rice. Steam the sorghum grain first, then top it with your favorite stir-fry ingredients to pack a nutritious punch. Every ¼ cup of sorghum flour is packed with 3g of fiber and 4g of protein.

**Soy:** Soy is a species of legume native to East Asia, widely grown for its edible bean, which has numerous uses. Soy foods are good sources of protein, and many are also good sources of fiber, calcium, potassium, magnesium, copper, and manganese.

**Spices:** Only 100 percent pure spices are gluten-free. Companies that use wheat flour to bulk up their spices exist, although they are few and far between. Thankfully, United States and Canadian labeling laws require these companies to disclose if wheat is used as a bulking agent. It is also prudent to look for gluten in the form of flour or dried soy sauce flakes in any premade spice mixes.

**Stearic Acid:** Stearic acid is used as a food additive, surfactant, and softening agent. It is obtained from fats and oils.

**Sucralose:** Sucralose is an artificial, non-caloric sugar substitute, making it an ideal sugar substitute for diabetics. When sold as a sweetener, it is often mixed with maltodextrin or dextrose. It is highly heat-stable, so it works well in baking.

**Sucrose:** Sucrose is another name for table sugar and is the most commonly found form of sugar. Sucrose is made from sugar cane and is gluten-free.

**Sunflower Seeds:** Sweet, nutty sunflower seeds are an excellent source of essential fatty acids, vitamins, and minerals. Besides being eaten as popular snacks, they are also used in the kitchen to prepare a variety of recipes.

**Sweet Rice Flour:** Sweet rice flour has thickening properties, but it is better used in gluten-free flour mixes for baked goods. Sweet rice flour is ground from short-grain glutinous rice, also known as "sticky rice." Don't worry, though—"glutinous rice" does not mean that it contains gluten!

**Tapioca Flour:** Tapioca flour helps to bind recipe ingredients and improves the texture of baked goods. It's slightly sweet and very starchy, so you only need a little bit of it in baked goods. You'll want to combine it with other gluten-free flours like brown rice or quinoa flour. Tapioca helps add crispness to crusts and chewiness to baked goods. It is an extremely smooth flour, which makes it a great thickener in sauces, pies, and soups and as a replacement for cornstarch.

**Taro Root:** Taro root is gluten-free and a good alternative carbohydrate to potato. Taro can be used in a similar way to a potato, but provides better nutritional value and a much lower glycemic index. Taro contains about three times more fiber and 30 percent less fat than potatoes. The low glycemic index of taro means that the blood sugar levels don't rise rapidly, making it a suitable food for diabetics and individuals with blood disorders.

**Tartaric Acid:** Tartaric acid is most commonly used to mix with sodium bicarbonate to create baking powder. It occurs naturally in many fruits and has a distinct sour taste.

**Tartrazine:** Tartrazine is a synthetic yellow dye primarily used as food coloring.

**Teff:** Teff is the smallest grain in the world. This African superfood is a great source of dietary fiber, protein, iron, amino acids, vitamin C, and calcium. It can be ground into flour to make an excellent gluten-free flour alternative and can be used to make pie crusts, cookies, breads, and an assortment of other baked goods. Teff can also be eaten whole, steamed, boiled, or baked as a side dish or a main course. Teff benefits blood sugar management, weight control, and colon health.

**Titanium Dioxide:** Titanium dioxide is a naturally occurring compound used as a food coloring.

**Tofu:** Plain tofu contains three ingredients: soybeans, water, and a curdling agent. As all of these ingredients are gluten-free, plain, unprepared tofu typically does not contain gluten. However, some varieties of flavored tofu are not gluten-free.

**Vanilla Bean:** Vanilla bean is grown from orchids in the genus "Vanilla" and is one of the world's most popular aromas and flavors.

**Vanilla Extract:** Vanilla extract is a solution made from crushed vanilla pods and ethanol. It is a very popular ingredient in Western desserts, especially baked goods.

**Wheat Starch:** Surprise! Although wheat starch is made from wheat, **some** wheat starch is processed so that the proteins, including gluten, are taken out of the final product. This means it passes the Food and Drug Administration (FDA) regulations as being gluten-free (when the final product has 20 parts per million or less of gluten). The label also has to say that the wheat has been processed to allow this food to meet the FDA requirements for gluten-free foods. It is important to note that **wheat starch is only safe for a person with celiac disease if the product is labeled "gluten-free,"** so be sure to read the labels thoroughly!

**Whey Protein:** Whey is the liquid that is left over after milk has been curdled and strained to make cheeses and yogurts. Whey is then dehydrated into a powder. It is the primary ingredient in most protein powders and is sold as a nutritional supplement to promote muscle growth and repair. Whey protein is found in a variety of flavors and added to liquid for ingestion. If you buy whey protein powder, be sure the mix doesn't contain "glutamine peptides," which are hydrolyzed wheat protein. Although the hydrolyzing process may remove most of the gluten, it is best if a celiac does not ingest it unless the mix has been tested to be gluten-free.

**White Rice Flour:** White rice flour is 100 percent stone ground from premium white rice. It is wonderful for gluten-free baking, as it results in light and fluffy cakes, pie crusts, and breads. It is also great for thickening sauces, gravies, and soups.

**Xanthan Gum:** Xanthan Gum is made from a microorganism called Xanthomonas Campestri and works best in baking and hot food preparations. It is a powerful thickening agent and is also used to prevent ingredients from separating. It is a crucial ingredient in most gluten-free baking. In gluten-free doughs, xanthan gum makes products more elastic and thick and gives baked products a better rise.

**Xylitol:** Xylitol is a sugar alcohol used as a sugar substitute. It does not affect blood sugar levels very much, making it a suitable alternative sweetener for diabetics.

**Yam:** Yams are a common name for sweet potatoes in the U.S. even though they are completely unrelated to each other. The yam is native to Africa and Asia. Yams are starchier and drier than sweet potatoes.

**Yuca:** Also known as cassava (and not to be confused with yucca), yuca is a dense, starchy food that is rich in carbohydrates. It's a good source of fiber, folate, vitamin C, and potassium. Like other starchy vegetables, it can be served fried, boiled, grilled, or mashed. When dried to a powder, it is known as tapioca.

# Recipe Index

## Chapter 8: Family Suppers

## Chapter 9: Simple Side Dishes

# Acknowledgments

It truly takes a village to write a cookbook, or at least it did for me. There were so many people who helped along the way, whether it was assisting with recipe development, food styling, washing dishes, or just offering moral support and a hug. I'm beyond grateful to everyone.

To Blair Raber, the founder of our Celiac Disease Program at Children's National who not only helped for days with testing recipes but also trekked through the aisles at Home Depot with me picking out slabs of tile and flooring to create the beautiful backdrops you see in the book. She went above and beyond by taking over my backyard to spray paint wooden planks and trays to help bring them to life. Every time I look at the photos in this book, I get a mental image of Blair outside in the freezing cold weather spray painting with her hair in a messy scrunchie! She's not only the hardest worker I've ever met but is also truly an incredible friend, mentor, and colleague.

The Gluten-Free Ingredients Glossary, Dr. Bear Facts, and all of the nutritional data was compiled by Kate Raber and Joyana McMahon from our Education Team at Children's National. While these nutritional boxes seem like a small addition to the recipes, their content is incredibly valuable to families managing both celiac disease and type 1 diabetes and who need these crucial values to keep their kids healthy.

A huge thank you to our Medical Director, Dr. Benny Kerzner, for ensuring that all of the medical information in the book is accurate. I also thank him for his great enthusiasm in wanting to try each recipe when I texted him newly-taken photos.

To the leadership team at Children's National, especially Dr. Kurt Newman, Elizabeth Flury, David Ashman, Kathy Gorman, Dr. Tony Sandler, Dr. Ian Leibowitz, and Shelley Cooke: Thank you for always believing in and encouraging our Celiac Disease Program team. Your endless support has helped us soar to new heights, and we can't wait to see what the future holds for our Program.

To my CNMC Celiac Disease Program Family (Dr. Benny Kerzner, Blair Raber, Lori Stern, Joyana McMahon, Kate Raber, Shayna Coburn, Kathleen Walters, Dr. Ilana Kahn, Maggie Parker, Maegan Sady, and Will Suslovic) and our Celiac Disease Program Advisory Board: I'm so lucky to work with the greatest people on Earth. Thanks for your creativity, energy, and enthusiasm in working with me to make the world a better place one gluten-free cupcake at a time.

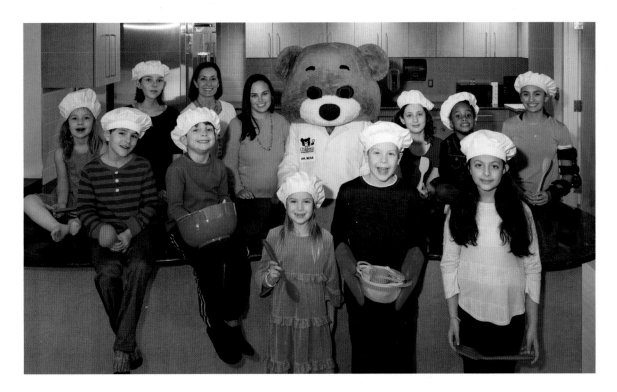

Thank you to Anthony Mattero, Naseeb Gill, and Jesse Uram at CAA-GBG and our editorial team at Post Hill Press for taking a chance on us and helping to build our vision for a truly delicious and inclusive gluten-free world.

A gigantic thank you to the following kiddos for helping with photos for the book: Ava Zaks, Rowen Smith, Ruthie Meytin, Maggie Nelson, Miles Nelson, Maisie Nelson, Julia Buchta, Caroline Wilkes, Jake Renzi, Sam Renzi, David Goren, Shahana Zafnia, CJ DeGier, and Keira DeGier. Thank you so much for being our "Gluten-Free Detectives" and helping other kids understand the gluten-free diet. And thank you to Kenson Noel for the beautiful photographs of the kids with food labels in the Diabetes Care Complex Kitchens, and to Elizabeth Morrow and Megan Laurent for helping to orchestrate the shoot. To Sweta Zaks: You know what you did. We'll keep it between us to keep the magic alive....

To my lifelong best friend, Julie Neimark, who spent her entire winter break cooking, cleaning, taste-testing, and entertaining my munchkins so I could work on the book—thank you. She always knew the right moment to uncork a bottle of buttery, oaky chardonnay! And thanks also to Brenda Mendes Cota, our wonderful au pair, who jumped in to help so many times and even shared one of her favorite traditional Brazilian desserts for the book.

A gigantic thank you to Jackie Kestler for helping with cooking and recipe development, and to Heather Isaacs for sharing her incredible ability to make the recipes in the book look beautiful. And, to Julianne Lepore and Amy Block for always responding immediately to my text messages requesting a "Jeffrey" to come help. If you're a fan of Ina Garten, you know what I mean.

Perhaps the biggest thank you goes to my family. To my grandmother Lela Mae: Thank you for teaching me to churn butter, make pies and snickerdoodles, and for the very important lesson to never let the men in my life have an empty belly. Even though you'll never hold a copy of this book on Earth, I know that you are cheering me on in the kitchen and in life from heaven.

To my parents, Alan and Connie Maltin: Thank you for raising me to love and appreciate food and for never letting me order off of the kid's menu. I genuinely believe that a child's love of food stems from how their parents feed them. I am beyond grateful that you forbade us to eat "kid junk food" and pushed us to eat real food, even if I made you crazy by demanding veal every night for dinner.

To my amazing husband, Eric: Thank you for your constant willingness to order gluten-free meals to share in restaurants so I can try everything and for being my gluten-free foodie co-pilot. Thank you for being a gluten-free advocate for me and our kids and always being the first one to speak up for us in a restaurant. We are so lucky to have you.

To my sons, Brandon and Leo: You are the sunshines of my life. I am so proud of how you have both taken ownership of your diets. I love how you know that a food sensitivity doesn't make you abnormal, it makes you special and superbly awesome.

To all of our patients and families at the Celiac Disease Program at Children's National Medical Center: This book is for you. I sincerely hope that you read it, cook it, and—most importantly—enjoy it.